CLINICAL
NEUROSURGERY

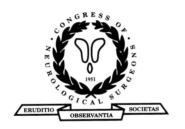

LIPPINCOTT
WILLIAMS
&WILKINS

Copyright © 2001
THE CONGRESS OF NEUROLOGICAL SURGEONS

Accurate indications, adverse reactions, and dosage schedules for drugs are provided in this book, but it possible that they may change. The reader is urged to review the package information data of the manufacturers of the medications mentioned.

Printed in the United States of America
(ISBN 0-7817-3627-7)

CLINICAL
NEUROSURGERY

Volume 48

Proceedings

OF THE
CONGRESS OF NEUROLOGICAL SURGEONS

San Antonio, Texas
2000

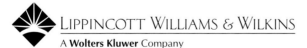
LIPPINCOTT WILLIAMS & WILKINS
A **Wolters Kluwer** Company
Philadelphia · Baltimore · New York · London
Buenos Aires · Hong Kong · Sydney · Tokyo

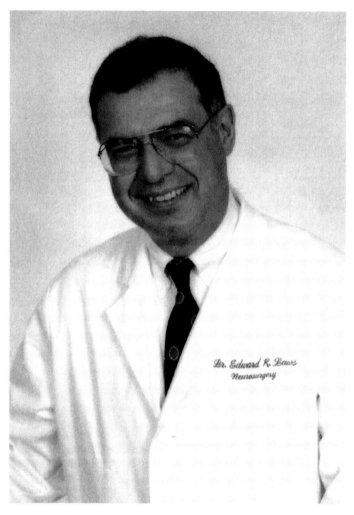

EDWARD R. LAWS, M.D.

Preface

The 50th Annual Meeting of the Congress of Neurological Surgeons was held at the Henry B. Gonzalez Convention Center in San Antonio, Texas, from September 25 to September 28, 2000. Volume 48 of *Clinical Neurosurgery* represents the official compendium of the platform presentations from that meeting.

The Annual Meeting Chairman, Dr. Vincent Traynelis, and the Scientific Program Chairman, Dr. Douglas Kondziolka, organized and led this outstanding, well-attended meeting. This year's Honored Guest, Dr. Edward R. Laws, presented his outstanding work with glioma and pituitary tumor surgery. The Presidential Address by Dr. Daniel Barrow provided an inspirational message to all neurosurgeons in training and in practice.

Crystal blue skies and moderate temperatures attended this year's event in The Alamo City, and members of the Congress were treated to a superb scientific and social program. My congratulations go out to all participants of the multiple meeting committees for their outstanding work this year. In particular, I would like to thank the contributors to *Clinical Neurosurgery* for their timely cooperation in submitting their manuscripts and to my Associate Editors for their dedication and care in completing their assignments. Once again, I would like to express my gratitude to Vicki Vaughn at Lippincott Williams & Wilkins for ably seeing this project through to completion. And last, but not least, I wish to acknowledge the dedicated work of my secretary, Brenda Gropman, for her excellent assistance. I have enjoyed this second year as Editor and look forward to seeing you all next September in San Diego, California, for our 51st Annual Meeting.

Matthew A. Howard III, M.D.
Editor

Charles S. Cobbs, M.D.
Associate Editor

J. Paul Elliott, M.D.
Associate Editor

Guy M. McKhann II, M.D.
Associate Editor

Honored Guests

1952—Professor Herbert Olivecrona, Stockholm, Sweden
1953—Sir Geoffrey Jefferson, Manchester, England
1954—Dr. Kenneth G. McKenzie, Toronto, Canada
1955—Dr. Carl W. Rand, Los Angeles, California
1956—Dr. Wilder G. Penfield, Montreal, Canada
1957—Dr. Francis C. Grant, Philadelphia, Pennsylvania
1958—Dr. A. Earl Walker, Baltimore, Maryland
1959—Dr. William J. German, New Haven, Connecticut
1960—Dr. Paul C. Bucy, Chicago, Illinois
1961—Professor Eduard A. V. Busch, Copenhagen, Denmark
1962—Dr. Bronson S. Ray, New York, New York
1963—Dr. James L. Poppen, Boston, Massachusetts
1964—Dr. Edgar A. Kahn, Ann Arbor, Michigan
1965—Dr. James C. White, Boston, Massachusetts
1966—Dr. Hugh A. Kravenbühl, Zurich, Switzerland
1967—Dr. W. James Gardner, Cleveland, Ohio
1968—Professor Normal M. Dott, Edinburgh, Scotland
1969—Dr. Wallace B. Hamby, Cleveland, Ohio
1970—Dr. Barnes Woodhall, Durham, North Carolina
1971—Dr. Elisha S. Gurdjian, Detroit, Michigan
1972—Dr. Francis Murphey, Memphis, Tennessee
1973—Dr. Henry G. Schwartz, St. Louis, Missouri
1974—Dr. Guy L. Odom, Durham, North Carolina
1975—Dr. William A. Sweet, Boston, Massachusetts
1976—Dr. Lyle A. French, Minneapolis, Minnesota
1977—Dr. Richard C. Schneider, Ann Arbor, Michigan
1978—Dr. Charles G. Drake, London, Ontario, Canada
1979—Dr. Frank H. Mayfield, Cincinnati, Ohio
1980—Dr. Eben Alexander, Jr., Winston-Salem, North Carolina
1981—Dr. J. Garber Galbraith, Birmingham, Alabama
1982—Dr. Keiji Sano, Tokyo, Japan
1983—Dr. C. Miller Fisher, Boston, Massachusetts
1984—Dr. Hugo V. Rizzoli, Washington, DC
        Dr. Walter E. Dandy (posthumously), Baltimore, Maryland
1985—Dr. Sidney Goldring, St. Louis, Missouri
1986—Dr. M. Gazi Yasargil, Zurich, Switzerland
1987—Dr. Thomas W. Langiftt, Philadelphia, Pennsylvania

1988—Professor Lindsay Symon, London, England
1989—Dr. Thoralf M. Sundt, Jr., Rochester, Minnesota
1990—Dr. Charles Byron Wilson, San Francisco, California
1991—Dr. Bennett M. Stein, New York, New York
1992—Dr. Robert G. Ojemann, Boston, Massachusetts
1993—Dr. Albert L. Rhoton, Jr., Gainesville, Florida
1994—Dr. Robert F. Spetzler, Phoenix, Arizona
1995—Dr. John A. Jane, Charlottesville, Virginia
1996—Dr. Peter J. Jannetta, Pittsburgh, Pennsylvania
1997—Dr. Nicholas T. Zervas, Boston, Massachusetts
1998—Dr. John M. Tew
1999—Dr. Duke S. Samson
2000—Dr. Edward R. Laws

Officers of the Congress
of
Neurological Surgeons
2000

DANIEL L BARROW, M.D.
President

ISSAM A. AWAD
President-Elect

STEVEN M. PAPADOPOULOS   MARK N. HADLEY
Vice-President   *Secretary*

EXECUTIVE COMMITTEE

DAVID ADELSON, M.D.   JOEL D. MACDONALD, M.D.
MARK H. CAMEL, M.D.   TIMOTHY B. MAPTSONE, M.D.
RICHARD G. ELLENBOGEN, M.D.   STANLEY B. MARTIN, M.D.
ISABELLE GERMANO, M.D.   NELSON M. OYESIKU, M.D.
SAMUEL HASSENBUSCH, M.D.   GERALD E. RODTS, JR., M.D.
DAVID JIMENEZ, M.D.   WARREN R. SELMAN, M.D.
DOUGLAS S. KONDZIOLKA, M.D.   VINCENT TRAYNELIS, M.D.
LYAL LEIBROCK, M.D.   CRAIG VAN DER VEER, M.D.
MICHAEL L. LEVY, M.D.

Editors-in-Chief
Clinical Neurosurgery

Volume	Date	Editor-in-Chief
1	1953	Raymond K. Thompson, M.D.
2	1954	Raymond K. Thompson, M.D. & Ira J. Jackson, M.D.
3	1955	Raymond K. Thompson, M.D. & Ira J. Jackson, M.D.
4	1956	Ira J. Jackson, M.D.
5	1957	Robert G. Fisher, M.D.
6	1958	Robert G. Fisher, M.D.
7	1959	Robert G. Fisher, M.D.
8	1960	William H. Mosberg, Jr., M.D.
9	1961	William H. Mosberg, Jr., M.D.
10	1962	William H. Mosberg, Jr., M.D.
11	1963	John Shillito, Jr., M.D., & William H. Mosberg, Jr., M.D.
12	1964	John Shillito, Jr., M.D.
13	1965	John Shillito, Jr., M.D.
14	1966	Robert G. Ojemann, M.D. & John Shillito, Jr., M.D.
15	1967	Robert G. Ojemann, M.D.
16	1968	Robert G. Ojemann, M.D.
17	1969	Robert G. Ojemann, M.D.
18	1970	George T. Tindall, M.D.
19	1971	George T. Tindall, M.D.
20	1972	Robert H. Wilkins, M.D.
21	1973	Robert H. Wilkins, M.D.
22	1974	Robert H. Wilkins, M.D.
23	1975	Ellis B. Keener, M.D.
24	1976	Ellis B. Keener, M.D.
25	1977	Ellis B. Keener, M.D.
26	1978	Peter W. Carmel, M.D.
27	1979	Peter W. Carmel, M.D.
28	1980	Peter W. Carmel, M.D.
29	1981	Martin H. Weiss, M.D.
30	1982	Martin H. Weiss, M.D.
31	1983	Martin H. Weiss, M.D.
32	1984	John R. Little, M.D.
33	1985	John R. Little, M.D.
34	1986	John R. Little, M.D.
35	1987	Peter McL. Black, M.D., Ph.D.
36	1988	Peter McL. Black, M.D., Ph.D.
37	1989	Peter McL. Black, M.D., Ph.D.
38	1990	Warren R. Selman, M.D.
39	1991	Warren R. Selman, M.D.

Contributors

Cristian Achim M.D., Ph.D.
Department of Pathology
    (Neuropathology)
University of Pittsburgh
Pittsburgh, Pennsylvania

Ossama Al-Mefty, M.D.
Department of Neurosurgery
University of Arkansas for
    Medical Sciences
Little Rock, Arkansas

Julian E. Bailes, Jr, M.D.
Department of Neurosurgery
West Virginia University
Morgantown, West Virginia

H. Hunt Batjer, M.D.
Department of Neurosurgery
Northwestern University Medical
    Center
Chicago, Illinois

Mitchel S. Berger, M.D.
Department of Neurological
    Surgery
University of California, San
    Francisco
San Francisco, California

Oliver Bogler, Ph.D.
Department of Neurosurgery
Henry Ford Health System
Hermelin Brain Tumor Center
Detroit, Michigan

David W. Cahill, M.D., F.A.C.S.
Chairman and Professor
Department of Neurosurgery
University of South Florida
College of Medicine
Tampa, Florida

P. Catalano, M.D.
Department of Otolaryngology
Lahey Clinic
Burlington, Massachusetts

Susan M. Chang, M.D.
Associate Professor
Department of Neurosurgery
University of California, San
    Francisco
San Francisco, California

P. Costantino, M.D.
Department of Otolaryngology
St. Luke's-Roosevelt Hospital
    Center
New York, New York

David Croteau, M.D. F.R.C.P.(C)
Department of Neurosurgery
Henry Ford Health System
Hermelin Brain Tumor Center
Detroit, Michigan

Franco DeMonte M.D.,
    F.R.C.S.C., F.A.C.S.
Associate Professor and Director
    of Training
Department of Neurosurgery
The University of Texas
M.D. Anderson Cancer Center
Houston, Texas

James M. Ecklund, M.D.,
   F.A.C.S., L.T.C., M.C., U.S.A.
Chief and Program Director
National Capital Consortium
(Walter Reed Army Medical
   Center
National Naval Medical Center)
Washington, DC

Michael G. Fehlings, M.D., Ph.D.,
   F.R.C.S.(C)
Professor of Surgery
Division of Neurosurgery
Robert O. Lawson Chair in Neural
   Repair and Regeneration
University of Toronto
University Health Network
Head, Spinal Program
Toronto Western Hospital
Toronto, Ontario, Canada

Peter C. Gerszten, M.D., M.P.H.
Assistant Professor
Department of Neurologic Surgery
UMPC-HS Presbyterian
   University Hospital
Pittsburgh, Pennsylvania

Regis W. Haid, M.D.
Associate Professor
Department of Neurosurgery
Emory University
School of Medicine
Atlanta, Georgia

Stephen J. Haines, M.D.
Department of Neurological
   Surgery
Medical University of South
   Carolina
Charleston, South Carolina

D. Hiltzik, M.D.
Mount Sinai School of Medicine
New York, New York

John A. Jane, Jr, M.D.
Department of Neurosurgery
University of Virginia
Health Sciences Center
Charlottesville, Virginia

Hae-Dong Jho, M.D., Ph.D.
Professor Neurological Surgery
Director, Minimally Invasive
   Innovative
   Microneurogurgery
Department of Neurological
   Surgery
University of Pittsburgh
Pittsburgh, Pennsylvania

Chandrasekar Kalavakonda, M.D.
Mid-Atlantic Brain & Spine
   Institutes
Washington, DC, and Annandale,
   Virginia
Assistant Professor of
   Neurosurgery
Sri Ramachandra Medical College
   and Research Institute
Chennai, India

Michael G. Kaplitt, M.D., Ph.D.
Fellow Functional and
   Stereotactic Neurosurgery
Division of Neurosurgery
Department of Surgery
Toronto Western Hospital
University Health Network
Toronto, Ontario, Canada

Douglas Kondziolka, M.D., M.Sc.,
   FRCS(C)
Professor, Department of
   Neurological Surgery
Director, Neurotransplantation
   Research Program
University of Pittsburgh
Pittsburgh, Pennsylvania

Edward R. Laws, Jr, M.D.,
F.A.C.S.
Department of Neurosurgery
University of Virginia
Health System
Charlottesville, Virginia

W. Lawson, M.D.
Department of Otolaryngology
Mount Sinai Medical Center
New York, New York

Geoffery Ling, M.D., Ph.D.,
L.T.X., M.C., U.S.A.
Associate Professor and Director
Critical Care Medicine
Uniformed Services
University of Health Sciences
Bethesda, Maryland

Andres M. Lozano, M.D., Ph.D.
Division of Neurosurgery
Department of Surgery
The Toronto Western Hospital
Toronto, Ontario, Canada

L. Dade Lunsford, M.D., F.A.C.S.
Chairman, Department of
Neurological Surgery
Professor of Neurological Surgery,
Radiology, and Radiation
Oncology
University of Pittsburgh School
of Medicine
Pittsburgh, Pennsylvania

Paul C. McCormick, M.D., M.P.H.
Professor of Clinical Neurosurgery
Columbia University College of
Physicians and Surgeons
The New York Presbyterian
Hospital
New York, New York

Paula McGrath, R.N.
Department of Neurologic Surgery
UMPC-HS Presbyterian
University Hospital
Pittsburgh, Pennsylvania

Mark R. McLaughlin, M.D.
Neurological and Neurosurgical
Associates
Springfield, Massachusetts

Tom Mikkelsen, M.D., F.R.C.P.(C)
Departments of Neurology and
Neurosurgery
Henry Ford Health System
Co-Director, Hermelin Brain
Tumor Center
Detroit, Michigan

Ross R. Moquin, M.D., C.D.R.,
U.S.N.
Associate Program Director
National Capital Consortium
(Walter Reed Army Medical
Center
National Naval Medical Center)
Washington, DC

Ajay Niranjan, M.B.B.S., M.S.,
M.Ch.
Research Assistant Professor
Department of Neurological
Surgery
University of Pittsburgh School
of Medicine
Pittsburgh, Pennsylvania

Thomas C. Origitano, M.D., Ph.D.,
F.A.C.S.
Professor and Chair
Department of Neurological
Surgery
Loyola University Medical
Center
Maywood, Illinois

Richard G. Perrin, M.D.
Wellesley Hospital
Toronto, Ontario, Canada

Joseph M. Piepmeier, M.D.
Professor and Vice-Chairman
Department of Neurosurgery
Yale University School of Medicine
New Haven, Connecticut

Sandra A. Rempel, Ph.D.
Department of Neurosurgery
Henry Ford Health System
Hermelin Brain Tumor Center
Detroit, Michigan

Gerald E. Rodts, Jr, M.D.
Associate Professor
Department of Neurosurgery
Emory University
School of Medicine
Atlanta, Georgia

Mark L. Rosenblum, M.D.
Chairman, Department of
    Neurosurgery
Henry Ford Health System
Co-Director, Hermelin Brain
    Tumor Center
Detroit, Michigan

Paul R. Sanberg, Ph.D., D.Sc.
Director, Center for Aging and
    Brain Repair
University of South Florida
College of Medicine
Tampa, Florida

Raymond Sawaya, M.D.
The University of Texas
MD Anderson Cancer Center
Texas Medical Center
Houston, Texas

Meic H. Schmidt, M.D.
Clinical Instructor
Department of Neurological
    Surgery
University of California, San
    Francisco
San Francisco, California

Laligam N. Sekhar, M.D.,
    F.A.C.S.
Mid-Atlantic Brain & Spine
    Institutes
Washington, DC, and Annandale,
    Virginia
Clinical Professor of
    Neurosurgery
The George Washington
    University Medical Center
Washington, DC

Lali H.S. Sekhon, M.B., B.S.,
    Ph.D., F.R.A.C.S.
Fellow in Complex Spine Surgery
Division of Neurosurgery
University of Toronto
Toronto Western Hospital
Toronto, Ontario, Canada

Chandranath Sen, M.D.
Chairman, Department of
    Neurosurgery
St. Luke's-Roosevelt Hospital
    Center
New York, New York

Mark E. Shaffrey, M.D.
Associate Professor
Vice-Chairman,
Department of Neurosurgery
University of Virginia
Health System
Charlottesville, Virginia

Volker K. H. Sonntag, M.D.
Vice Chairman
Division of Neurological Surgery
Director, Residency Program
Chairman, BNI Spine Section
Clinical Professor of Surgery
    (Neurosurgery)
University of Arizona
Phoenix, Arizona

Robert D. Strang, M.D.
University of Arkansas for
    Medical Sciences
Department of Neurosurgery
Little, Rock, Arkansas

Brian R. Subach, M.D.
Assistant Professor
Department of Neurosurgery
Emory University
School of Medicine
Atlanta, Georgia

Nicholas Theodore, M.D.
Chief Resident
Division of Neurological Surgery
Barrow Neurological Institute
St. Joseph's Hospital and Medical
    Center
Phoenix, Arizona

Vincent C. Traynelis, M.D.
Professor of Neurosurgery
Department of Neurosurgery
The University of Iowa
Iowa City, Iowa

A. Triana, M.D.
Department of Neurosurgery
Mount Sinai Medical Center
New York, New York

Elizabeth Tyler-Kabara, M.D.,
    Ph.D.
Department of Neurological
    Surgery
University of Pittsburgh
Pittsburgh, Pennsylvania

M. Urken, M.D.
Department of Otolaryngology
Mount Sinai Medical Center
New York, New York

Craig A. Van Der Veer, M.D.
Charlotte Neurosurgical
    Associates
Charlotte, North Carolina

William C. Welch, M.D., FACS
Associate Professor
Department of Neurologic
    Surgery
UPMC-HS Presbyterian
    University Hospital
Pittsburgh, Pennsylvania

Alison E. Willing, Ph.D.
Assistant Professor
Department of Neurosurgery
University of South Florida
College of Medicine
Tampa, Florida

Biography

Edward R. Laws, was born in New York City on April 29, 1938. He received his bachelor's degree from Princeton University with honors in Economics and Sociology in the Special Program in American Civilization, and he then attended the Johns Hopkins University School of Medicine in Baltimore, Maryland, receiving an M.D. in 1963. He did his surgical internship and neurosurgical residency at Johns Hopkins under A. Earl Walker. After completing his residency in 1971, he joined the faculty at the Johns Hopkins medical school with a primary appointment in pediatric neurosurgery. In 1972, he joined the staff of the Mayo Clinic in Rochester, Minnesota, where ultimately he became Professor of Neurosurgery and developed major interests in pituitary surgery and epilepsy surgery along with a continuing interest in the metabolism and pathophysiology of primary brain tumors. In 1987 he became Professor and Chairman of the Department of Neurosurgery at the George Washington University in Washington, D.C., and in 1992 joined the faculty of the University of Virginia as Professor of Neurosurgery and Professor of Medicine, establishing a Neuro-Endocrine Center there. During this surgical career he has operated upon more than 5000 brain tumors, of which 3600 have been pituitary lesions.

Dr. Laws has served as President of the Congress of Neurological Surgeons, Editor of *Neurosurgery,* Chairman of the Board of Trustees of the Foundation for International Education in Neurosurgery, Secretary of the World Federation of Neurological Societies, Director of the American Board of Neurological Surgery, President of the American Association of Neurological Surgeons, and President of the Pituitary Society. He has authored over 400 scientific papers and book chapters, and with Andrew Kaye is co-editor of the encyclopedic volume *Brain Tumors.*

Currently he is a member of the Executive Committee of the Board of Regents of the American College of Surgeons and is Chair of Residency Review Committee for Neurosurgery. He remains actively involved in brain tumor and neuroendocrine research.

Dr. Laws and his wife Margaret (Peggy) have four daughters and three grandchildren.

Bibliography

ORIGINAL REPORTS (Peer Reviewed)

1. Udvarhelyi GB, O'Connor JS, Walker AE, Laws ER Jr., Krainin S: A histochemical study of tumors of the central nervous system. **Proc IV Int'l Cong Neuropath** 1: 95–102, 1962.
2. O'Connor JS, Laws ER Jr: Histochemical survey of brain tumor enzymes. **Arch Neurol** 9: 641–651, 1963.
3. Laws ER Jr: Route of absorption of DDAVP after oral administration to rats. **Toxicol Appl Pharmacol** 8: 193–196, 1966.
4. Laws ER Jr: What to do after a pesticide accident. **Pest Control** 34: 8–19, 1966.
5. Gaines TB, Kimbrough R, Laws ER Jr: Toxicology of Abate in laboratory animals. **Arch Environ Health** 14: 282–288, 1967.
6. Laws ER Jr, Morales FR, Hayes WJ Jr, Joseph CR: Toxicology of Abate in Volunteers. **Arch Environ Health** 14: 289–291, 1967.
7. Laws ER Jr, Curley A, Biros FJ: Men with intensive occupational exposure to dichlorodiphenyl trichloromethane: a clinical and chemical study. **Arch Environ Health** 16: 766–775, 1967.
8. Laws ER Jr, Sedlack VA, Miles JW, Joseph CR, Lacomba JR, Rivera AD: Field study of the safety of Abate for treating potable water and observations on the effectiveness of a control programme involving both Abate and malathion. **Bull WHO** 38: 439–445, 1968.
9. O'Connor JS, Laws ER Jr: Changes in histochemical staining of brain tumor blood vessels associated with increasing malignancy. **Acta Neuropathol** 14: 161–173, 1969.
10. Niedermeyer E, Laws ER Jr, Walker AE: Depth electroencephalography findings in epileptics with generalized spike-wave complexes. **Arch Neurol** 21: 51–58, 1969.
11. Laws ER Jr, Niedermeyer E, Walker AE: Diagnostic significance of scalp and depth electroencephalography findings in patients with temporal and frontal lobe epilepsy, **Johns Hopkins Med Journal** 126: 146–153, 1970.
12. Laws ER Jr, O'Connor JS: ATPase in human brain tumors. **J Neurosurg** 33: 167–171, 1970.
13. Laws ER Jr: Evidence of antitumorigenic effects of dichlorodiphenyl trichloromethane. **Arch Environ Health** 23: 181–184, 1971.
14. Laws ER Jr, Maddrey WC, Curley A, Burse VW: Long-term occu-

pational exposure to DDT: effect on the human liver, **Arch Environ Health** 27: 318–321, 1973.

15. Powell DF, Baker HL Jr, Laws ER Jr: The primary angiographic findings in pituitary adenomas. **Radiology** 110: 589–595, 1974.

16. Campbell JK, Baker HL Jr, Laws ER Jr: Computer assisted axial tomography (EMI Scan) in neurologic investigation. **Trans Am Neurol Assoc** 99: 117–120, 1974.

17. Ebersold MJ, Laws ER Jr, Stonnington HH, Stillwell GK: Transcutaneous electrical stimulation for treatment of chronic pain relief: a preliminary report. **Surgical Neurol** 4: 96–99, 1975.

18. Laws ER Jr: Junior neuroemergencies—an injured skull. **Emergency Medicine** 1: 219–235, 1975.

19. Laws ER Jr, Kern EB: Complications of transsphenoidal surgery. **Clin Neurosurg** 23: 401–416, 1976.

20. Stonnington HH, Stillwell GK, Ebersold MJ, Thorsteinsson G, Laws ER Jr: Transcutaneous electrical stimulation for chronic pain relief: a pilot study. **Minnesota Medicine** pp 681–683, 1976.

21. Saez RJ, Campbell RJ, Laws ER Jr: Chemotherapeutic trials on human malignant astrocytomas in organ culture. **J Neurosurg** 46: 320–327, 1977.

22. Ebersold MJ, Laws ER Jr and Albers JW: Measurements of autonomic function before, during and after transcutaneous stimulation in patients with chronic pain and in control subjects. **Mayo Clinic Proc** 52: 228–232, 1977.

23. Rosenbaum TJ, Houser OW, Laws ER Jr: Pituitary apoplexy producing internal carotid artery occlusion. Case report. **J Neurosurg** 47: 599–604, 1977.

24. Kern EB, Laws ER Jr, Randall RV, Westwood WB: A transseptal, transsphenoidal approach to the pituitary. An old approach, a new technique in the management of pituitary tumors and related disorders. **Trans Amer Acad Ophthalmol and Otolaryngol** 84: 997–1010, 1977.

25. Laws ER Jr, Mokri B: Occult hydrocephalus: results of shunting correlated with diagnostic tests. **Clin Neurosurg** 24:316–333, 1977.

26. Laws ER Jr, Trautman JC, Hollenhorst RW Jr: Transsphenoidal decompression of the optic nerve and chiasm. **J Neurosurg** 46: 717–722, 1977.

27. Sim FH, Stauffer RN, Dahlin DC, Laws ER Jr: Primary bone tumors simulating lumbar disk syndrome. **Spine** 2: 65–74, 1977.

28. Salassa RM, Laws ER Jr, Carpenter PC, Northcutt RC: Transsphenoidal removal of pituitary microadenoma in Cushing's disease. **Mayo Clinic Proc** 53: 24–28, 1978.

29. Messick JM, Laws ER Jr, Abboud CF: Anesthesia for transsphenoidal surgery of the hypophyseal region. **Anesthesia and Analgesia** 57: 206–215, 1978.

30. Tyson JE, Archer DF, Friesen HG, Laws ER Jr, Naftolin F, Robyn C: Symposium: Pituitary tumors: approaches to diagnosis and treatment. **Contemp OB/GYN** 11: 84–143, 1978.

31. Kern EB, Laws ER Jr, Randall RV, Westwood WB: A transseptal, transsphenoidal approach to the pituitary. **Postgraduate Medicine** 63: 97–108, 1978.

32. Kern EB, Laws ER Jr: The transseptal approach to the pituitary gland. **Rhinology** 16: 59–78, 1978.

33. Goellner JR, Laws ER Jr, Soule EH, Okazaki H: Hemangiopericytoma of the meninges. Mayo Clinic Experience. **American Journal of Clinical Pathology** 70: 375–380, 1978.

34. Annegers JF, Coulam CB, Abboud CF, Laws ER Jr, Kurland LT: Pituitary adenoma in Olmsted County, Minnesota, 1935–1977. **Mayo Clinic Proc** 53: 641–643, 1978.

35. Donat JF, Okazaki H, Gomez MR, Reagan TJ, Baker HL Jr, Laws ER Jr: Pineal tumors—a 53-year experience. **Archives of Neurology** 35: 736–740, 1978.

36. Fode NC, Laws ER Jr, Sharbrough FW: The assessment of patients with temporal lobe epilepsy: results in 38 patients treated surgically. **J Neurosurg Nursing** 10: 130–135, 1978.

37. Kern EB, Laws ER Jr, Randall RV: Transseptal, transsphenoidal pituitary surgery. **Minerva Endocrinologica** 3: 187–198, 1978.

38. Coulam CB, Annegers JF, Abboud CF, Laws ER Jr, Kurland LT: Pituitary adenoma and oral contraceptives: a case control study. **Fertility and Sterility** 31: 25–28, 1979.

39. Laws ER Jr: Transsphenoidal tumor surgery for intrasellar pathology. **Clin Neurosurg** 26: 391–397, 1979.

40. Laws ER Jr, Onofrio BM, Pearson BW, McDonald TJ, Dirrenberger RA: Successful management of bilateral carotid-cavernous fistulae with transsphenoidal approach. **Neurosurg** 4: 162–167, 1979.

41. Laws ER Jr, Piepgras DG, Randall RV, Abboud CF: Neurosurgical management of acromegaly—results in 82 patients treated between 1972 and 1977. **J Neurosurg** 50: 454–461, 1979.

42. Kern EB, Pearson BW, McDonald TJ, Laws ER Jr: The transseptal approach to lesion of the pituitary and parasellar regions. **The Laryngoscope,** Suppl No. 15 89: 1–34, 1979.

43. Laws ER Jr, Ivins JC: Atlanto-occipital instability as a result of pituitary adenoma: case report with successful management by cervico-occipital fusion. **Johns Hopkins Med Journ** 145: 136–183, 1979.

44. Simeone FA, Kjellberg RN, Laws ER Jr: Therapy of recurrent acromegaly. **Neurosurg** 4: 573–574, 1979.
45. Annegers JF, Laws ER Jr, Kurland LT, Grabow JD: Head trauma and subsequent brain tumors. **Neurosurg** 4: 203–206, 1979.
46. Eagan RT, Childs DS Jr, Layton DD Jr, Laws ER Jr, Bisel HF, Holbrook MA, Fleming TR: Dianhydrogalactitol and radiation therapy—treatment of supratentorial gliomas. **JAMA** 241: 2046–2050, 1979.
47. McDonald TJ, Kern EB, Laws ER Jr, Pearson BW: Surgical approaches to the pituitary gland with emphasis on the transseptal route. **Head & Neck Surgery** 1: 498–504, 1979.
48. Abboud CF, Laws ER Jr: Clinical endocrinological approach to hypothalamic-pituitary disease. **J Neurosurg** 51: 271–291, 1979.
49. Fode NC, Laws ER Jr, Sundt TM Jr: Communicating hydrocephalus after subarachnoid hemorrhage: results of shunt procedures. **J Neurosurg Nursing** 11: 253–256, 1979.
50. Laws ER Jr: The neurosurgeon and neuroendocrinology. **Clin Neurosurg** 27: 3–18, 1980.
51. Kern EB, Laws ER Jr: A speculum for transseptal, transsphenoidal pituitary surgery. **Rhinology** 18: 155–156, 1980.
52. Kern EB, Pearson BW, McDonald TJ, Laws ER Jr: Transseptal approach to lesions of pituitary and parasellar regions. **Year Book of Surgery** 224–225, 1980.
53. Martin JB, Reichlin S, Besser GM, Krieger DT, Laws ER Jr: Symposium on pituitary tumors. **Trans Am Neurol Assoc** 105: 241–275, 1980.
54. Laws ER Jr: Transsphenoidal microsurgery in the management of craniopharyngioma. **J Neurosurg** 52: 661–666, 1980.
55. Campbell WM, McDonald TJ, Unni KK, Laws ER Jr: Nasal and paranasal presentations of chordomas. **Laryngoscope** 90: 612–618, 1980.
56. Annegers JF, Grabow JD, Groover RV, Laws ER Jr, Elveback LR, Kurland LT: Seizures after head trauma: a population study. **Neurology** 30: 683–689, 1980.
57. Lantz EJ, Forbes GS, Brown ML, Laws ER Jr: Radiology of cerebrospinal fluid rhinorrhea. **AJNR** 1: 391–398, 1980.
58. Gorenstein A, Kern EB, Facer FW, Laws ER Jr: Nasal gliomas. **Arch Otolaryngol** 106: 536–540, 1980.
59. Annegers JF, Grabow JD, Kurland LT, Laws ER Jr: The incidence, causes, and secular trends of head trauma in Olmsted County, Minnesota, 1935–1974. **Neurology** 30: 912–919, 1980.
60. Laws ER Jr, Abboud CF, Kern EB: Perioperative management of

patients with pituitary microadenomas. **Neurosurg** 7: 566–570, 1980.

61. Fode NC, Laws ER Jr, Abboud CF, Randall RV, Kempers RD: Prolactin secreting pituitary adenoma: a review and study of their implications for fertility in women. **J Neurosurg Nursing** 12: 210–213, 1980.

62. Harner SG, Laws ER Jr: The middle cranial fossa approach to the temporal bone. **Minnesota Medicine** 63: 250–255, 1980.

63. Lantz EJ, Forbes GS, Brown ML, Laws ER Jr: Radiology of cerebrospinal fluid rhinorrhea. **AJR** 135: 1023–1030, 1980.

64. Laws ER Jr, Abboud CF, Hayles AB: The practical management of pituitary replacement therapy related to sellar and parasellar surgery. **Clin Neurosurg** 28: 108–115, 1981.

65. Deen HG Jr, Laws ER Jr: Multiple primary brain tumors of different cell types. **Neurosurg** 8: 20–25, 1981.

66. Davis DH, Laws ER Jr, McDonald TJ, Salassa TJ, Phillips LH II: Intraventricular tension pneumocephalus as a complication of paranasal sinus surgery: **Case Report Neurosurg** 8: 574–576, 1981.

67. Kern EB, Laws ER Jr: Transnasal pituitary surgery. **Head and Neck Surgery** 7: 1–19, 1981.

68. Atassi H, Laws ER Jr, Veneziale CM: Can androgens alone fully restore seminal vesicle epithelium? **Proc Soc Exp Biol Med** 167: 94–97, 1981.

69. Stoffer SS, McKeel DW Jr, Randall RV, Laws ER Jr: Pituitary prolactin hyperplasia with autonomous prolactin secretion and primary hypothyroidism. **Fertility Sterility** 36: 682–688, 1982.

70. Auger RG, Piepgras DG, Laws ER Jr, Miller RH: Microvascular decompression of the facial nerve for hemifacial spasm: clinical and electrophysiologic observations. **Neurology** 41: 346–350, 1981.

71. White KT, Fleming TR, Laws ER Jr: Single metastasis to the brain: surgical treatment in 122 consecutive patients. **Mayo Clinic Proc** 56: 424–428, 1981.

72. Coulam CB, Laws ER Jr, Abboud CF, Randall RV: Primary amenorrhea and pituitary adenomas. **Fertility Sterility** 35: 615–619, 1981.

73. Yasuoka S, Peterson HA, Laws ER Jr, MacCarty CS: Pathogenesis and prophylaxis of post-laminectomy deformity of the spine after multiple level laminectomy: difference between children and adults. **Neurosurg** 9: 145–152, 1981.

74. Harner SG, Laws ER Jr: Diagnosis of acoustic neurinoma. **Neurosurg** 9: 373–379, 1981.

75. Harner SG, Laws ER Jr: Posterior fossa approach for removal of acoustic neurinomas. **Arch Otolaryng** 107: 590–593, 1981.
76. Abay EO, Laws ER Jr, Grado GL, Bruckman JE, Forbes GS, Gomez MR, Scott M: Pineal tumors in children and adolescents—treatment by CSF shunting and radiotherapy. **J Neurosurg** 55: 889–895, 1981.
77. Laws ER Jr, Cortese DA, Kinsey JH, Eagan RT, Anderson RE: Photoradiation therapy in the treatment of malignant brain tumors: a phase I (feasibility) study. **Neurosurg** 9: 672–678, 1981.
78. Johnson RE, Campbell RJ, Laws ER Jr: The cytotoxic effect of ethylnitrosourea on the developing rat cerebellum—morphologic observations. **Acta Neuropathol (Berl)** 55: 257–261, 1981.
79. Laws ER Jr, Ebersold MJ: Pituitary apoplexy—an endocrine emergency. **World J Surg** 6: 686–688, 1982.
80. Jackson IT, Hide TAH, Gomuwka PK, Laws ER Jr, Langford K: Treatment of cranio-orbital fibrous dysplasia. **J Maxillo-facial Surg** 10: 138–141, 1982.
81. Tenny RT, Laws ER Jr, Younge BR, Rush JA: The neurosurgical management of optic glioma. **J Neurosurg** 57: 452–458, 1982.
82. Wharen RE Jr, Scheithauer BW, Laws ER Jr: Thrombosed arteriovenous malformations of the brain. **J Neurosurg** 57: 520–526, 1982.
83. Harner SG, Laws ER Jr: Translabyrinthine repair for cerebrospinal fluid otorhinorrhea. **J Neurosurg** 57: 258–261, 1982.
84. Randall RV, Scheithauer BW, Laws ER Jr, Abboud CF: Pseudoprolactinomas. **Trans Am Clin Climatol Assoc** 94: 114–121, 1982.
85. Salassa RM, Laws ER Jr, Carpenter PC, Northcutt RC: Cushing's disease—50 years later. **Trans Am Clin Climatol Assoc** 94: 122–129, 1982.
86. Randall RV, Laws ER Jr, Abboud CF, Ebersold MJ, Kao PC, Scheithauer BW: Transsphenoidal microsurgical treatment of prolactin-producing pituitary adenomas: results in 100 patients. **Mayo Clinic Proc** 58: 108–121, 1983.
87. Ebersold MJ, Laws ER Jr, Scheithauer BW, Randall RV: Pituitary apoplexy treated by transsphenoidal surgery. A clinicopathological and immunocytochemical study. **J Neurosurg** 58: 315–320, 1983.
88. Fode NC, Laws ER Jr, Northcutt RC: Pituitary tumors and hypertension: implications for neurosurgical nurses. **J Neurosurg Nursing** 15: 33–35, 1983.
89. Laws ER Jr, Fode NC, Randall RV, Abboud CF, Coulam CB: Pregnancy following transsphenoidal resection of prolactin-secreting pituitary tumors. **J Neurosurg** 58: 685–688, 1983.

90. Wharen RE Jr, Anderson RE, Laws ER Jr: Quantitation of hematoporphyrin derivative in human gliomas, experimental central nervous system tumors, and normal tissue. **Neurosurg** 12: 446–450, 1983.

91. Wirth FP, Laws ER Jr, Piepgras DG, Scott RM: Surgical treatment of incidental intracranial aneurysms. **Neurosurg** 12: 507–511, 1983.

92. Gharib H, Frey HM, Laws ER Jr, Randall RV, Scheithauer BW: Coexistent primary empty sella syndrome and hyperprolactinemia. **Arch Intern Med** 143: 1383–1386, 1983.

93. Trautman JC, Laws ER Jr: Visual status after transsphenoidal surgery at the Mayo Clinic, 1971–1982. **Am J Ophthalmol** 96: 200–208, 1983.

94. Jackson IT, Laws ER Jr, Martin RD: A craniofacial approach to advanced recurrent cancer of the central face. **Head Neck Surg** 5: 474–488, 1983.

95. Harner SG, Laws ER Jr: Clinical findings in patients with acoustic neurinoma. **Mayo Clinic Proc** 58: 721–728, 1983.

96. Wold LE, Laws ER Jr: Cranial chordomas in children and young adults. **J Neurosurg** 59: 1043–1047, 1983.

97. Jackson IT, Laws ER Jr, Martin RD: The surgical management of orbital neurofibromatosis. **Plast Reconst Surg** 71: 751–758, 1983.

98. Scheithauer BW, Kovacs K, Randall RV, Horvath E, Okazaki H, Laws ER Jr: Hypothalamic neuronal hamartoma and adenohypophyseal neuronal choristoma: their association with growth hormone adenoma of the pituitary gland. **J Neuropath Experimental Neurol** 42: 648–663, 1983.

99. Agrez MV, Wharen RE Jr, Anderson RE, Laws ER Jr, Ilstrup DM, Cortese DA, Shorter RG, Lieber MM: Hematoporphyrin derivative: quantitative uptake in dimethylhydrazine-induced murine colorectal carcinoma. **J Surg Onc** 24: 173–176, 1983.

100. Horvath E, Kovacs K, Scheithauer BW, Randall RV, Laws ER Jr, Thorner MO, Tindall GT, Barrow DL: Pituitary adenomas producing growth hormone, prolactin, and one or more glycoprotein hormones: a histologic, immunohistochemical, and ultrastructural study of four surgically removed tumors. **Ultrastructural Pathol** 5: 171–183, 1983.

101. Laws ER Jr: Transspehnoidal surgery for tumors of the clivus. **Head Neck Surg** 92: 100–101, 1984.

102. Laws ER Jr: The pituitary before and after adrenalectomy for Cushing's syndrome. **World J Surg** 8: 386–387, 1984.

103. Asa SL, Scheithauer BW, Bilbao JM, Horvath E, Ryan N, Kovacs

K, Randall RV, Laws ER Jr, Singer W, Linfoot JA, Thorner MO, Vale W: A case for hypothalmic acromegaly: a clinicopathological study of six patients with hypothalamic gangliocytomas producing growth hormone-releasing factor. **J Clin Endo Met** 58: 796–803, 1984.

104. Young WF Jr, Okazaki H, Laws ER Jr, Weinshilboum RM: Human brain phenol sulfotransferase: biochemical properties and regional localization. **J Neurochem** 43: 706–715, 1984.

105. Nelson EL, Melton LJ III, Annegers JF, Laws ER Jr, Offord KP: Incidence of skull fractures in Olmsted County, Minnesota. **Neurosurg** 15: 318–324, 1984.

106. Laws ER Jr, Taylor WF, Clifton MB, Okazaki H: Neurosurgical management of low-grade astrocytoma of the cerebral hemospheres. **J Neurosurg** 61: 665–673, 1984.

107. Young WF Jr, Abboud CF, Laws ER Jr, VanLoon JA, Weinshilboum RM: Erythrocyte catechol-O-methyltransferase, platelet monoamine oxidase, and platelet phenol sulfotransferase activities in patients with prolactin-secreting pituitary adenomas. **J Clin Endocrinol Metab** 59: 1207–1210, 1984.

108. Anderson RE, Wharen R, Laws ER Jr, et al: Parameters of hematoporphyrin derivative cell killing efficiency: decomposition of hematoporphyrin derivative at high power densities. **Prog Clin Biol Res** 170: 483–500, 1984.

109. Harner SG, Laws ER Jr, Onofrio BM: Hearing preservation after removal of acoustic neurinoma. **Laryngoscope** 94: 1431–1434, 1984.

110. Randall, RV, Scheithauer BW, Laws ER Jr: Hormone-containing non-secreting pituitary tumors: Clinically silent monohormonal pituitary adenomas. **Trans Am Clin Climatol Assoc** 96: 98–103, 1984.

111. Scheithauer BW, Randall RV, Laws ER Jr, Kovacs KT, Horvath E, Whitaker MD: Prolactin cell carcinoma of the pituitary. **Cancer** 55: 598–604, 1985.

112. Petersen RC, Mokri B, Laws ER Jr: Surgical treatment of idiopathic hydrocephalus in elderly patients. **Neurology** 35: 307–311, 1985.

113. Molinatti PA, Scheithauer BW, Randall RV, Laws ER Jr: Metastasis to pituitary adenoma. **Arch Pathol Lab Med** 109: 287–289, 1985.

114. Marsh WR, Laws ER Jr: Shunting and irradiation of pineal tumors. **Clin Neurosurg** 32: 540–573, 1985.

115. Hubbard JL, McDonald TJ, Pearson BW, Laws ER Jr: Spontaneous cerebrospinal fluid rhinorrhea: Evolving concepts in diag-

nosis and surgical management based on the Mayo Clinic experience from 1970 through 1981. **Neurosurg** 16: 314–321, 1985.

116. Young WF Jr, Laws ER Jr, Sharbrough FW, Weinshilboum RM: Human phenol sulfotransferase: Correlation of brain and platelet activities. **J Neurochem** 44: 1131–1137, 1985.

117. Laird FJ, Harner SG, Laws ER Jr, Reese DF: Meningiomas of the cerebellopontine angle. **Otolaryngol Head Neck Surg** 93: 163–167, 1985.

118. Laws ER Jr: Tradition in Neurosurgery: doing well what has been done before. **Neurosurg** 16: 739–753, 1985.

119. Laws ER Jr, Scheithauer BW, Carpenter SM, Randall RV, Abboud CF: The pathogenesis of acromegaly: Clinical and immunocytochemical analysis in 75 patients. **J Neurosurg** 63: 35–38, 1985.

120. Earnest F, Baker HL Jr, Kispert DB, Laws ER Jr: Magnetic resonance imaging vs. computed tomography: advantages and disadvantages. **Clin Neurosurg** 32: 540–573, 1985.

121. Kaplan HC, Baker HL Jr, Houser OW, Laws ER Jr, Abboud CF, Scheithauer BW: CT of sella turcica after transsphenoidal resection of pituitary adenomas. **AJNR** 6: 723–732, 1985.

122. Randall RV, Scheithauer BW, Laws ER Jr, Abboud CF, Ebersold MJ, Kao PC: Pituitary adenomas associated with hyperprolactinemia: A clinical and immunohistochemical study of 97 patients operated on transsphenoidally. **Mayo Clin Proc** 60: 753–762, 1985.

123. Laws ER Jr, Fode NC, Redmond MJ: Transsphenoidal surgery following unsuccessful prior therapy. **J Neurosurg** 63: 823–829, 1985.

124. Brennan MD, Jackson IT, Keller EE, Laws ER Jr, Sather AH: Multidisciplinary management of acromegaly and it deformities. **JAMA** 253: 683–683, 1985.

125. Meyer FB, Marsh WR, Laws ER Jr, Sharbrough FW: Temporal lobectomy in children with epilepsy. **J Neurosurg** 64: 371–376, 1986.

126. Ransohoff J, Kelly PJ, Laws ER Jr: The role of intracranial surgery for the treatment of malignant gliomas. **Semin Oncol** 13: 27–37, 1986.

127. Laws ER Jr, Taylor WF, Bergstralh EJ, Okazaki H, Clifton MB: The neurosurgical management of low-grade astrocytoma. **Clin Neurosurg** 33: 575–588, 1986.

128. Scheithauer BW, Kovacs KT, Randall RV, Horvath E, Laws ER Jr: Pathology of excessive production of growth hormone. **Clin Endocrinol Metab** 15: 655–681, 1986.

129. Wass JAH, Laws ER Jr, Randall RV, Sheline GE: The treatment of acromegaly. **Clin Endocrinol Metab** 15: 683–707, 1986.
130. Selman WR, Laws ER Jr, Scheithauer BW, Carpenter SM: The occurrence of dural invasion in pituitary adenomas. **J Neurosurg** 64: 402–407, 1986.
131. Kooistra KL, Rodriguez M, Powis G, Yaksh TL, Harty GJ, Hilton JF, Laws ER Jr: Development of experimental models for meningeal neoplasia using intrathecal injection of 9L gliosarcoma and Walker 256 carcinosarcoma in the rat. **Cancer Res** 46: 317–323, 1986.
132. Scheithauer BW, Horvath E, Kovacs K, Laws ER Jr, Randall RV, Ryan N: Plurihormonal pituitary adenomas. **Semin Diag Pathol** 3: 69–82, 1986.
133. Ebersold MJ, Quast LM, Laws ER Jr, Scheithauer BW, Randall RV: Long-term results in transsphenoidal removal of nonfunctioning pituitary adenomas. **J Neurosurg** 64: 713–719, 1986.
134. Ormson MJ, Kispert DB, Sharbrough FW, Houser OW, Earnest F, Scheithauer BW, Laws ER Jr: Cryptic structural lesions in refractory partial epilepsy: MR imaging and CT studies. **Radiology** 160: 215–219, 1986.
135. Young WF Jr, Laws ER Jr, Sharbrough FW, Weinshilboum RM: Human monoamine oxidase—lack of brain and platelet correlation. **Arch Gen Psychiatry** 43: 604–609, 1986.
136. Auger RG, Piepgras DG, Laws ER Jr: Hemifacial spasm: results of microvascular decompression of the facial nerve in 54 patients. **Mayo Clin Proc** 61: 640–644, 1986.
137. Hardie NA, Molgaard CA, Laws ER Jr, O'Fallon WM, Kurland LT: Incidence and effectiveness of cerebrospinal fluid shunts in Olmsted County, Minnesota, 1956–1981. **Neuroepidem** 5: 95–104, 1986.
138. Bahn RS, Scheithauer BW, vanHeerden JA, Laws ER Jr, Horvath E, Gharib H: Nonidentical expressions of multiple endocrine neoplasia, Type I, in identical twins. **Mayo Clin Proc** 61: 689–696, 1986.
139. Waren RE Jr, So S, Anderson RE, Laws ER Jr: Hematoporphyrin derivative photocytotoxicity of human glioblastoma in cell culture. **Neurosurg** 19: 495–501, 1986.
140. Scheithauer BW, Kovacs KT, Laws ER Jr, Randall RV: Pathology of invasive pituitary tumors with special reference to functional classification. **J Neurosurg** 65: 733–744, 1986.
141. Laws ER Jr, Kelly PJ, Sundt TM Jr: Clip-grafts in microvascular decompression of the posterior fossa. Technical note. **J Neurosurg** 64: 679–681, 1986.

142. Halper J, Scheithauer BW, Okazaki H, Laws ER Jr: Meningio-angiomatosis: A report of six cases with special reference to the occurrence of neurofibrillary tangles. **J Neuropath Exp Neurol** 45: 426–446, 1986.

143. Ivnik RJ, Sharbrough FW, Laws FR Jr: Effects of anterior temporal lobectomy on cognitive function. **J Clin Psych** 43: 128–137, 1987.

144. Hubbard JL, Houser OW, Laws ER Jr: Trapped fourth ventricle in an adult: radiographic findings and surgical treatment. **Surg Neurol** 28: 301–306, 1987.

145. Laws ER Jr: The evolution and current results of the neurosurgical management of pituitary adenomas. **Clinical Neuroscience** 1: 5–9, 1987.

146. Dobyns EB, Michels VV, Groover RV, Mokri B, Trautmann JC, Forbes GS, Laws ER Jr: Familial cavernous malformations of the central nervous system and retina. **Ann Neurol** 21: 578–583, 1987.

147. Meyer FB, Carpenter SM, Laws ER Jr: Intrasellar arachnoid cysts. **Surg Neurol** 28: 105–110, 1987.

148. Larson TC, Houser OW, Laws ER Jr: Imaging of cranial chrodomas. **Mayo Clin Proc** 62: 886–893, 1987.

149. Abernathey CD, Anderson RE, Kooistra KL, Laws ER Jr: Activity of phthalocyanine photosensitizers against human glioblastoma in vitro. **Neurosurg** 21: 468–473, 1987.

150. Branch CL Jr, Laws ER Jr: Metastatic tumors of the sella turcica masquerading as primary pituitary tumors. **J Clin Endocrinol Metab** 65: 469–474, 1987.

151. Hubbard JL, Scheithauer BW, Abboud CF, Laws ER Jr: Prolactin-secreting adenomas: the preoperative response to bromocriptine treatment and surgical outcome. **J Neurosurg** 67: 816–821, 1987.

152. Jack CR Jr, Mokri B, Laws ER Jr, Houser OW, Baker HL Jr, Petersen RC: MR findings in normal-pressure hydrocephalus: significance and comparison with other forms of dementia. **J Comput Assist Tomogr** 11: 923–931, 1987.

153. Smalley SR, Schray MF, Laws ER Jr, O'Fallon J: Adjuvant radiation therapy after surgical resection of solitary brain metastasis. Association with patterns of failure and survival. **Int J Radiation Onc Biol Phys** 13: 1611–1616, 1987.

154. Scheithauer BW, Laws ER Jr, Kovacs KT, Horvath E, Randall RV, Carney JA; Pituitary adenomas of the multiple endocrine neoplasia Type I syndrome. **Semin Diag Pathol** 4: 205–211, 1987.

155. Talley PW, Laws ER Jr, Scheithauer BW: Metastases to central nervous system neoplasms. **J Neurosurg** 68: 811–816, 1988.
156. Abboud CF, Laws ER Jr: Diagnosis of pituitary tumors. **Endocrinol Metabol Clin North Am** 17: 241–280, 1988.
157. Pioro EP, Scheithauer BW, Laws ER Jr, Randall RV, Kovacs KT, Horvath E: Combined thyrotroph and lactotroph cell hyperplasia simulating prolactin-secreting pituitary adenoma in long-standing primary hypothyroidism. **Surg Neurol** 29: 218–226, 1988.
158. Nichols DA, Laws ER Jr, Houser OW, Abboud CF: Comparison of magnetic resonance imaging and computed tomography in the preoperative evaluation of pituitary adenomas. **Neurosurg** 22: 380–385, 1988.
159. Abernathey CD, Kooistra KL, Wilcox GL, Laws ER Jr: New xenograft model for assessing experimental therapy of central nervous system tumors: human glioblastoma in the intrathecal compartment of the nude mouse. **Neurosurg** 22: 877–881, 1988.
160. Horvath E, Kovacs KT, Smyth HS, Killinger DW, Scheithauer BW, Randall RV, Laws ER Jr, Singer W: A novel type of pituitary adenoma: morphological features and clinical correlations. **J Clin Endocrin Metabol** 66: 111–1118, 1988.
161. Young WF Jr, Scheithauer BW, Gharib H, Laws ER Jr, Carpenter PC: Cushing's syndrome due to primary multinodular corticotrope hyperplasia. **Mayo Clin Proc** 63: 256–262, 1988.
162. Ivnik RJ, Sharbrough FW, Laws ER Jr: Anterior temporal lobectomy for the control of complex partial seizures: information for counseling patients. **Mayo Clin Proc** 63: 783–793, 1988.
163. Daumas-Duport C, Scheithauer BW, Chodkiewicz JP, Laws ER Jr, Vedrenne C: Dysembryoplastic neuroepithelial tumor: a surgically cruable tumor of young patients with intractable partial seizures. **Neurosurg** 23: 545–556, 1988.
164. Wiederholt WC, Melton LJ III, Annegers JF, Grabow JD, Laws ER Jr, Ilstrup DM: Short-term outcomes of skull fracture: a population based study of survival and neurologic complications. **Neurology** 39: 96–102, 1989.
165. Bernstein JJ, Goldberg WJ, Laws ER Jr: Human malignant astrocytoma xenografts migrate in rat brain: a model for central nervous system cancer research. **J Neurosci Res** 21: 134–142, 1989.
166. Bernstein JJ, Goldberg WJ, Laws ER Jr: Immunohistochemistry of human malignant astrocytoma cells xenografted to rat brain: **Apolipoprotein E. Neurosurg** 24: 541–546, 1989.
167. Shaw EG, Scheithauer BW, Gilbertson DT, Nichols DA, Laws ER Jr, Earle JD, Daumas-Duport C, O'Fallon Jr, Dinapoli RP: Post-

operative radiotherapy of supratentorial low-grade gliomas. **Int J Radiation Onco Biol Phys** 16: 663–668, 1989.

168. Camacho A, Abernathey CD, Kelly PJ, Laws ER Jr: Colloid cysts: experience with the management of 84 cases since the introduction of computed tomography. **Neurosurg** 24: 693–700, 1989.

169. Hubbard JL, Scheithauer BW, Kispert DB, Carpenter SM, Wick MR, Laws ER Jr: Adult cerebellar medulloblastoma: the pathological radiographic and clinical disease spectrum. **J Neurosurg** 70: 536–544, 1989.

170. Halper J, Colvard DS, Scheithauer BS, Jiang N-S, Press MF, Graham ML II, Reihl E, Laws ER Jr, Spelsberg TC: Estrogen and progesterone receptors in meningiomas: comparison of nuclear binding, dextran-coated charcoal and immunoperoxidase staining assays. **Neurosurg** 25: 546–553, 1989.

171. Mahaley MS Jr, Mettlin C, Natarajan N, Laws ER Jr, Peace BB: National survey of patterns of care for brain-tumor patients. **J Neurosurg** 71: 826–836, 1989.

172. Smalley SR, Schomberg PJ, Scheithauer BW, Laws ER Jr, O'Fallon JR: Radiotherapeutic considerations in the treatment of hemangioblastomas of the central nervous system. **Int J Radiat Oncol Biol Phys** 18: 1165–1171, 1990.

173. Berg KK, Scheithauer BW, Felise I, Kovacs KT, Horvath E, Klee GG, Laws ER Jr: Pituitary adenomas that produce adrenocorticotropic hormone and alpha-subunit: clinicopathological, immunohistochemical, ultrastructural and immunoelectron microscopic studies in nine cases. **Neurosurg** 26: 397–403, 1990.

174. Al-Rodhan NRF, Laws ER Jr: Meningioma: a historical study of the tumor and its surgical management. **Neurosurg** 26: 832–847, 1990.

175. Bernstein JJ, Goldberg WJ, Laws ER Jr, Conger D, Morreale V, Wood LR: C6 glioma cell invasion and migration of rat brain after neural homografting: ultrastructure. **Neurosurg** 26: 622–628, 1990.

176. Mahaley MS Jr, Mettlin C, Natarajan N, Laws ER Jr, Peace BB: Analysis of patterns of care of brain tumor patients in the United States: a study of the brain tumor section of the AANS and the CNS and the Commission on Cancer of the ACS. **Clin Neurosurg** 36: 347–352, 1990.

177. Laws ER Jr: The conservative management of primary gliomas of the brain. **Clin Neurosurg** 367–374, 1990.

178. Garton GR, Schomberg PJ, Scheithauer BW, Shaw EG, Ilstrup DM, Blackwell CR, Laws ER Jr, Earle JD: Medulloblastoma—

Prognostic factors and outcome of treatment: review of Mayo Clinic experience. **Mayo Clin Proc** 65: 1077–1086, 1990.

179. Goldberg W, Laws ER Jr, Bernstein JJ: Individual C6 glioma cells migrate in adult rat after homografting. **Int J Dev Neuro Sci** 9: 427–436, 1991.

180. Pait TG, Dennis MW, Laws ER Jr, Rizzoli HV, Azzam CJ: The history of the neurosurgical engine. **Neurosurg** 28: 111–129, 1991.

181. Bernstein JJ, Laws ER Jr, Levine KV, Wood LR, Tadvalkar G, Goldberg WJ: C6 Glioma-astrocyte cell and fetal astrocyte migration into artificial basement membrane: a permissive substrate for neural tumors but not fetal astrocytes. **Neurosurg** 28: 652–657, 1991.

182. Kelly DF, Bernstein JJ, Laws ER Jr: Methylprednisolone: therapeutic time window in experimental spinal cord injury in rats. **Surg Forum** 42: 512–514, 1991.

183. Goldberg WJ, Dickens BF, Tadvalkar G, Bernstein JJ, Laws ER Jr, Weglicki WB: Free radical-induced injury to C6 glioma cells. **Neurosurg** 29: 532–537, 1991.

184. Laws ER Jr: The advantages of collegiality in medicine. **Bull NY Acad Med** 68: 297–302, 1992.

185. Kao PC, Laws ER Jr, Zimmerman D: Somatomedian C/Insulin-like growth factor I levels after treatment of acromegaly. **Ann Clin Lab Science** 22: 95–99, 1992.

186. Goldberg WL, Levine KV, Tadvalker G, Laws ER Jr, Bernstein JJ: Mechanisms of C6 glioma cell and fetal astrocyte migration into hydrated collagen I gels. **Brain Res** 581: 81–90, 1992.

187. Laws ER Jr: Craniopharyngioma: diagnosis and treatment. **Endocrinologist** 2: 184–188, 1992.

188. Wilson WR, Laws ER Jr: Transnasal septal displacement approach for secondary transsphenoidal pituitary surgery. **Laryngoscope** 102: 951–953, 1992.

189. Dina TS, Feaster SH, Laws ER Jr, Davis DO: MR of the pituitary gland postsurgery: serial MR studies following transsphenoidal resection. **AJNR** 14: 763–769, 1993.

190. Smalley SR, Laws ER Jr, O'Fallon Jr, Shaw EG, Schray MF: Resection for solitary brain metastasis: role of adjuvant radiation and prognostic variables in 229 patients. **J Neurosurg** 77: 531–540, 1992.

191. Bernstein JJ, Goldberg W, Laws ER Jr: Human specific c-neu proto-oncogene protein expression in human malignant astrocytomas before and after xenografting into rat brain. **J Neurosurg** 78: 240–251, 1993.

192. Blevins LS Jr, Hall GS, Madoff DH, Laws ER Jr, Wand GS:

Acromegaly and Cushing disease in a patient with synchronous pituitary adenomas. **Am J Med Sci** 304: 294–297, 1992.

193. Khan A, Wilson WR, Laws ER Jr: Transseptal transsphenoidal approach for pituitary surgery. **J Med Sci** 2: 1–4, 1992.

194. Bjornsson J, Wold LE, Ebersold MJ, Laws ER Jr: Chordoma of the mobile spine. A Clinicopathologic analysis of 40 patients. **Cancer** 71: 753–740, 1993.

195. Thapar K, Kovacs K, Laws ER Jr., Muller PJ: Pituitary adenomas: current concepts in classification, histopathology, and molecular biology. **Endocrinologist** 3: 39–57, 1993.

196. Bill DC, Meyer FB, Laws ER Jr, Davis DH, Ebersold MJ, Scheithauer BW, Ilstrup DM, Abboud CF: A restrospective analysis of pituitary apoplexy. **Neurosurgery** 33: 602–609, 1993.

197. Laws ER Jr, Goldberg WJ, Bernstein JJ: Migration of human malignant astrocytoma cells in the mammalian brain—Scherer revisted. **Intl J Development Neuroscience** 11: 691–697, 1993.

198. Laws ER Jr, Thapar K: Brain tumors. **Cancer** 43: 263–271, 1993.

199. Laws ER Jr. The contributions of neurosurgeons to medical history. **Acta Neurochir** 124: 172–175, 1993.

200. Friend KE, Chiou YK, Laws ER Jr, Lopes MBS, Shupnik MA: Pit-1 mRNA is differentially expressed in human pituitary adenomas. **J Clin Endocrinol Metabol** 77: 1281–1286, 1993.

201. Davis DH, Laws ER Jr, Ilstrup DM, Speed JK, Caruso M, Shaw EG, Abboud CF, Scheithauer BW, Root LM, Schlick C: Results of surgical treatment for growth-hormone secreting pituitary adenomas. **J Neurosurg** 79: 70–75, 1993.

202. Bernstein JJ, Goldberg WJ, Laws ER Jr: Migration of fresh human malignant astrocytoma cells into hydrated gel waters in vitro. **J Neuro-Oncol** 18: 151–161, 1994.

203. Haile-Mariam T, Laws ER Jr, Tuazon CU: Gram negative meningitis related to transsphenoidal surgery. **Clin Inf Dis** 18: 553–556, 1994.

204. Friend KE, Chiou YK, Lopes MBS, Laws ER Jr, Shupnik MA: Estrogen receptor expression in human pituitary: correlation with immunohistochemistry and morphology in macroadenomas. **J Clin Endocrinol Metabol** 78: 1497–1504, 1994.

205. Thapar K, Kovacs K, Laws ER Jr: Estrogen receptor gene expression in craniopharyngiomas: an in-situ hybridization study. **Neurosurgery** 35: 1012–1017, 1994.

206. Lee JH, Laws ER Jr, Guthrie BL, Dina TS, Nochomovitz LE: Lymphocytic hypophysitis: occurrence in two men. **Neurosurgery** 34: 159–163, 1994.

207. Laws ER Jr, Thaper K: Treatment of craniopharyngioma: Growth, Genetics and Hormones Vol. 10, 3: 6–10, 1994.
208. Nyquist P, Laws ER Jr: Novel Features of tumors that secrete both growth hormone and prolactin in acromegaly. **Neurosurgery** 35: 179–184, 1994.
209. Laws ER Jr: The binding influence of the Journal of Neurosurgery on the evolution of Neurosurgery. **J Neurosurg** 81: 317–321, 1994.
210. Smith MV, Laws ER Jr: Magnetic resonance imaging measurements of pituitary stalk compression and deviation in patients with nonprolactin-secreting intrasellar and parasellar tumors: lack of correlation with serum prolactin level. **Neurosurgery** 34: 834–839, 1994.
211. Laws ER Jr: Transsphenoidal removal of craniopharyngioma. **Pediatr Neurosurg 21,** (suppl 1): 57–63, 1994.
212. Kane LA, Leinung MC, Carpenter PC, Laws ER Jr, Zimmerman D: Pituitary adenomas in childhood and adolescence. **J Clin Endocrinol Metabol** 79: 1135–1140, 1994.
213. Partington MD, Davis DH, Laws ER Jr, Scheithauer BW: Pituitary adenomas in childhood and adolescence: Results of transsphenoidal surgery. **J Neurosurg** 80: 209–216, 1994.
214. Thapar K, Kovacs K, Laws ER Jr: The classification and molecular biology of pituitary adenomas. **Adv Tech Stan Neurosurg** 22: 3–53, 1995.
215. Laws ER Jr, Thapar K: Surgical management of pituitary adenoma. **J Clin Endocrinol Metabol** 9: 391–406, 1995.
216. Kelly DF, Laws ER Jr, Fosset D: Delayed hyponatremia after transsphenoidal surgery for pituitary adenoma. Report of nine cases. **J Neurosurg** 83: 363–367, 1995.
217. Baskin DS, Laws ER Jr, Post KD: Endocrinologically active pituitary microadenomas. **Perspec Neurol Surg** 6: 89–106, 1995.
218. Leinung MC, Kane LA, Scheithauer BW, Carpenter PC, Laws ER Jr, Zimmerman D: Long term follow-up of transsphenoidal surgery for the treatment of Cushing's disease in childhood. **J Clin Endocrinol Metabol** 80: 2475–2479, 1995.
219. Laws ER Jr: Radical resection in the treatment of gliomas. **Clin Neurosurg** 42: 480–487, 1995.
220. Shaffrey CI, Munoz EL, Sutton CL, Alston SR, Shaffrey ME, Laws ER Jr: Tumoral calcium pyrophosphate deposition disease mimicking a cervical spine neoplasm: case report: **Neurosurg** 37: 335–339, 1995.
221. Thapar K, Kovacs K, Scheithauer BW, Stefaneanu L, Horvath

E, Pernicone PJ, Murray D, Laws ER Jr: Proliferative activity and invasiveness among pituitary adenomas and carcinomas: an analysis using the MIB-1 antibody. **Neurosurgery** 38: 99–107, 1996.

222. Alexander JM, Bikkal HA, Zervas NT, Laws ER Jr, Klibanski A: Tumor specific expression and alternate splicing of mRNAs encoding activin/TGFβ receptors in human pituitary adenomas. **J Clin Endocrinol Metabol** 81: 785–790, 1996.

223. Sawin PD, Follett KA, Chen Wen B, Laws ER Jr: Symptomatic intrasellar hemangioblastoma in a child treated with subtotal resection and adjuvant radiosurgery. **J Neurosurg** 84: 1046–1050, 1996.

224. Laws ER Jr: Diagnosis and management of craniopharyngioma in children and adolescents. **Curr Opin Endocrinol Diabetes** 3: 110–114, 1996.

225. Thapar K, Scheithauer B, Kovacs K, Pernicone PJ, Laws ER Jr: p53 expression in pituitary adenomas and carcinomas: correlation with invasiveness and tumor growth fractions. **Neurosurgery** 38: 765–771, 1996.

226. Laws ER Jr, Bertram E: Epilepsy surgery in children and adolescents. **Neurosurg Focus** 1(5): 1, 1996.

227. Kamiryo T, Laws ER Jr: A burr hole button device to secure the electrode cable in depth electrode placement. **Neurosurg Focus** 1(5): 5, 1995.

228. Laws ER Jr, Thorner MO, Vance ML: Bromocriptine therapy for prolactin-secreting pituitary tumors. **Neurosurg Focus** 1(1): 4, 1996.

229. Laws ER Jr: Referral guidelines: carpal tunnel syndrome. **Neurosurg Focus** 3(1): 11, 1997.

230. Schoen SR, Khan A, Wilson WR, Laws ER Jr: Minimizing upper lip and incisor teeth paraesthesias in approaches to transsphenoidal surgery. **Otolaryngol Head Neck Surg** 116: 656–661, 1997.

231. Quigg M, Bertram EH, Jackson TK, Laws ER Jr: Volumetric MRI evidence of bilateral hippocampal atrophy in mesial temporal lobe epilepsy. **Epilepsia** 38: 588–594, 1997.

232. Lopes MB, Salomon I, Nagy N, Decaestecker C, Pasteels J-L, Laws ER Jr, Kiss R: Computer-assisted microscope analysis of Feulgen-stained nuclei in gonadotroph adenomas and null-cell adenomas of the pituitary gland. **Endocrine Pathol** 8: 109–120, 1997.

233. Laws ER Jr, Jane JA Sr, Pait TG: Pitfalls and successes of peer review in neurosurgery. **J Neurosurg** 87: 972–976, 1997.

234. Kamiryo T, Laws ER Jr: Stereotactic frame-based error in MR guided stereotactic procedures: a methodology for measurement of error and standardization of technique. **Stereotactic Funct Neurosurg** 67: 198–209, 1997.

235. Kamiryo T, Laws ER Jr: A stereotactic gauge for defining the cranial entry point. **Stereotactic Funct Neurosurg** 67: 210–212, 1997.

236. McCarthy BJ, Davis F, Freels S, Surawicz TS, Damek D, Laws ER Jr: Factors associated with survival in patients with meningioma. **Neurosurg Focus** 2: 1–8, 1997.

237. Kamiryo T, Laws ER Jr: Identification and localization of intracerebral vessels by microvascular doppler in stereotactic pallidotomy and thalamotomy: technical note. **Neurosurgery** 40: 877–879, 1997.

238. Laws ER Jr: Management of prolactin macroadenoma with visual loss: indications for surgery. **J Clin Neurosci** 4: 64–65, 1997.

239. Lanzino G, DiPierro CG, Laws ER Jr: One century after the description of the "sign": Joseph Babinski and his contribution to neurosrugery. **Neurosurgery** 40: 822–828, 1997.

240. Kamiryo T, Laws ER Jr: A burr hole button to secure the electrode cable in depth electrode placement: technical note. **J Neurosurg** 86: 905–906, 1997.

241. Young JN, Shaffrey CI, Laws ER Jr, Lovell LR: Lumbar disc surgery in a fixed compensation population: a model for influence of secondary gain on surgical outcome. **Surg Neurol** 48: 552–559, 1997.

242. Pajewski TN, Vance ML, Jacger JM, Laws ER: Perioperative ACTH changes predict outcome during transsphnoidal microsurgery for Cushing's disease. **J Neurosurg Anaesth** 9: 38, 1997.

243. Thapar K, Kovacs K, Stefaneanu L, Scheithauer B, Killinger DW, Lloyd R, Smyth HS, Barr A, Thorner MO, Gaylinn B, Laws ER Jr: Overexpression of the growth hormone-releasing hormone gene in acromegaly—associated pituitary tumors: an event associated with neoplastic progression and aggressive behavior. **Am J Pathol** 151: 769–784, 1997.

244. Thapar K, Kovacs K, Stefaneanu L, Scheithauer BW, Horvath E, Lloyd RV, Li J, Laws ER Jr: Antiproliferative effect of the somatostatin analogue octreotide on growth hormone—producing pituitary tumors: results of a multicenter randomized trial. **Mayo Clin Proc** 72: 893–900, 1997.

245. diPierro C, Jackson TR, Kamiryo T, Laws ER Jr: Optimization of the accuracy of MRI-guided stereotaxis: a methodology with vali-

dation based on the AC-PC line. **Neurosurg Focus** 2(3): 1–7, 1997.

246. Simmons N, Laws ER Jr: Glioma occurrence after sellar irradiation. **Neurosurg** 42: 172–178, 1998.

247. Lanzino, diPierro CG, Laws ER Jr: Sutureless repair of major intracranial vessels with the Sundt Clip-Graft: Technical Note. **Acta Neurochir (Wien)** 140: 491–493, 1998.

248. McCarthy BJ, Davis FG, Freels S, Surawicz TS, Damek DM, Grutsch J, Menek HR, Laws ER Jr: Factors associated with survival in patients with meningioma. **J Neurosurg** 88: 831–839, 1998.

249. Skalabrin EJ, Laws ER Jr, Bennett JP Jr: Pallidotomy improves motor responses and widens the levodopa therapeutic window in Parkinson's disease. **Movement Disorders** 13: 775–81, 1998.

250. Zhu Z, McCutcheon IE, Lopes MBS, Laws ER Jr, Brunner JM, Fuller GN, Langford LA, Ang LW, Friend KE: Sulfonylurea receptor mRNA expression in pituitary macroadenomas. **Endocrine** 8: 7–12, 1998.

251. Larner J, Shaffrey ME, Jane JA Sr, Laws ER Jr: A Phase 1-2 trial of Lovastatin for anaplastic astrocytoma and glioblastoma multiforme. **Am J Clin Oncol** 21: 580–583, 1998.

252. Laws ER Jr: A neurosurgical way of life. **J Neurosurg** 89: 901–10, 1998.

253. Laws ER Jr: Central nervous system tumors: what have we learned and where are we going. **Cancer** 48: 327–9, 1998.

254. Skinner MM, Nass R, Lopes MB, Laws ER Jr, Thorner MO: Growth hormone secretagogue receptor expression in human pituitary tumors. **J Clin Endocrinol Metabol** 83: 4314–20, 1998.

255. Shupnik MA, Pitt Lk, Soh AY, Anderson A, Lopes MB, Laws ER Jr: Selective expression of estrogen receptor α and β isoforms in human pituitary tumors. **J Clin Endocrinol Metabol** 83: 3965–3972, 1998.

256. Morita A, Meyer FB, Laws ER Jr: Symptomatic pituitary metastases. **J Neurosurg** 89: 69–73, 1998.

257. Lopes MBS, Lanzino G, Cloft HI, Winston DC, Vance ML, Laws ER Jr: Primary fibrosarcoma of the sella unrelated to previous radiation therapy. **Mod Pathol** 11: 579–584, 1998.

258. Surawicz TS, Davis F, Freels S, Laws ER Jr, Menck HR: Brain Tumor survival: results from the National Cancer Data Base. **J Neurooncol** 40: 151–160, 1998.

259. Kaptain GJ, Shaffrey CI, Alden TD, Young JN, Laws ER, Whitehill R: Secondary gain influences the outcome of lumbar but not cervical disc surgery. **Surg Neurol** 52: 217–25, 1999.

260. Kaptain GJ, Simmons NE, Lopes MB, Vance ML, Laws ER Jr: Estrogen receptors in prolactinomas: A clinico-pathological study. **Pituitary** 1(2): 91–8, 1999.

261. Hirano H, Lopes, Laws ER Jr, Asakura T, Goto M, Carpenter J, Karns LR, VandenBerg SR: The IGF-1 content and pattern of expression correlates with histopathologic grade in differently infiltrating astrocytomas. **Neuro-Oncol** 1(2): 98–116, 1999.

262. Laws ER Jr, Thapar K: Pituitary Surgery. **Endocrinol Metabol Clin North Am** 28: 119–131, 1999.

263. diPierro C, Francel PC, Jackson TK, Kamiryo T, Laws ER Jr: Optimizing accuracy in MRI-guided stereotaxis: a technique with validation based on the AC-PC line. **J Neurosurg** 90: 94–100, 1999.

264. Kamiyro T, Laws ER Jr: An accurate adjustable applicator for MRI-based stereotactic procedures using the Leksell G Frame. **Neurosurg** 45: 397–400, 1999.

265. Semple PL, Laws ER Jr: Complications of contemporary transsphenoidal surgery for Cushing's disease. **J Neurosurg** 91: 175–179, 1999.

266. Elias WJ, Chadduck JB, Alden TD, Laws ER Jr: Frameless stereotaxy for transsphenoidal surgery. **Neurosurg** 45: 271–277, 1999.

267. Laws ER Jr: Vascular complications of transsphenoidal surgery. **Pituitary** 2: 163–170, 1999.

268. Laws ER Jr, Shaffrey MS: The inherent invasiveness of cerebral gliomas—implications for clinic management. **Int J Dev Neurosci** 17/5–6, 413–420, 1999.

269. Laws ER JR, Vance ML: Radiosurgery for pituitary tumors and craniopharyngiomas. **Neurosurg Clin N Am** 10: 327–336, 1999.

270. Laws ER Jr: Neurosurgery's man of the century: Harvey Cushing—The man and his legacy. **Neurosurg** 45, 977–982, 1999.

271. Laws ER: From child to adult. **Childs Nerv Syst** 15: 620–623, 1999.

272. Simmons NE, Elias WJ, Henson SL, Laws ER Jr: Small cell lung carcinoma causing epidural hematoma: case report. **Surg Neurol** 51: 56–59, 1999.

273. Theodou E, Kontogeorgos G, Scheithauer BW, Tzanis S, Mariatos P, Laws ER Jr: Intrasellar chordomas mimicking pituitary adenoma. **J Neurosurg** 92: 976–983, 1999.

274. Duff JM, Meyer FB, Ilstrup DM, Laws ER Jr, Schleck CD, Scheithauer BW: Long-term outcomes for surgically resected craniopharyngiomas. **Neurosurg** 46: 291–305, 2000.

275. Simmons NE, Do HM, Lipper MH, Laws ER Jr: Cerebral atrophy in Cushing's disease. **Surg Neurol** 53: 72–76, 2000.

276. Kamiryo T, Jackson TE, Laws ER Jr: A methodology designed to

increase accuracy and safety in stereotactic brain surgery. **Minim Invas Neurosurg** 43: 1–3, 2000.

277. Laws ER, Vance ML, Thapar K: Pituitary surgery for the management of acromegaly. **Hom Res** 53(suppl 3): 71–75, 2000.

278. Laws ER Jr: The decade of the brain: 1990 to 2000. **Neurosurg** 47: 1257–1260, 2000.

279. Kaptain GJ, Vincent DA, Sheehan JP, Laws ER Jr: Clival encephalocele: Case illustration. **J Neurosurg** 93: 513, 2000.

280. Laffey TA Jr, Leech RW, Scheithauer BW, Blick K, Kovacs K, Horvath E, Young WF Jr, Lloyd RV, Ebersold M, Laws ER Jr, DeBault LE: Pituitary adenomas: a DNA flow cytometric study of 192 clinicopathologically characterized tumors. **Endocrine Pathol** (in press), 2001.

281. Steele CB, Surawicz TS, Clutter G, Phillips JL, Ries L, Gershamn ST, Perey C, Gurney JGl, Bushhouse SA, Laws ER Jr: Surveillance of primary intracranial and central nervous system tumors. **Cancer** (submitted), 2001.

282. Reitmeyer M, Vance ML, Lopes MB, Laws ER Jr: Metastatic ACTH-producing carcinoid presenting as a pituitary tumor. **Endocrine Practice** (submitted), 2001.

283. Pajewski TN, Vance ML, Jaeger JM, Laws ER: Perioperative neuroendocrine changes predict outcome during transsphenoidal surgery for Cushing's disease. **JCEM,** submitted, 2001.

284. Kaptain GJ, Vincent DA, Laws ER Jr: Cranial base reconstruction after transsphenoidal surgery with bioabsorbable implants: technical note. **Neurosurg** 48: 232–234, 2001.

BOOKS

1. Laws ER Jr, Randall RV, Kern EB, Abboud CF (eds): *Management of Pituitary Adenomas and Related Lesions with Emphasis on Transsphenoidal Microsurgery;* New York, Appleton-Century-Crofts, 1982, 376 pp.

2. Fox WL: *Dandy of John Hopkins.* Baltimore, Williams & Wilkins, 1984. Sponsored by the Congress of Neurological Surgeons and edited by Laws ER Jr and Carmel PW.

3. Laws ER Jr (ed): *The Diagnosis and Management of Orbital Tumors.* Mount Kisco, New York, Futura, 1988, 316 pp.

4. Hayes WJ Jr, Laws ER Jr (eds): *Handbook of Pesticide Toxicology,* 3 volumes, San Diego, Academic Press, 1991.

5. Boden SD, Wiesel SW, Laws ER Jr, Rothman RH (eds): *The Aging Spine.* Philadelphia, Saunders, 1991, 347 pp.

6. Karim ABMF, Laws ER Jr (eds): *Glioma—Principles and Practice in Neuro-Oncology.* Heidelberg, Springer-Verlag, 1991, 310 pp.

7. Kaye AH, Laws ER Jr (eds): *Brain Tumors.* London, Churchill-Livingstone, 1995, 990 pp.
8. Laws ER Jr, Udvarhelyi GB (eds): *A Early Walker's Genesis of Ideas in Neuroscience.* Park Ridge, AANS Publications, 1998.
9. Salcman M, Heros R, Laws ER, Sonntag V (eds): *Kempe's Atlas of Neurosurgical Technique.* (In press), 2001.
10. Kaye AH, Laws ER (eds): *Brain Tumors,* 2nd Edition. London, Harcourt, 2001.

BOOK CHAPTERS

1. Laws ER Jr, Curley A, Biros FJ: Men with intensive occupational exposure to DDT: A clinical and chemical study, in Kay K, Hipskind MM, Schafer M, et al. (eds): *Adverse Effects of Common Environmental Pollutants.* New York, MSS Information Corp., 1972, pp. 60–69.
2. Laws ER Jr, Morales FR, Hayes WJ Jr, Joseph CR: Toxicology of abate in volunteers, in Kay K, Hipskind MM, Schafter M, et al. New York, MSS Information Corp., 1972, pp. 70–72.
3. Ray CD, Laws ER Jr: Craniocerebral injury: classification physical mechanism and underlying pathology, in Ballenger WF II, Rutherford RB, Zuidema GD (eds): *The Management of Trauma.* Philadelphia, W.B. Saunders Co., 1973, pp. 180–183.
4. Laws ER Jr: The neurosurgical management of meningomyelocele, in Freeman JM (ed): *Practical Management of Meningomyelocele.* Baltimore, University Park Press, 1974, pp. 31–50.
5. Laws ER Jr: The management of hydrocephalus, in Freeman JM (ed): *Practical Management of Meningomyelocele.* Baltimore, University Park Press, 1974, pp. 51–67.
6. Laws ER Jr, Udvarhelyi GB: The brain scan in pediatric neurosurgery, in Wagner H, James E (eds): *Pediatric Nuclear Medicine.* Philadelphia, W.B. Saunders Co., 1974, pp. 133–143.
7. Laws ER Jr: Transsphenoidal approach to lesions in and about the sella turcica, in Schmidek HH, Sweet WH (eds): *Current Techniques in Operative Neurosurgery.* Grune & Stratton, Inc., 1977, Chapter 12, pp. 161–172.
8. Laws ER Jr: Brain, in Beahrs OH, Copeland MM (eds): *Manual for Staging of Cancer, American Joint Committee on Cancer Staging and End-Results Reporting.* Philadelphia, J.B. Lippincott Co., 1977.
9. Laws ER Jr, Ray CD: Craniocerebral injury: classification, physical mechanism and underlying pathology, in Zuidema GD, Rutherford RB, Ballinger WF II (eds): *The Management of Trauma.* Philadelphia, W.B. Saunders Co., 1979, Chapter 8, pp. 183–194.

10. Laws ER Jr, Houser OW: Diagnostic roentgenology of pituitary lesions, in Tindall GT, Collins WF (eds): *Clinical Management of Pituitary Disorders.* New York, Raven Press, 1979, Chapter 5, pp. 133–145.

11. Laws ER Jr, Kern EB: Complications of transsphenoidal surgery, in Tindall GT, Collins WF (eds): *Clinical Management of Pituitary Disorders.* New York, Raven Press, 1979, Chapter 5, pp. 435–445.

12. Laws ER Jr: Transsphenoidal microsurgery in the management of acromegaly, in Smith JL (ed): *Smith's Neuro-Ophthalmology Focus, 1980.* New York, Masson Publishing Co., pp. 289–293.

13. Pearson BW, Kern EB, McDonald TJ, Laws ER Jr: Anatomical aspects of the transseptal approach to the sphenoid sinus, in Post KS, Jackson IMD, Reichlin S (eds): *The Pituitary Adenoma.* 1980, Chapter 17, pp. 365–377.

14. Laws ER Jr, Kern EB: Pituitary tumors treated by transnasal microsurgery—7 years of clinical experience with 539 patients, in *Proceedings, Pituitary Workshop,* Tokyo, Japan, 1980, pp. 25–34.

15. Laws ER Jr, Houser OW: Diagnostic roentgenology of pituitary lesions with emphasis on angiography, in *Proceedings, Pituitary Workshop,* Tokyo, Japan, 1980, pp. 55–60.

16. Hodgson SF, Randall RV, Laws ER Jr: Empty sella syndrome, in Youmans JR (ed): *Neurological Surgery—A Comprehensive Reference Guide to the Diagnosis and Management of Neurosurgical Problems.* Philadelphia, Saunders, 1982, 3170–3178.

17. Laws ER Jr: Complications of transsphenoidal microsurgery for pituitary adenoma, in Brock M (ed): *Modern Neurosurgery 1.* Heidelberg, Springer-Verlag Berlin, 1982, pp. 181–186.

18. Laws ER Jr, Kern EB, McDonald TJ, Pearson BW: Surgery of the pituitary gland, in Brackmann DE (ed): *Neurological Surgery of the Ear and Skull Base.* New York, Raven Press, 1982, pp. 123–126.

19. Laws ER Jr, Kohler P, Acker J, Kovacs KT, Sheline G: Panel II: The pretreatment pituitary patient, in Givens JR (ed): *Hormone-Secreting Pituitary Tumors.* Chicago, Year Book Medical Publishers, Inc., 1982, pp. 145–162.

20. Laws ER Jr, Randall RV, Abboud CF: Surgical treatment of acromegaly: results in 140 patients, in Givens JR (ed): *Hormone-Secreting Pituitary Tumors.* Chicago, Year Book Medical Publishers, Inc., 1982, pp. 225–228.

21. Randall RV, Laws ER Jr, Abboud CF: Postoperative evaluation of pituitary status, in Givens R (ed): *Hormone-Secreting Pituitary Tumors.* Chicago, Year Book Medical Publishers, Inc., 1982, pp. 329–348.

22. Annegers JF, Coulam CB, Laws ER Jr: Pituitary tumors: epidemi-

ology, in Givens JR (ed): *Hormone-Secreting Pituitary Tumors.* Chicago, Year Book Medical Publishers, Inc., 1982, pp. 393–403.

23. Laws ER Jr: Transsphenoidal approach to lesions in and about the sella turcica: in Schmidek HH, Sweet WH (eds): *Operative Neurosurgical Techniques—Indications, Methods and Results.* New York, Grune & Stratton, Inc., 1982, pp. 327–341.
24. Houser OW, Baker HL Jr, Gomez MR, Laws ER Jr: Computed tomography of intracranial neoplasms in the young, in Amador LV (ed): *Brain Tumors in the Young.* Springfield, IL, Charles C Thomas 1983, Chapter 7, pp. 161–176.
25. Laws ER Jr: Brain, in Beahrs OH, Myers MH (eds): *Manual for Staging of Cancer, American Joint Committee on Cancer, 2nd ed.* Philadelphia, J.B. Lippincott Co., 1983, pp. 219–226.
26. Laws ER Jr: Transsphenoidal microsurgery in the management of pituitary adenoma, in *Neurosurgeons, Proceedings of the 3rd annual meeting of the Japanese Congress of Neurological Surgeons,* 1983, Vol. 3, pp. 79–82.
27. Laws ER Jr: Specialized uses of CT scanning, in *Neurosurgeons, Proceedings of the 3rd annual meeting of the Japanese Congress of Neurological Surgeons,* 1983, Vol. 3, pp. 245–248.
28. Laws ER Jr: Non-functioning pituitary tumors. Special tape presentation for "Topics in Neurosurgery", 1983.
29. Laws ER Jr: Low grade gliomas. Special tape presentation for Neurosurgery Review, 1983 Vol. 1282, Issue 6.
30. Laws ER Jr: Craniopharyngioma. *Neurosurgery Review,* 1983, Vol. 1383, Issue 11.
31. Randall RV, Laws ER Jr, Trautman JC: Results of transsphenoidal microsurgery for pituitary adenoma in 892 patients, in Camanni F, Muller EE (eds): *Pituitary Hyperfunction: Physiopathology and Clinical Aspects.* New York, Raven Press, 1984, pp. 417–419.
32. Randall RV, Laws ER Jr, Abboud CF: Clinical presentation of craniopharyngiomas: A brief review of 300 cases, in Givens JR (ed). *The Hypothalamus.* Chicago, Illinois, Year Book Medical Publishers, 1984, pp. 321–333.
33. Laws ER Jr, Randall RV, Abboud CF, Hayles AB: Craniopharyngioma—The transsphenoidal microsurgical approach, in Givens JR (ed): *The Hypothalamus.* Chicago, Illinois, Book Medical Publishers 1984, pp. 335–347.
34. Abboud CF, Randall RV, Laws ER Jr: Clinical manifestations of suprasellar germinomas, in Givens JR (ed): *The Hypothalamus.* Chicago, Illinois, Year Book Medical Publishers, 1984, pp. 355–359.
35. Laws ER Jr: Surgical management of pituitary adenomas, in

Hickey RC (ed): *Current Problems in Cancer.* Chicago, Illinois, Year Book Medical Publishers, 1984, pp. 335–347.

36. Laws ER Jr, Abay EO III, Forbes GS, Grado GL, Bruckman JE, Scott M: Conservative management of pineal tumors—Mayo Clinic Experience, in Neuwelt EA (ed): *Diagnosis and Treatment of Pineal Region Tumors.* Baltimore, Williams & Wilkins, 1984, pp. 323–331.

37. Houser OW, Baker HL Jr, Reese DF, Earnest F IV, Laws FR Jr: Diagnosis of pituitary microadenoma by computed tomography, in Belchetz PE (ed): *Management of Pituitary Disease.* London, Chapman and Hall, Ltd., 1984, pp. 234–250.

38. Laws ER Jr: The neurosurgical management of acromegaly, in Black PMcL, Zervas NT, Ridgway EC, Martin JB (eds): *Secretory Tumors of the Pituitary Gland.* New York, Raven Press, 1984, pp. 169–173.

39. Anderson RE, Wharen RE Jr, Jones CA, Laws ER Jr: Parameters of hematoporphyrin derivative tumor cell killing efficiency: Decomposition of hematoporphyrin derivative at high power densities, in *Porphyrin Localization and Treatment of Tumors,* New York, Alan R. Liss, Inc., 1984, pp. 483–500.

40. Wharen RE Jr, Laws ER Jr: Thrombosed arteriovenous malformations of the brain. An important entity in the differential diagnosis of intractable focal seizure disorder, in Year Book of Diagnostic Radiology, 1984.

41. Laws ER Jr: Acromegaly and Gigantism, in Wilkins RH, Rengachary SS (eds): *Neurosurgery.* New York, New York, McGraw-Hill Book Company, 1985, pp. 864–867.

42. Laws ER Jr: Cranial chordomas, in Wilkins RH, Rengachary SS (eds): *Neurosurgery.* New York, New York, McGraw-Hill Book Company, 1985, pp. 927–930.

43. Laws ER Jr: Pituitary adenomas, in Johnson RT (ed): *Current Therapy in Neurologic Disease 1985/1986.* Philadelphia, B.C. Decker, Inc., 1985, pp. 220–225.

44. Laws ER Jr, Ebersold MJ, Piepgras DG, Abboud CF, Randall RV, Scheithauer BW: The role of surgery in the management of prolactinoma, in MacLeod RM, Thorner MO, Scapagnini U (eds): *Prolactin, Basic and Clinical Correlates.* New York, Springer-Verlag, 1985, pp. 849–853.

45. Laws ER Jr: Growth hormone-secreting pituitary tumor, in Long DM (ed): *Current Therapy in Neurosurgical Surgery 1985/1986.* Philadelphia, B.C. Decker, Inc., 1985, pp. 55–57.

46. Laws ER Jr, Wharen RE Jr, Anderson RE: Photodynamic therapy of brain tumors, in Jori G, Perria C (eds): *Photodynamic Therapy*

of Tumors and Other Diseases. Italy, Libreria Progetto Editore Padova, 1985, pp. 311–316.

47. Laws ER Jr: The surgical management of pituitary adenomas, in Sinha KK (ed): *Progress in Clinical Neurosciences, Vol. 2.* Ranchi, India, Catholic Press, 1986, pp. 11–19.

48. Wharen RE Jr, Anderson RE, Laws ER Jr: Photoradiation therapy with hematoporphyrin derivative in the management of brain tumors, in Fasano VA (ed): *Advanced Intraoperative Technologies in Neurosurgery.* Wien, Springer-Verlag, 1986, pp. 211–227.

49. Laws ER Jr, Randall RV, Abboud CF: Special problems in the therapeutic management of acromegaly, in Ludecke DK, Tolis G (eds): *Growth Hormone, Growth Factors and Acromegaly.* New York, Raven Press, 1987, pp. 259–266.

50. Laws ER Jr, Bergstralh EJ, Taylor WF: Cerebellar astrocytoma in children, in Homburger F (ed): *Progress in Experimental Tumor Research.* Basel, Switzerland, S. Karger, 1987, pp. 122–127.

51. Laws ER Jr: Craniopharyngiomas in children and young adults, in Homburger F (ed): *Progress in Experimental Tumor Research.* Basel, Switzerland, S. Karger, 1987, pp. 335–340.

52. Laws ER Jr, Scheithauer BW, Groover RV: Pituitary adenomas in childhood and adolescence, in Homburger F (ed): *Progress in Experimental Tumor Research.* Basel, Switzerland, S. Karger, 1987, pp. 359–361.

53. Marsh WR, Laws ER Jr: Intracranial ependymomas, in Homburger F (ed): *Progress in Experimental Tumor Research.* Basel, Switzerland, S. Karger, 1987, pp. 175–180.

54. Laws ER Jr, Carpenter SM, Scheithauer BW, Randall RV: Long-term results of transsphenoidal surgery for the management of acromegaly, in Robbins RJ, Melmed S (eds): *Acromegaly.* New York, Plenum Publishing Corporation, 1987.

55. Laws ER Jr: Craniopharyngiomas: Diagnosis and Treatment, in Sekhar LN, Schramm VL Jr (eds): *Tumors of the Cranial Base: Diagnosis and Treatment.* New York, Futura Publishing Co., Inc., 1987, pp. 347–372.

56. Laws ER Jr: Cerebellar astrocytoma in children, in Kageyama N (ed): *Proceedings of the First International Symposium on Pediatric Neuro-oncology.* Nagoya, University of Nagoya Press, 1987, pp. 125–127.

57. Laws ER Jr: Neurosurgical management of ependymomas, in Kageyama N (ed): *Proceedings of the First International Symposium on Pediatric Neuro-oncology.* Nagoya, University of Nagoya press, 1987, pp. 151–155.

58. Laws ER Jr: Craniopharyngioma, in Kageyama N (ed): *Proceedings*

of the First International Symposium on Pediatric Neuro-oncology. Nagoya, University of Nagoya Press, 1987, pp. 265–266.

59. Laws ER Jr: Pituitary surgery, in Molitch ME (ed): *Pituitary Tumors: Diagnosis and Management.* Philadelphia, W.B. Saunders Company, 1987, pp. 647–665.

60. Wharen RE Jr, Anderson RE, Laws ER Jr: Photoradiation therapy of malignant brain tumors, in Cerullo LJ (ed): *Application of Lasers in Neurosurgery.* Chicago, Year Book Medical Publishers, 1988, pp. 156–171.

61. Laws ER Jr, Wharen RE Jr, Anderson RE: The treatment of brain tumors by photoradiation, in Pluchino F, Broggi G (eds): *Advanced Technology in Neurosurgery.* Heidelberg, Springer-Verlag, 1988, pp. 46–60.

62. Laws ER Jr: Transsphenoidal approach to lesions in and about the sella turcica, in Schmidek HH, Sweet WH (eds): *Operative Neurosurgical Techniques—Indications, Methods and Results.* New York, Grune & Stratton, Inc., 1988, pp. 309–319.

63. Laws ER Jr: Brain, in Beahrs OH, Henson De, Hutter RVP, Myers MH (eds): *Manual for Staging of Cancer, third edition, American Joint Committee on Cancer.* Philadelphia, J. B. Lippincott Co., 1988, pp. 249–254.

64. Berg KK, Scheithauer BW, Klee GG, Laws ER, Kovacs K, Horvath E: Alpha subunit in pituitary adenomas: a radioimmunoassay and immunohistochemical study, in Landolt AM, Heitz PU, Zapf J, Girard J, del Pozo E (eds): *Advances in Pituitary Adenoma Research.* Oxford, Pergamon Press, 1988, pp. 397–411.

65. Laws ER Jr: Cushing's disease—neurosurgical viewpoint, in van Heerden JA (ed): *Common Problems in Endocrine Surgery.* Chicago, Year Book Medical Publishers, 1989, pp. 18–22.

66. Laws ER Jr: Prolactinoma, in Long DM (ed): *Current Therapy in Neurological Surgery—2.* Philadelphia, B.C. Decker, Inc., 1989, pp. 119–121.

67. Laws ER Jr: Hypophysectomy, in Youmans JR (ed): *Neurological Surgery, third edition.* Philadelphia, Saunders, 1989, Vol. 6, pp. 4358–4368.

68. Guthrie BL, Laws ER Jr: Supratentorial low-grade gliomas, in Rosenblum ML, Winn HR, Mayberg M (eds): *The Role of Surgery in Brain Tumor Management.* Neurosurgery Clinics of North America, 1990, 1: 37–48.

69. Laws ER Jr, Wharen RE Jr, Anderson RE: Photoradiation therapy for malignant gliomas, in Wilkins RH, Rengachary SS (eds): *Neurosurgical Update I.* New York, McGraw-Hill, 1990, 260–265.

70. Laws ER Jr: Complications of surgery for ACTH secreting pituitary

tumors, in Ludecke DK, Chrousos GP, Tolis G (eds): *ACTH, Cushing's Syndrome and Other Hypercortisolemic States.* New York, Raven Press, 1990, pp. 275–280.

71. Laws ER Jr: Diagnosis and treatment of poisoning, in Hayes WJ Jr, Laws ER Jr. (eds): *Handbook of Pesticide Toxicology. Vol. 1, General Principles.* San Diego, Academic Press, 1991, pp. 361–403.

72. Al-Rodhan NRF, Laws ER Jr: The History of intracranial meningiomas, in Al-Mefty O (ed): *Meningiomas.* New York, Raven Press, 1991, pp. 1–8.

73. Laws ER Jr: Craniopharyngiomas: Indications for and results of transsphenoidal surgery, in Barden CW (ed): *Current Therapy in Endocrinology and Metabolism.* Philadelphia, B. C. Decker, Inc., 1991, pp. 30–32.

74. Laws ER Jr: Meningiomas of the temporal bone, in Al-Mefty O (ed): *Meningiomas.* New York, Raven Press, 1991, pp. 539–542.

75. Guthrie BL, Carabell SC, Laws ER Jr: Radiation therapy for intracranial meningiomas, in Al-Mefty O (ed): *Meningiomas.* New York, Raven Press, 1991, pp. 255–262.

76. Laws ER Jr: Diagnosis and treatment of poisoning, in Hayes WJ Jr, Laws ER Jr. (eds): *Handbook of Pesticide Toxicology.* New York, Academic Press, 1991, pp. 361–404.

77. Laws ER Jr: Complications of transsphenoidal surgery, in Samii M (ed): *Surgery of the Sellar Region and Paranasal Sinuses.* Berlin, Springer-Verlag, 1991, pp. 336–340.

78. Wharen RE Jr, Anderson RE, Laws ER Jr: Photoradiation therapy of brain tumors, in Salcman M (ed): *Neurobiology of Brain Tumors.* Baltimore, Williams & Wilkins, 1991, pp. 341–357.

79. Laws ER Jr: Pituitary tumors, in Little JR, Awad IA (eds): *Reoperative Neurosurgery.* Baltimore, Williams and Wilkins, 1992, pp. 105–112.

80. Laws ER Jr: Pituitary tumors—therapeutic considerations: surgical, in Barrow DL, Selman W (eds): *Neuroendocrinology, Concepts in Neurosurgery,* Vol. 5, Wilkins & Wilkins, 1992, pp. 395–400.

81. Laws ER Jr: Surgical management of pituitary adenomas, in Niederhuber JE (ed): *Current Therapy in Oncology.* New York, BC Decker-Mosby, 1993, pp. 279–282.

82. Laws ER Jr: Structural lesions as a cause of focal epilepsy: Pathology, incidence and results, in Continuing Education Program, The 51st Annual Meeting of the Japan Neurological Society, Kagoshima, 1992, 1993, pp. 17–26.

83. Laws ER Jr: Surgical management of pituitary tumors, in Mazzaferri EL, Samaan N (eds): *Endocrine Tumors.* Boston, Blackwell, 1993, pp. 215–222.

84. Laws ER Jr: Transsphenoidal surgery, in Apuzzo M (ed): *Brain Surgery, Complication Avoidance and Management.* 1993, pp. 357–361.

85. Laws ER Jr: Cushing's Neurosurgical Trainees, in Black PM, Moore MR, Rossitch E Jr: *Cushing at the Brigham.* Park Ridge, AANS Publishing Co, 1993.

86. Laws ER Jr: Results of transsphenoidal microsurgical management of acromegaly, in Wass, JAH (ed): *Treating Acromegaly: 100 years on.* Bristol, Journal of Endocrinology, Ltd., 1994, pp. 59–64.

87. Laws ER Jr: Vascular complications of transsphenoidal surgery, in Takakura K, Sasaki T (eds): *Cerebrovascular Surgery.* Tokyo, University of Tokyo Press, 1994, pp. 259–260.

88. Thapar K, Kovacs K, Laws ER Jr: The classification and molecular biology of pituitary adenomas, in *Advances and Technical Standards in Neurosurgery, Vol 22,* New York, Springer, 1995, 3–53.

89. Laws ER Jr: Transsphenoidal approach to pituitary tumors, in Schmidck HH, Sweet WH (eds): *Operative Neurosurgical Techniques, 3rd Edition.* Phila., Sanders, 1995, pp. 283–292.

90. Thapar K, Laws ER Jr: Tumors of the central nervous system, in Murphy GP, Lawrence W Jr, Lenhard RE Jr (eds): *American Cancer Society Textbook of Clinical Oncology, 2nd Edition.* Atlanta, American Cancer Society, 1995, pp. 378–410.

91. Thapar K, Laws ER Jr: Tumors of the pituitary gland, in Murphy GP, Lawrence W Jr, Lenhard Re Jr (eds): *American Cancer Society Textbook of Clinical Oncology, 2nd Edition.* Atlanta, American Cancer Society, 1995, pp. 411–427.

92. Kaye AH, Laws ER Jr: Historical perspective, in Kaye AH, Laws ER Jr (eds): *Brain Tumors.* London, Churchill Livingstone, 1995, pp. 3–9.

93. Thapar K, Laws ER Jr: Pituitary tumors, in Kaye AH, Laws ER Jr (eds): *Brain Tumors.* London, Churchill Livingstone, 1995, pp. 759–777.

94. Thapar K, Rutka JT, Laws ER Jr: Brain edema, increased intracranial pressure, vascular effects and other epiphenomena of brain tumors, in Kaye AH, Laws ER Jr (eds): *Brain Tumors.* London, Churchill Livingstone, 1995, pp. 163–190.

95. Sindou M, Hallacq P, Ojemann RG, Laws ER Jr: Aggressive vs. conservative treatment of parasagittal meningiomas involving the superior sagittal sinus, in Al-Mefty O, Origitano TC, Harkey HL (eds): *Controversies in Neurosurgery.* Thieme, New York, 1995, pp. 80–89.

96. Laws ER Jr: Surgical aspects and general management of astrocytomas, in Apuzzo MLJ (ed): *Benign Cerebral Glioma.* Vol II, Park Ridge, AANS, 1995, pp. 381–396.

97. Laws ER Jr: Acromegaly and gigantism, in Wilkins RA, Rengachary SS (eds): *Neurosurgery, 2nd Edition,* Vol. I, New York, McGraw-Hill, 1996, pp. 1317–1320.

98. Laws ER Jr, Wharen RE Jr, Anderson RE: Photoradiation therapy for malignant gliomas, in Wilkins RH, Rengachary SS (eds): *Neurosurgery, 2nd Edition,* Vol. II, New York, McGraw-Hill, 1996, pp. 1973–1978.

99. Thapar K, Laws ER Jr: Parasellar lesions other than pituitary adenomas, in Powell M, Lightman SL (eds): *The Management of Pituitary Tumors.* London, Churchill Livingstone, 1996, pp. 175–222.

100. Ater JL, Tarbell NJ, Laws ER Jr: Optic nerve, chiasmal and hypothalamic region tumors, in Levin VA (ed): *Cancer in the Nervous System.* New York, Churchill Livingstone, 1996, pp. 139–152.

101. Laws ER Jr: Commentary: Spinal cord Meningioma, in *The Tumor Board.* New York, Lippincott-Raven, 1996, p. 622.

102. Laws ER Jr, Thapar K: Recurrent Pituitary Adenomas, in Landolt AM, Vance ML, Reilly P (eds): *Pituitary Adenomas—Biology, Diagnosis and Treatment.* New York, Churchill Livingstone, 1996.

103. Laws ER Jr, Chenelle AG, Thapar K: Recurrence after transsphenoidal surgery for pituitary adenomas: clinical and basic science aspects, in von Werder K, Fahlbusch R (eds): *Pituitary Adenomas: From Basic Research to Diagnosis and Therapy.* Amsterdam, Elsevier, 1996, pp. 3–9.

104. Laws ER Jr: Pituitary Adenoma, in John RT, Griffin JW (eds): *Current Therapy in Neurologic Disease, 5th Edition,* St. Louis, Mosby, 1997.

105. Laws ER Jr: Surgical management of pituitary apoplexy, in Welch KMA, Caplan LR, Reis DJ, Siesjo B, Weir B (eds): *Primer on Cerebrovascular Diseases.* New York, Academic Press, 1997, pp. 508–510.

106. Laws ER Jr: Craniopharyngioma: transsphenoidal surgery, in Bardin CW (ed): *Current Therapy in Endocrinology and Metabolism, 6th Edition.* St. Louis, Mosby, 1997, pp. 35–37.

107. Laws ER Jr: Pituitary and brain tumors (consultant), in Murphy GP, Morris LB: *The American Cancer Society's Informed Decisions: The Complete Book of Cancer Diagnosis Treatment and Recovery.* Atlanta, Viking Press, 1997.

108. Laws ER Jr, Bruner J: Central nervous system: brain and spinal cord, in Fleming ID, Cooper JR, Henson De, Hutter RV, Kennedy BJ, Murphy GP, O'Sullivan B, Sobin LH, Yarbro JW (eds): *AJCC Cancer Staging Manual 5th edition.* Philadelphia, Lippincott, 1997, pp. 281–283.

109. Thapar K, Laws ER Jr: Vascular tumors: hemangioblastomas, hemangiopericytomas and cavernous hemangiomas, in Scheaves R, Jenkins PJ, Wass JAH (eds): *Clinical Endocrine Oncology.* Oxford, Blackwell, 1997, pp. 264–270.

110. Laws ER Jr: "Schools" of Neurosurgery: their development and evolution, in Greenblatt SH (ed): *A History of Neurosurgery.* Park Ridge, IL, Amer. Assn of Neurological Surgeons, 1997, pp. 519–528.

111. Laws ER Jr: Outcome measurements for intrinsic brain and pituitary tumors, in Swash M (ed): *Outcomes in Neurological and Neurosurgical Disorders.* Cambridge, Cambridge University Press, 1998, pp. 219–226.

112. Thapar K, Laws ER Jr: Current management of prolactin-secreting tumors, in Salcman M (ed): Current Techniques in Neurosurgery—Philadelphia, Springer, 1998, pp. 176–191.

113. Polin RS, Laws ER Jr, Shaffrey ME: Hypophysectomy for intractable pain from metastatic carcinoma. A historical perspective, in Burchiel K. *Pain.* Thieme, 1998, 821–826.

114. Thapar K, Laws ER Jr: Growth-hormone secreting pituitary tumors: operative management, in Krisht A, Tindall G (eds): *Pituitary Disorders—Comprehensive Management.* Baltimore, Lippincott-Williams & Wilkins, 1999, pp. 243–258.

115. Laws ER Jr, Thapar K: The results of surgical therapy for acromegaly on CD ROM, in Giustina A (eds): *A CD ROM On Acromegaly,* 1999.

116. Laws ER Jr: Boron neutron capture therapy, Chapter 19, in Bernstein M, Berger M (eds): *Neuro-Oncology: The Essentials.* New York, Thieme, 1999, 205–209.

117. Thapar K, Laws ER Jr: Transsphenoidal surgery for recurrent pituitary tumors, in Kaye AH, Black PM (eds): *Operative Neurosurgery,* 2000.

118. Laws ER Jr: Epilepsy operations, in Heros R, Salcman M (eds): *Kempe's Operative Neurosurgery Vol. 1. Current Medicine,* (in press), 2000.

119. Laws ER Jr, Thapar K: Unusual lesions in the sella turcica, in Kaye A, Black P (eds): *Operative Neurosurgery.* London, Harcourt Brace, 2000.

120. Laws ER Jr, Thapar K, Vance ML: Pituitary adenomas with invasion of the skull base: biology, surgery and radiotherapy, in Fahlbusch R, Buchfelder M (eds): *The Centre of the Skull Base.* Reinbeck, Einhorn Presse-Verlag, 2000, pp. 159–162.

121. Laws ER: The development of neuro-oncology in the second half

of the 20th century, in Barrow D (ed): *Fifty Years of Neurosurgery*. Congress of Neurological Surgeons, 2000, pp. 169–177.

122. Thapar K, Laws ER Jr: Pituitary Surgery, in Thapar K, Kovacs K, Scheithauer BW, Lloyd R (eds): *Diagnosis and Management of Pituitary Tumors*. Totowa, NJ, Humana, 2001, (in press).

123. Thapar K, Laws ER Jr: Management of extrasellar pituitary lesions, in Thapar K, Kovacs K, Scheithauer BW, Lloyd R (eds): *Diagnosis and Management of Pituitary Tumors*. Totowa, NJ, Humana 2001, (in press).

124. Laws ER Jr: Transsphenoidal surgery for chordomas and chondrosarcomas, in Harsh G IV, Janecka I, Mankin H, Ojemann R, Suit H, McKenna M (eds): *Chordomas and Chondrosarcomas*. New York, Thieme, 2001, (in press).

125. Ater N, Tarbell NJ, Laws ER Jr: Optic nerve, chiasmal and hypothalamus region tumors, in Levin VA (ed): *Cancer in the Nervous System. 2nd Edition*. New York, Churchill Livingstone, 2001, in press.

126. Laws ER: Brain tumor affecting growth and development, in Brook CDG (ed).

127. Shaffrey Me, Laws ER: Brain tumors, in Rakel RE, Bope ET (eds): *Conn's Current Therapy 2001*. New York, Saunders, 2001, pp. 1006–1009.

Contents

GENERAL SCIENTIFIC SESSION I

I

General Scientific
Session I
Brain Tumor Management:
Present and Future

1

Cerebral Gliomas: How Tumor Biology Affects Management

JOSEPH M. PIEPMEIER, M.D.

INTRODUCTION

In 1952, Kernohan published the first classification system for gliomas (predominantly astrocytomas) that placed these tumors into grades according to specific histologic findings including anaplasia, necrosis, and vascularity (1). Kernohan's four-tiered classification was the first system that recognized what clinicians had long ago realized, that lower grade gliomas eventually evolve into higher grade lesions.

Over the past 50 years we have further defined the clinical, radiological, and epidemiological factors that are associated with the biology of gliomas. Although we have yet to identify what causes these tumors, we have a better understanding of the genetic mutations associated with malignant progression and the biological barriers to effective treatment (2).

This chapter will discuss some of the ways that advances in the understanding of biology of gliomas affects management. Specifically, it will address epidemiology, the malignant phenotype (proliferation, neovascularity, migration), immune suppression, the blood-brain barrier, and the genetics of gliomas.

EPIDEMIOLOGY OF GLIOMAS

We know from population-based studies that gliomas occur more frequently in males (7.2/100,000) than females (5.05/100,000) and that the incidence of specific histological subtypes are age dependent (3). For example low-grade gliomas including astrocytomas, oligodendrogliomas, and mixed oligoastrocytomas are found predominantly in patients aged 30 to 40 years. Anaplastic astrocytomas generally arise around ages 40 to 50 years, whereas glioblastomas are the most common gliomas and occur in patients over 50 years of age. Epidemiology teaches us that the relative risk of a glioma increases with age and the risk that the lesion will be a high-grade tumor also increases with age (3).

CURRENT TREATMENT

One of the fundamental principles of direct treatment strategy for malignancies is the observation that cells are more susceptible to radiation and chemotherapy when they are actively dividing. This relative increase in sensitivity is applicable to malignant gliomas. The benefit of aggressive surgery for gliomas has never been tested in a randomized clinical trial, nor is it likely that it will be. It is the experience of many neurosurgeons that maximal surgery can prolong survival as well as relieve mass effect while providing the pathologist with adequate samples for diagnostic purposes. The value of radiotherapy and chemotherapy was tested in a randomized clinical trial by the Brain Tumor Study Group (BTSG) in the 1970s (4). BTSG 69-01 showed that nitrosourea alone without radiotherapy produced a 15% survival at 1-year. Radiotherapy alone (60Gy) without chemotherapy increased 1-year survival to 34.6%. The addition of radiotherapy and nitrosurea was associated with a 50% 1-year survival.

The conclusions of this study indicated that patients randomized to receive radiotherapy did better than those who did not receive it. However, when adjusted for prognostic variables, there was no significant difference between the median survival for patients who received radiotherapy alone and those who received radiotherapy and chemotherapy. While median survival was not changed, the addition of chemotherapy did increase the 18-month survival (27%) compared with radiotherapy alone (15%). One can conclude from these data that there are a subset of patients with malignant gliomas who befit from the addition of chemotherapy. The most important findings in this and other clinical trials is the overwhelming significance of age, performance status, length of symptoms, and the presence of seizures. These "biological" factors are so important that they must be considered when comparing treatment groups.

MALIGNANT PHENOTYPE

The World Health Organization classifies all gliomas as malignant regardless of their degree of anaplasia. This is because gliomas are not encapsulated and characteristically infiltrate into the surrounding brain. Gliomas also are characterized by their variable degree of proliferative capacity, the ability to induce neovascularization, the capacity to suppress the immune response while the blood-brain barrier provides a mutable protective mechanism to prevent access by chemotherapy. While each of these biological characteristics presents an obstacle to treatment, each also offers a potential target for therapy.

As we better understand the biology of these lesions, we also increase the opportunity to find effective treatment.

PROLIFERATION

It is common practice by neuropathologists to obtain a quantitative measure of the proliferating capacity of a glioma through a labeling index. This is typically performed by immunohistochemistry with an antibody (MIB-1) that binds to cells actively involved in the cell cycle (5). Within a selected field of view at a set magnification, the numbers of immunopositive (labeled) cells is expressed as a numerator and the number of unlabeled cells makes up the denominator. The resulting labeling index is presented as a percentage derived from the region of the tumor where labeling is maximally present (5). In general, low-grade gliomas have a labeling index <1%; however, this can range up to 5%. Anaplastic gliomas generally have a labeling index ranging from 5 to 8% whereas glioblastomas commonly have a labeling index > 10%. However, there is variability of the labeling index within each tumor grade, and the labeling index may not be a reliable marker for prognosis.

The presence of proliferating cells i a glioma is a response top genetic mutations leading to the loss of control over the mechanisms that regulate the cell cycle. The absence of normal regulatory cycle control is associated with amplification of oncogenes as well as deletion of tumor suppresser genes. For example, it is well recognized that glioblastoma is a single diagnosis that can arise from at least two distinct pathways. "primary" glioblastomas occur in older patients (55–60 years) with a short clinical history (6, 7). At the time of biopsy these lesions do not contain evidence of an antecedent low-grade tumor. These tumors are characterized by specific genetic mutations like amplification of MDM2 (murine double minute 2) and EGFR (epidermal growth factor receptor) genes, loss of tumor suppresser genes like CDK2NA as well as LOH10 (loss of heterozygosity chromosome 10) (6, 7). In contrast, secondary glioblastomas arise in younger patients (40 years), have a relatively longer clinical history, and occur as a result of transition from a low-grade glioma. The hallmark of high-grade transition from a low-grade glioma is mutation of the tumor suppressor gene, p53 (6, 7). The other genetic mutation associated with secondary glioblastomas is amplification or overexpression of PDGF (platelet derived growth factor).

A separate and distinct set of genetic alterations are found in oligodendrogliomas. These tumors are associated with loss of alleles on chromosome 1p and 19q (8). In fact, these tumors rarely have p53 mutation. However, as oligodendrogliomas gain anaplastic features, they also gain the genetic profile associated with malignant astrocytomas including CDK2NA deletion, amplification of EGFR and LOH10. These findings suggest that although tumors composed of oligodendroglial cells are characterized by 1p and 19q deletions, their progression to anaplasia follows a pathway similar to astroglial tumors.

Glioma genetics have important impact on treatment. Specifically, the finding of 1p, 19q deletions in anaplastic oligodendrogliomas identifies tumors that respond well to chemotherapy. The reasons for this finding remain obscure; however, recently, a small subset of glioblastomas also have been shown to contain a 1p deletion (personal communication, Greg Cairncross). These tumors are unique because their outcome is significantly better than expected based on the histological tumor grade. These findings not only influence treatment and prognosis, but also they represent the potential for changing how gliomas are classified. Since tumors with similar histopathological findings can have very different outcomes and because these variations may be identified by specific genetic "fingerprints," the future classification of gliomas may require an assessment of genetic mutations. These may be more informative than histology in directing treatment and establishing prognosis.

NEOVASCULARITY AND THE BLOOD-BRAIN BARRIER

Gliomas create their own blood supply (9). This is accomplished in part, by the secretion of vascular growth factors such as vascular endothelial growth factor (VEGF) and fibroblastic growth factor (FGF). Tumor induced vessels do not contain endothelial tight junctions that maintain the blood-brain barrier, hence neovascularization commonly results in enhancement on MRI and CT imaging (10). A robust production of new vessels is a characteristic of advanced grade of glioma. Therefore, enhancement on MRI or CT imaging is generally a finding suggesting a worse prognosis. Inhibition of neovascularization presents an attractive target for treatment. At this time, clinical trials with putative angiogenic inhibitors have not achieved success.

Another strategy for manipulating tumor biology for treatment is the use of agents that transiently open the blood-brain barrier. This strategy is based on the proposition that if more agent (chemotherapy) can be delivered to areas where the barrier remains intact, then the infiltrative tumor cells that escape surgery and radiation therapy can be more effectively treated. Mannitol and Cereport (RMP7) are the two agents that have received the most clinical investigation. In general, these studies have shown that if the tumor is chemosensitive (e.g., primary CNS lymphoma) then the increased concentration of delivered agent is also effective. It is more difficult to demonstrate similar responses with malignant gliomas (11).

A reverse strategy also has been utilized to take advantage of the blood-brain barrier. If the barrier can prevent access by chemotherapy to infiltrative tumor cells following systemic application, then agents that cannot cross the barrier will remain within the tumor when given directly into the lesion. Direct infusion of chemotherapy into the tumor (convection-enhanced delivery) has been shown to distribute relatively high concentrations of agents in a pattern that replicates the infiltrative topography of glioma cells (12). New clinical trials with convection delivery are in progress.

MIGRATION

The most vexing problem that precludes surgical cure of most gliomas is the observation that the vast majority of these lesions include isolated tumor cells that have migrated into the brain. Infiltration of tumor cells is best illustrated by the large area of signal change surrounding the solid tumor mass as shown on T2-weighted MRI (10, 13). Glioma cells produce enzymes (proteases) that degrade the surrounding extracellular matrix, and the tumor cells can produce matrix proteins that are more permissive for migration. For example, brain derived by hyaluronic acid binding (BEHAB) protein is at tumor-specific protein found during gestation in the immature CNS during a period of glial proliferation and migration (14). BEHAB is not present in the adult CNS but can be found in infiltrative gliomas. Since BEHAB is tumor specific, it presents an attractive target for antimigration therapy. Similarly, inhibitors of tumor-derived proteases (metaloprotease inhibitors) also can be used to restrict tumor cell migration (15). Unfortunately, by the time most gliomas are detected, significant migration already has occurred. For glioblastoma, tumor cells can be grown in culture from brain tissue that has no radiological or histopathological evidence of involvement (16). Consequently, the importance of antimigration therapy will be realized when restricting further migration can be coupled with other forms of therapy.

IMMUNOTHERAPY

Perhaps the most promising areas where glioma biology directs treatment is in the field of immunotherapy. It is well recognized that malignant gliomas escape an immune response by hiding behind the blood-brain barrier and by producing proteins that suppress systemic immunity. However, if gliomas can be made to be more immunogenic or if a tumor vaccine can be produced, then access to all tumor cells including those that infiltrate into the brain can be achieved through the patient's immune response.

Several strategies have been investigated for immunotherapy. These include extracting tumor tissue or portions of tumor cells homogenates and exposing them as antigens to cytokines, lymphocytes, or dendritic cells. Laboratory studies and animal models have shown that these immune cells will attack the tumor, reduce the size of implanted tumors, and that the immune memory is sufficient to suppress tumor growth when the animal is rechallenged with a tumor implant (17–19). These studies have been sufficiently successful that several clinical trials have been established and are currently recruiting patients.

However, major challenges to effective immunotherapy remain. The threat of an autoimmune response exists since the antigens that are found on tumor cells also may coexist on normal glia. In addition, obtaining a sufficient number of immune cells within the tumor may prove to be problematic Finally, immune therapy can induce high amounts of brain edema. Consequently, careful study and toxicity issues remain to be resolved before these therapies can enter randomized clinical trials.

CONCLUSION

We are entering an era when more effective glioma therapy can be achieved. This optimistic outlook is based on the premise that research focused on glioma biology will form the basis for strategies to identify more effective therapy. The time has past when tumors are classified only by the tumor cell morphology, and the future will include genetic fingerprinting. We better understand how the loss of tumor suppressor genes releases gliomas from normal regulatory mechanisms of growth control. Antiangiogenesis and antimigration therapies will inhibit the properties that allow gliomas to progress to a higher grade before this progression further impairs the patient's function. Perturbation of the blood-brain barrier or better access to the tumor or convection-enhanced delivery of compounds directly into the tumor will find wider application as more effective agents are found. Finally, the identification of an effective tumor vaccine will likely be the mechanisms where the concept of "cure" becomes a reality.

REFERENCES

1. Kernohan J, Sayre G: Tumors of the nervous system. Section X-Fascicles 35 and 37. *Atlas of Tumor Pathology*. Washington DC, Armed Forces Institute of Pathology, 1952.
2. Manuelidis L: Genomic stability and instability in different neuroepithelial tumors. A role for chromosome structure? **J Neurooncol** 18:225–239, 1994.
3. Giles G, Gonzales M: Epidemiology of brain tumors and factors in prognosis, in Kay A, Laws E (eds). *Brain Tumors*. Edinburgh, Churchill Livingstone, 1995, pp 47–68.

4. Walker M, Green S, Byar D, et al.: Randomized comparisons of radiotherapy and nitrosoureas for the treatment of malignant gliomas after surgery. **N Engl J Med** 303:1323–1329, 1980.
5. Heesters M, Koustall J, Go K, Molenaar W: Analysis of proliferation and apoptosis in brain gliomas: Prognostic and clinical value. **J Neurooncol** 44:255–266, 1999.
6. Kleihues P, Ohgaki H: Primary and secondary glioblastomas: From concept to clinical diagnosis. **Neuro-oncol** 1:44–51, 1999.
7. Fults D, Brockenmeyer D, Tullos M, Pedone C, Cawthon R: p53 mutation and loss of heterozygosity on chromosomes 17 and 10 during human astrocytomas progression. **Cancer Res** 52:674–679, 1992.
8. Cairncross JG, Ueki K, Zlatescu MC, et al.: Specific genetic predictors of chemotherapeutic response and survival in patients with anaplastic oligodendrogliomas. **J Natl Cancer Inst** 90:1473–1479, 1998.
9. Folkman J: Angiogenesis and its inhibitors, in DeVita V, Hellman S, Rosenberg S (eds): *Important Advances in Oncology 1985*. Philadelphia: Lippincott, 1985, pp 42–62.
10. Byrne T, Piepmeier J, Yoshida D: Imaging and clinical features of gliomas, in Tindall G, Cooper P, Barrow D (eds): *The Practice of Neurosurgery*. Baltimore: Williams and Wilkins, 1995, pp 637–648.
11. Doolittle N, Miner M, Hall W, et al.: Safety and efficacy of a multi-center study using intraarterial chemotherapy in conjunction with osmotic opening of the blood-brain barrier for the testament of malignant brain tumors. **Cancer** 88:637–647, 2000.
12. Laske D, Ilercil O, Akbasak A, Youle R, Oldfield E: Efficacy of direct intratumoral therapy with targeted protein toxins for solid human gliomas in nude mice. **J Neurosurg** 80:520–526, 1994.
13. Kelly P, Daumas-Duport C, Scheithauer B, Kall B, Kispert D: Stereotactic histologic correlations of computed tomography and magnetic resonance imaging defined abnormalities in patients with glial neoplasms. **Mayo Clin Proc** 62:450–459, 1987.
14. Jaworski D, Kelly G, Piepmeier J, Pedersen P, Hockfield S: BEHAB, the CNS specific hyaluronan-binding protein, is expressed in glioma and in intracranial grafts of glioma cell lines. **Cancer Res** 56:2293–2298, 1996.
15. Yoshida D, Piepmeier J, Bergenheim T, Henriksson R, Teramoto A: Suppression of matrix metalloproteinase-2 medicated cell invasion in U87MG human glioma cells by anti-microtubile agent: in vitro study. **Br J Cancer** 77:21–25, 1998.
16. Silbergeld D, Chicoine M: Isolation and characterization of human malignant glioma cells from histological normal brain. **J Neurosurg** 86:525–531, 1997.
17. Quattrocchi K, Miller C, Berbard C, et al.: Pilot study of local autologous tumor infiltrating lymphocytes for the treatment of recurrent malignant gliomas. **J Neurooncol** 45:141–157, 1999.
18. Plautz G, Miller D, Barnett G, et al.: T cell adoptive immunotherapy of newly diagnosed gliomas. **Clin Cancer Res** 6:209–2218, 2000.
19. Heimberger A, Crotty L, Archer G, et al.: Bone marrow derived dendritic cells pulsed with tumor homogenate induces immunity against syngeneic intracerebral gliomas. **J Neuroimmunol** 1:16–25, 2000.

2

Fifty Years of Neurosurgery Argue in Favor of Glioma Resection

RAYMOND SAWAYA, M.D.

INTRODUCTION

Much progress has taken place in the surgical management of gliomas over the past 50 years and even more so over the past 10 years with the advances in imaging technology and in surgical adjuncts. Operative mortality has declined steadily from 41.1% in 1949 to current levels of 2 to 3% *(Table 2.1)*. This improvement in outcome is due to the advent of modern neuroanesthesia, the latest prophylactic measures, improved neuroimaging definition, microsurgical techniques, cortical mapping, state-of-the-art navigational devices, and an interactive psychodynamic between physician and patient.

Paul Bucy reported a patient whose glioblastoma was operated upon in 1958 and who received subsequent radiotherapy (1). The patient was considered cured 26 years later.

Yet, an exhaustive review of the literature on malignant glioma resection prior to 1990 (2) concluded that during the previous 50 years there was little justification for dogmatic statements concerning the relationship between increasing patient survival times and aggressive surgical management in adults with supratentorial intermediate or high-grade astrocytomas.

Basis for the Controversy

Why is the role of surgery in glioma treatment still considered controversial? The reasons for this include the following:

1. *The overall poor prognosis of patients with malignant gliomas.* Glioblastomas are highly aggressive and resistant tumors that tend to have a short time to recurrence, even when extensively resected. It is difficult to remove such infiltrating tumors, and there are risks of producing new neurological deficits with extensive resections. Patients with glioblastoma multiforme (GBM) have a median survival time of approximately 1 year, measured from the time of diagnosis (3, 4).

TABLE 2.1
Operative Mortality of Craniotomy for Resection of Malignant Gliomas

Authors (ref. no.)	Year	Number of resections	Mortality (%)
Davis et al. (32)	1949	187	41.1
Grant (33)	1956	350	38.0
Roth and Elvidge (34)	1960	399	21.5
Hitchcock and Sato (35)	1964	222	19.0
Jelsma and Bucy (36)	1967	122	27.9
Leibel et al. (37)	1975	147	17.0
Fadul et al. (38)	1988	104	3.3
Salcman et al. (39)	1994	509	2.7

2. *The lack of a published randomized trial.* To date, no one has published a prospective series in which glioma patients are randomized to well-defined protocols for either aggressive or conservative surgical treatment (5). It will be difficult to conduct such a study because adhering to the protocol could interfere with the neurosurgeon's wish to select the optimal extent of resection for a given glioma patient based on the size and location of the tumor, as well as the patient's medical and neurological condition.

3. *Insufficient scientific validity of the conclusions of current studies.* During the past decade, studies of surgical treatment for gliomas concluding that extensive surgical resection produces an increased survival in glioma patients have generally been retrospective in nature, making them subject to numerous sources of variation and bias *(Table 2.2)*. Note

TABLE 2.2
Analysis of the Effect of Extent of Resection of Gliomas on Survival

Authors (ref. no.)	Year	No. of resections	Prospective study	Confounding factors adjusted for	Effect on survival
Prados et al. (8)	1992	357	No	No	No*
Curran et al. (7)	1992	103	No	No	No*
Kreth et al. (9)	1993	115	No	No	No*
Devaux et al. (16)	1993	218	No	Yes	Yes
Lai et al. (40)	1993	116	No	Yes	Yes
Kelly & Hunt (10)	1994	128	No	No	N/A[†]
Albert et al. (6)	1994	60	Yes	Yes	Yes
Nitta & Sato (11)	1995	101	No	No	N/A[†]
Kiwit et al. (12)	1996	80	No	Yes	Yes

*Insufficient statistical power to support conclusion.
[†] Not applicable.

that the only prospective study listed is that of Albert and coworkers (6). These studies are difficult to compare because they differ with respect to classification criteria, patient selection, and distributions of covariates (5). They also suffer from a variety of statistical and design flaws. Thus, the conclusions reached are frequently not supported by adequate statistical power.

4. *Statistical flaws in studies to date.* Relevant studies since 1991 on the effect of extent of resection on survival of glioma patients are shown in Table 2.2. Five of the 9 studies (7–11) failed to provide an adjustment for confounding from known prognostic factors (such as patient age, neurological performance status, and histological grade of glioma). Two of these studies used univariate instead of multivariate analysis, rendering their conclusions ambiguous (10, 11). The other three studies (7–9) inappropriately employed stepwise variable selection in their analyses, which not only provided no confounding adjustment but also caused the studies to have insufficient statistical power for the conclusions drawn.

5. *The lack of confirmation of extent of resection with imaging data.* With the relatively recent advent of modern imaging methods, some investigators have employed pre- and postoperative computed tomography (CT) or magnetic resonance (MR) imaging scans to estimate extent of resection, an improvement over relying on the surgeon's opinion for this parameter (6, 12, 13). Nevertheless, since 1989, as shown in Table 2.3, only half of 10 glioma patient series have employed postoperative radiological imaging in their estimation of extent of resection.

TABLE 2.3
Treatment and Results in Surgical Series of Glioma Patients from the Past Decade

Authors (ref. no.)	Year	Resection verified by postoperative imaging	% patients receiving GTR*
Winger et al. (41)	1989	No	12.6
Vecht et al. (14)	1990	No	6.2
Ciric et al. (42)	1990	Yes	71.0
Curran et al. (7)	1992	No	14.0
Kreth et al. (9)	1993	No	Not stated
Devaux et al. (16)	1993	Yes	Not stated
Iacoangeli et al. (43)	1993	Yes	35.0
Albert et al. (6)	1994	Yes	18.0
Berger 1994 (17)	1994	Yes	Not stated
Barker et al. (15)	1998	No	12

*GTR, gross total resection.

6. *The lack of complete resections in recent studies.* Over the past decade, in some series of glioma surgeries (Table 2.3) the number of GTRs has been limited to a mere 6.2% (14) or 12% (15) of the total. Other series fail to mention how many GTRs were performed (9, 16, 17). Only a few series such as that of Barker and coworkers (15) give a firm definition of GTR (even though that definition indicates that a GTR is > 90%) and also perform postoperative imaging confirmation of extent of resection.

7. *Histological contamination.* If patients with anaplastic astrocytomas (AAs), which carry a longer expectancy of survival, are included in the study along with glioblastoma multiforme patients, the median survival time observed for patients in such series will vary depending upon the number of AA patients included.

MEASURES OF EFFECTIVENESS IN GLIOMA RESECTION

The measures of effectiveness of surgical treatment of gliomas are, in fact, multiple and include: extent of resection, relief of mass effect, enhanced tolerance to radiotherapy, prolonged survival, diagnostic accuracy, mortality rate, morbidity rate, and research discoveries. These measures will be examined below.

Extent of Resection and Prolonged Survival

Extent of resection was studied recently in relation to patient survival at The University of Texas M. D. Anderson Cancer Center (18). Between June 1993 and June 1999, 416 consecutive patients with histologically verified GBM underwent tumor resection at M. D. Anderson. Because most studies that have examined the role of surgery in the management of high-grade gliomas have lacked an objective measure of resected tumor volume, we prospectively collected data on tumor volume both pre- and postoperatively (shortly after surgery) from MRI scans by a computerized measurement method (13). Cumulative patient survival times were computed by the Kaplan-Meier method. Survival curves were compared using the log-rank test, and both univariate and multivariate analyses were performed using the Cox proportional hazards model.

Sixty-three percent of the patients were men; the median patient age was 53 years; 75% of patients had a preoperative Karnofsky Performance Scale (KPS) score of 80 or more; 91% of the gliomas were hemispheric in location; and 48% of tumors were located near eloquent brain, whereas 44% were within eloquent brain. The median preoperative tumor volume in this patient series was 34 cm^3, whereas the median postoperative tumor volume was 0.68 cm^3.

The mean extent of resection for glioma patients in this series was 89%. An extent of resection of 98% or more was obtained for 47% of patients. Resection of 98% or more of the tumor volume was found to be an independent variable associated with longer survival (median = 13.4 months; P < 0.0001) in patients with GBM *(Table 2.4)*. In patients with tumor resection of less than 98%, median survival time was only 8.8 months. Tumor removal of less than 94% may still provide diagnostic and symptomatic benefits, but there is no statistical survival benefit.

Relief of Mass Effect and Enhanced Tolerance to Radiotherapy

Many malignant gliomas tend to reach large sizes prior to detection (mean volume of 38.55 cm^3 seen in the M. D. Anderson series above) and frequently produce mass effects such as neurological deficits or seizures. Patients who underwent gross total resections (GTRs) of such tumors were shown to display better neurological performance scores than those receiving less aggressive surgical treatment (19, 20). Moreover, radiation oncologists expect patients undergoing gross total resection of malignant gliomas to experience fewer side effects from radiation therapy.

Diagnostic Accuracy

Does a stereotactic biopsy of a malignant glioma provide results equivalent to those obtained with a radical excision of the mass? In 1988, Coffey and coworkers (21) studied 64 patients with GBM and 27 who had anaplastic astrocytomas (AAs). Only 15 of 91 patients were treated surgically, and the rest had stereotactic biopsies. Nine of 64 patients with GBMs underwent surgical resection, showing 29.5 weeks median survival, and 6 of 27 patients undergoing surgical excision of AAs had a median survival of 74 weeks. Although the number of resec-

TABLE 2.4
Survival Time Relative to Degree of Tumor Resection in Glioma Patients

Extent of tumor resection	Median survival in months (95% CI*)	Rate ratio (95% of CI)	P value
≥ 85%	10.90 (9.7–12.2)	1.11 (0.8–1.5)	0.5
≥ 90%	11.43 (10.1–12.7)	1.27 (1.0–1.7)	0.08
≥ 94%	11.90 (10.3–13.4)	1.31 (1.0–1.7)	0.03
≥ 96%	13.10 (11.3–14.9)	1.56 (1.2–2.0)	0.0004
≥ 98%	13.40 (12.0–14.9)	1.74 (1.4–2.2)	< 0.0001
100%	13.60 (12.2–15.0)	1.78 (1.4–2.3)	< 0.0001

*CI, confidence interval.

tions was very limited, the extent of resection was not defined, multivariate analysis of the data was not performed, and the statistical power of the analysis was insufficient; the authors nevertheless concluded that cytoreductive surgery had no statistically significant effect on survival.

Despite its being championed by Dr. Lunsford, stereotactic biopsy appears to have significant limitations in terms of diagnostic accuracy, associated morbidity, and inability to provide relief from mass effect. To investigate this, at M. D. Anderson we performed a study of stereotactic biopsy versus resection of malignant gliomas (22). Between 1993 and 1998, a series of 81 consecutive patients with imaging studies suggestive of glioma were retrospectively reviewed. All patients underwent stereotactic biopsy (at hospitals other than M. D. Anderson), and tumors were analyzed volumetrically at M. D. Anderson based on pre- and postoperative MR images. No patients had received prior therapy for gliomas. All resections were performed at M. D. Anderson, and all stereotactic biopsy slides were reviewed there as well.

Characteristics of patients in this series included: a sex ratio of 49 males to 32 females, a mean age of 48 years (range, 15–81), and a median preoperative KPS score of 90. Sixty-seven percent of patients underwent stereotactic biopsy at nonacademic (nonuniversity-affiliated) centers, whereas 33% had their biopsy at an academic center. Most of the tumors resided in near-eloquent brain (51%) or eloquent brain (44%), and this was often given as the grounds for performing stereotactic biopsy. The median extent of resection reached in this series was 96%, and a gross total resection (> 95%) was achieved in 57% of patients. Major neurological morbidity was 12.3% (10 of 81 patients), and mortality was 1.2%. The median length of hospital stay was 4 days, and the median postoperative KPS score was 90.

There were significant discrepancies between diagnoses based on stereotactic biopsy samples and those based on resected specimens in 49% of cases. When the biopsy slides were reviewed preoperatively by neuropathologists at M. D. Anderson, this discrepancy was reduced to 38%. This 38% discrepancy would probably have affected therapeutic implications in 26% of cases and prognostic implications in 38% of cases. The most likely explanations for the discrepancies observed relate to the small quantity of tissue obtained from stereotactic biopsies and sampling error. Only a limited number of studies (with small sample sizes) have been published that report accuracy of diagnosis based on the stereotactic biopsy specimen relative to that based on the resected specimen *(Table 2.5)*. Moreover, none of the first five studies

TABLE 2.5
Accuracy of Stereotactic Biopsy of Glioma

Authors (ref. no.)	Year	Diagnostic accuracy	No. of patients with subsequent confirmation*
Broggi et al. (44)	1984	89%	36
Kleihues et al. (45)	1984	85%	52
Scerrati & Rossi (46)	1984	95%	19
Chandrasoma et al. (23)	1989	63%	30
Feiden et al. (47)	1991	89%	47
Jackson et al. (22)	2000	62%	81

*Confirmation of diagnosis based on specimen obtained by surgery or autopsy.

shown in Table 2.5 specified or restricted the time interval between biopsy and subsequent confirmation by surgical resection or autopsy. The overall diagnostic accuracy in the M. D. Anderson study (62%) most closely parallels that of Chandrasoma and coworkers (63%) (23), who have extensive experience with the use of stereotactic biopsy in the diagnosis of brain masses (24, 25).

In this series, we found that stereotactic biopsy was either performed inappropriately in patients with moderate to severe tumor-related mass effect or edema, resulted in additional morbidity, and/or yielded an incorrect diagnosis in 75% (61 of 81) of patients. Such biopsy adds additional risks of 0.9% and 4% of mortality and major morbidity, respectively (25–31). We thus question the routine use of stereotactic biopsy instead of, or in a staged approach to, the management of patients whose clinical and imaging studies highly suggest a glioma. Such biopsies are likely to be followed by a more definitive therapeutic procedure.

Morbidity and Mortality Rates

On average, the major complication incidence after craniotomy for resection of an intrinsic brain tumor is about 15%; when such tumors are located in eloquent brain regions, the rate can reach 26% (20). The incidence of mortality with craniotomy for resection of parenchymal brain tumors at M. D. Anderson is 1.7% (20). Operative mortality for malignant glioma resection now typically ranges from 2 to 3% (see Table 2.1).

Research Discoveries

There is a research advantage to performing large resections of malignant gliomas. Harvesting of the entire, frequently morphologically diverse, tumor permits its comprehensive molecular fingerprinting. When a sufficient number of tumors have been so categorized, this should lead us toward the appropriate type of molecular intervention and to more effective and individually tailored therapies. It is unlikely that a cure for gliomas will be developed unless intensely focused research is pursued toward this goal using human samples.

CONCLUSION

In this chapter we have reviewed the benefits expected from extensive resections of malignant gliomas. It is important to remember that the surgeon's judgment must play a major role in selecting patients who are most likely to benefit from more extensive resections. The surgeon's goal should be to maximize the benefits of the resection through use of proper tools while simultaneously minimizing operative risks.

In the absence of prospective studies that randomize glioma patients to either maximal or minimal tumor resection, we must collectively focus on obtaining valid data from well-designed and carefully executed prospective observational studies in which all known prognostic variables are comprehensively analyzed and reported. Such studies do not deprive patients of the benefits of resection, are clinically practical and ethically acceptable, and may provide a more realistic way of assessing the role of resection in glioma management.

ACKNOWLEDGMENT

I thank David M. Wildrick, Ph.D., for his editorial assistance in the preparation of this article.

REFERENCES

1. Bucy PC, Oberhill HR, Siqueira EB, Zimmerman HM, Jelsma RK: Cerebral glioblastomas can be cured. **Neurosurgery** 16:714–717, 1985.
2. Nazzaro JM, Neuwelt EA: The role of surgery in the management of supratentorial intermediate and high-grade astrocytoma in adults. **J Neurosurg** 73:331–344, 1990.
3. Shapiro WR, Green SB, Burger PC, et al.: Randomized trial of three chemotherapy regimens and two radiotherapy regimens in postoperative treatment of malignant glioma: Brain Tumor Cooperative Group Trial 8001. **J Neurosurg** 71:1–9, 1989.
4. Walker MD, Green SB, Byar DP, et al.: Randomized comparisons of radiotherapy and nitrosoureas for the treatment of malignant glioma after surgery. **N Engl J Med** 303:1323–1329, 1980.
5. Hess KR: Extent of resection as a prognostic variable in the treatment of gliomas. **J Neurooncol** 42:227–231, 1999.
6. Albert FK, Forsting M, Sartor K, Adams HP, Kunze S: Early postoperative magnetic resonance imaging after resection of malignant glioma: Objective evaluation of residual tumor and its influence on regrowth and prognosis. **Neurosurgery** 34:45–60, 1994.

7. Curran WJ, Jr., Scott CB, Horton J, et al.: Does extent of surgery influence outcome for astrocytoma with atypical or anaplastic foci (AAF)? A report from three Radiation Therapy Oncology Group (RTOG) trials. **J Neurooncol** 12:219–227, 1992.
8. Prados MD, Gutin PH, Phillips TL, et al.: Highly anaplastic astrocytoma: A review of 357 patients treated between 1977 and 1989. **Int J Radiat Oncol Biol Phys** 23:3–8, 1992.
9. Kreth FW, Warnke PC, Scheremet R, Ostertag CB: Surgical resection and radiation therapy versus biopsy and radiation therapy in the treatment of glioblastoma multiforme. **J Neurosurg** 78:762–766, 1993.
10. Kelly PJ, Hunt C: The limited value of cytoreductive surgery in elderly patients with malignant gliomas. **Neurosurgery** 34:62–67, 1994.
11. Nitta T, Sato K: Prognostic implications of the extent of surgical resection in patients with intracranial malignant gliomas. **Cancer** 75:2727–2731, 1995.
12. Kiwit JC, Floeth FW, Bock WJ: Survival in malignant glioma: analysis of prognostic factors with special regard to cytoreductive surgery. **Zentralbl Neurochir** 57:76–88, 1996.
13. Shi W-M, Wildrick DM, Sawaya R: Volumetric measurement of brain tumors from MR imaging. **J Neurooncol** 37:87–93, 1998.
14. Vecht CJ, Avezaat CJ, van Putten WL, Eijkenboom WM, Stefanko SZ: The influence of the extent of surgery on the neurological function and survival in malignant glioma. A retrospective analysis in 243 patients. **J Neurol Neurosurg Psychiatry** 53:466–471, 1990.
15. Barker FG, 2nd, Chang SM, Gutin PH, et al.: Survival and functional status after resection of recurrent glioblastoma multiforme. **Neurosurgery** 42:709–720, 1998.
16. Devaux BC, O'Fallon JR, Kelly PJ: Resection, biopsy, and survival in malignant glial neoplasms. A retrospective study of clinical parameters, therapy, and outcome. **J Neurosurg** 78:767–775, 1993.
17. Berger MS: Malignant astrocytomas: Surgical aspects. **Semin Oncol** 21:172–85, 1994.
18. Lacroix M, Abi-Said D, Fourney DR, et al.: A multivariate analysis of 416 patients with glioblastoma multiforme: Prognosis, extent of resection, and survival. **J Neurosurg** (August 2001) in press.
19. Ammirati M, Vick N, Liao YL, Ciric I, Mikhael M: Effect of the extent of surgical resection on survival and quality of life in patients with supratentorial glioblastomas and anaplastic astrocytomas. **Neurosurgery** 21:201–206, 1987.
20. Sawaya R, Hammoud M, Schoppa D, et al.: Neurosurgical outcomes in a modern series of 400 craniotomies for treatment of parenchymal tumors. **Neurosurgery** 42:1044–1056, 1998.
21. Coffey RJ, Lunsford LD, Taylor FH: Survival after stereotactic biopsy of malignant gliomas. **Neurosurgery** 22:465–473, 1998.
22. Jackson RJ, Fuller GN, Abi-Said D, et al.: Limitations of stereotactic biopsy in the initial management of gliomas. **Neuro-Oncology** (July 2001) in press.
23. Chandrasoma PT, Smith MM, Apuzzo ML: Stereotactic biopsy in the diagnosis of brain masses: Comparison of results of biopsy and resected surgical specimen. **Neurosurgery** 24:160–165, 1989.
24. Apuzzo ML, Sabshin JK: Computed tomographic guidance stereotaxis in the management of intracranial mass lesions. **Neurosurgery** 12:277–285, 1983.
25. Apuzzo ML, Chandrasoma PT, Cohen D, Zee CS, Zelman V: Computed imaging stereotaxy: Experience and perspective related to 500 procedures applied to brain masses. **Neurosurgery** 20:930–937, 1987.
26. Bernstein M, Parrent AG: Complications of CT-guided stereotactic biopsy of intra-axial brain lesions. **J Neurosurg** 81:165–168, 1994.

27. Hall WA: The safety and efficacy of stereotactic biopsy for intracranial lesions. **Cancer** 82:1749–1755, 1998.
28. Mundinger F: CT stereotactic biopsy for optimizing the therapy of intracranial processes. **Acta Neurochir Suppl (Wien)** 35:70–74, 1985.
29. Ostertag CB, Mennel HD, Kiessling M. Stereotactic biopsy of brain tumors. **Surg Neurol** 14:275–283, 1980.
30. Sawin PD, Hitchon PW, Follett KA, Torner JC: Computed imaging-assisted stereotactic brain biopsy: A risk analysis of 225 consecutive cases. **Surg Neurol** 49:640–649, 1998.
31. Sedan R, Peragut JC, Farnarier PH, Hassoun J, Sethian M: Intra-encephalic stereotactic biopsies (309 patients/318 biopsies). **Acta Neurochir Suppl** 33:207–210, 1984.
32. Davis L, Martin J, Goldstein SL, Ashkenazy M: A study of 211 patients with verified glioblastoma multiforme. **J Neurosurg** 6:33–44, 1949.
33. Grant FC: A study of the results of surgical treatment in 2,326 consecutive patients with brain tumor. **J Neurosurg** 13:479–488, 1956.
34. Roth JG, Elvidge AR: Glioblastoma multiforme: A clinical survey. **J Neurosurg** 17:736–750, 1960.
35. Hitchcock E, Sato F: Treatment of malignant gliomata. **J Neurosurg** 21:497–505, 1964.
36. Jelsma R, Bucy PC: The treatment of glioblastoma multiforme of the brain. **J Neurosurg** 27:388–400, 1967.
37. Leibel SA, Sheline GE, Wara WM, Boldrey EB, Nielsen SL: The role of radiation therapy in the treatment of astrocytomas. **Cancer** 35:1551–1557, 1975.
38. Fadul C, Wood J, Thaler H, Galicich J, Patterson RH, Posner JB: Morbidity and mortality of craniotomy for excision of supratentorial gliomas. **Neurology** 38:1374–1379, 1988.
39. Salcman M, Scholtz H, Kaplan RS, Kulik S: Long term survival in patients with malignant astrocytoma. **Neurosurgery** 34:213–220, 1994.
40. Lai DM, Lin SM, Tu YK, Kao MC, Hung CC: Therapy for supratentorial malignant astrocytomas: Survival and possible prognostic factors. **J Formos Med Assoc** 92:220–226, 1993.
41. Winger MJ, Macdonald DR, Cairncross JG: Supratentorial anaplastic gliomas in adults. The prognostic importance of extent of resection and prior low-grade glioma. **J Neurosurg** 71:487–493, 1989.
42. Ciric I, Rovin R, Cozzens JW, Eller TW, Vick NA, Mikhael MA: Role of surgery in the treatment of malignant cerebral gliomas, in Apuzzo MLJ, (ed): *Malignant Cerebral Glioma.* Park Ridge, IL, American Association of Neurological Surgeons, 1990, pp.141–153.
43. Iacoangeli M, Roselli R, Prezioso A, Scerrati M, Rossi GF: Staging of supratentorial hemispheric glioma using tumour extension, histopathological grade and extent of surgical resection. **Br J Surg** 80:1130–1133, 1993.
44. Broggi G, Franzini A, Giorgi C, Allegranza A: Diagnostic accuracy and multimodal approach in stereotactic biopsies of deep brain tumors. **Acta Neurochir Suppl** 33:211–212, 1984.
45. Kleihues P, Volk B, Anagnostopoulos J, Kiessling M: Morphologic evaluation of stereotactic brain tumour biopsies. **Acta Neurochir Suppl (Wien)** 33:171–181, 1984.
46. Scerrati M, Rossi GF: The reliability of stereotactic biopsy. **Acta Neurochir Suppl** 33:207–210, 1984.
47. Feiden W, Steude U, Bise K, Gundisch O: Accuracy of stereotactic brain tumor biopsy: Comparison of the histologic findings in biopsy cylinders and resected tumor tissue. **Neurosurg Rev** 14:51–56, 1991.

3

The Rationale for Rational Surgery for Fibrillary Astrocytomas

L. DADE LUNSFORD, M.D., F.A.C.S.,
AND AJAY NIRANJAN, M.B.B.S., M.S., M.CH.

INTRODUCTION

Surgery does not cure fibrillary astrocytomas of the brain. For this reason, this glial neoplasm remains a formidable challenge to both patients and physicians. Almost 125 years ago, the first craniotomy for a brain tumor was performed. Localization was based entirely on the presentation and neurological examination. The craniotomy technique was crude by modern standards, and the results predictable. This inauspicious beginning to the field of glial tumor management by surgeons and their neurological surgery descendants has not daunted our desire to perfect a surgical procedure that cures glial neoplasms. For 125 years, surgeons and, more recently, their medical oncology counterparts, have argued vociferously about the relative merits of surgical cytoreductive therapy. To be sure, many positive features have impacted upon the survival and quality of life of patients diagnosed with this difficult tumor. Most of us have dropped the erroneous depiction of these tumors as "benign," noting that historical median survivals of 7 years do not warrant this benign sobriquet (1–3).

Most of us, somewhere deep in our heart, acknowledge the fact that despite our best intentions, surgery alone is an unreliable and occasionally costly management strategy to patients. As surgeons, we are trained to perform delicate brain operations, and we have reveled in the development of new technologies that assist us in this effort. New imaging tools, image guidance, frameless stereotactic surgery, robotic microsurgery, preoperative and intraoperative functional mapping, intraoperative computed tomography (CT) and magnetic resonance imaging (MRI), and a myriad of other technical adjuncts pushes us to achieve that ever elusive goal: "total," "radical," or "complete" extirpation of a Grade II astrocytoma.

As surgeons, we need to be sure that we are not distracted by either the quantity or quality of this 125-year-old relentless argument. We do diagnose these tumors sooner, mainly because of the use of MRI in screening of patients with minor symptoms. We have impacted positively on survival times (although in truth we cannot as yet separate out the effect of earlier diagnosis on these statistics). However, we must refrain from the distraction of pointless arguments. Grade II fibrillary astrocytoma is a tumor of the young adults: 20s, 30s and rarely 40s. Such tumors do occur in the pediatric age group, and it is possible that both the biology, the tumor morphology, and the recovery potential of younger patients mitigate in favor of a more radical approach. What is still remarkable (even in the 21st century) is the inherent tendency of some neurosurgeons, neurologists, and oncologists to delay diagnosis in the belief that it is "benign," or "slow growing" tumor. For some physicians, suspected astrocytomas warrant a "go slow" approach. How do we justify such concepts in tumor patients whose median survival is 7 to 10 years with aggressive treatment including surgery (when indicated) and radiation therapy? How can we argue for "benign neglect" when such tumors gradually transform from a slower growth rate with lower mitotic index to an anaplastic form with higher mitotic index? (1–3) A rapid downhill spiral thereafter ensues with only 2 to 3 years of additional median survival.

DEFINITION OF THE TUMOR

Biology at the Time of Recognition

This tumor occurs most regularly in young adults. Its recognition usually is heralded by a seizure "out of the blue" or by a benign headache syndrome that leads the anxious patient to insist on getting an MRI scan. The MRI is often initially resisted by the primary care physician leading to diagnostic delay (and successful law suits) in some cases. New molecular studies under the direction of skilled neuropathologists lead us to a better understanding of the molecular changes that occur in these young patients. For the most part, this is a sporadic, noninheritance based neoplasm, but we do not as yet know whether this begins from a single cell or from multiple cells. We understand that tumor suppressor gene deletions may play a part, yet molecular studies looking for this gene deletion in low grade fibrillary astrocytomas are unrevealing. Does it begin from a single cell, which loses its normal genetic suppression and begins cell division in unregulated growth? This clearly represents important issues because every tumor cell has the potential for cell division in the absence of treatment. Surgical cytoreductive cure requires removal of every tumor cell, unless we are to assume that some magic number exists which allows the body to mount some form of internal defense or immune response. Surprisingly, the histopathology of these tumors rarely shows any evidence of an immune or inflammatory response, a feature sometimes seen in more aggressive glial neoplasm. Light microscopy studies clearly show a neoplasm consisting of hypercellularity but with little pleomorphism, very rare mitoses, absence of necrosis, and an absence of blood vessel endothelial change. The tumors themselves seem rather monotonous, especially when they are located in white matter structures, sampled during cytoreductive surgery. When they may involve the cortical mantle, we often find trapped neurons with tumor cell satellitosis.

We must be clear that low grade fibrillary astrocytoma is quite different than the WHO Grade I or pilocytic astrocytoma. The nonpilocytic fibrillary astrocytoma is a different breed. It must also be clear that we are not dealing with the oligodendroglioma, which is being increasingly diagnosed in the hope that it will be more sensitive to chemotherapeutic regimens, especially when the 1p/19q gene deletion is detected in the genetics laboratory. Both of these tumors behave biologically different, are morphologically different, and have clearly different survival rates. They have different response rates to currently available chemotherapeutic agents.

Tumor Morphology

Most fibrillary astrocytomas of the brain (at least those that are surgically approachable) occur in lobar locations. Because of their lobar location, they become eligible for direct surgical extirpative approaches, and lead to the concept of "radical" or even "complete" extirpation. Twenty-five years ago, we glimpsed the first CT scans that definitively changed our methods to recognize and ultimately to treat many of these patients. We saw an abnormal, low attenuation, noncontrast enhancing lobar signal abnormality, occasionally confused with a cerebrovascular accident. Most patients reported the recent onset of seizure or a progressive headache syndrome. By the time these patients came to surgery, their interval from development to recognition was already shortened. Once MRI became available, we had various pulse sequences as well as contrast agents to help us sort out the tumor morphology better. We got accurate multiplanar recognition of the tumor. Using long TR weighted images, we thought, could begin to recognize "tumor margins." This logically led us to believe that these tumors looked, smelled, and behaved like lung, liver, or renal tumors. If one did a good and aggressive operation, one could eradicate the tumor.

Our 50 years of neuropathologic studies thereby were discarded in one fell swoop of advanced neurodiagnostic imaging. This aberration was in part led by the charge of the radiologists, who maintained that they could determine the tumor boundaries based on neurodiagnostic imaging. We forgot that these tumors are infiltrative and that while they may have a core mass of uniformly neoplastic tissue, they are usually surrounded by a zone of brain adjacent to tumor which has a residual high volume of neoplastic cells. This region in turn is surrounded by a larger zone of normal brain infiltrated by tumor cells *(Fig. 3.1)*. This is, in fact, the nature of fibrillary astrocytoma, in contrast to pilocytic tumors or oligodendroglial tumors, or neurocytomas, or pleomorphic xanthoastrocytomas, or even the more benign and potentially curable dysembryoplastic neurepithelial tumor. It is the very nature of the tumor biology as well as the tumor morphology that should give responsible surgeons due pause as they begin to extol the virtues of radical resection, especially in critical or functional areas of the brain.

WHAT IS THE CORRECT ROLE OF SURGERY FOR FIBRILLARY ASTROCYTOMA?

Many small series report the extent of surgical excision as a prognostic variable (4–9). However this has not been confirmed in large studies employing more sophisticated multivariate analysis (10). Is surgery never indicated? Certainly not. Despite the earlier recognition of this tumor by imaging in younger patients who present at an earlier stage of disease, we are still left with a group of patients who have large tumors at the time of diagnosis. Those lobar tumors associated with significant clinical signs of mass effect, including focal neurological deficits, decline in cognitive function, or morning headache, display signs of increased intracranial pressure, and localized mass effect. Can we relegate such patients to an observation status or stereotactic

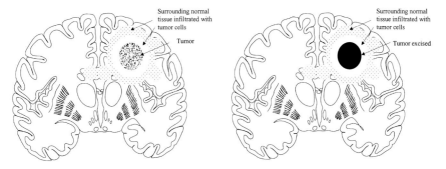

FIG. 3.1 Astrocutoma grade II. Tumor mass as seen on MR imaging (left). Surgical cytoreduction (even 99%) leaves residual tumor in the brain adjacent to tumor (right) and as many as $3–6 \times 10^8$ cells remain.

biopsy for histological diagnosis? In order to benefit from other potential adjuvant strategies as well as in order to actually define the true
histological nature and grade of the neoplasm, we must do cytoreductive surgery. An image-guided craniotomy, perhaps preceded by functional neurosurgical mapping and enhanced during surgery by speech,
language, or sensory mapping, is a necessary management strategy.
Failure to do so usually condemns the patient to rapid progression, diminished quality of life, and relatively poor likelihood of response to the
standard form of fractionated external beam radiation therapy.

It is important, however, to understand the meaning of our best efforts at cytoreductive surgery. *Table 3.1* slightly modifies the principles
of William Shapiro who noted the impact of various treatment strategies in the management of a 30–60 g tumor with 3–6 $\times 10^{10}$ cells at the
time of presentation (11). After 90% resection 3–6 $\times 10^9$ cells remain. After a 99% resection 3–6 $\times 10^8$ remain. These remaining cells are in the
brain adjacent to the tumor mass as well as scattered more widely in the
brain at a greater distance. Conventional fractionated radiation therapy
(55–60 Gy, 1.8 Gy per fraction) has the potential to have a two log kill
reducing the tumor cells to 10^6 or 10^7. It is entirely possible, of course,
that the remaining cells while viable, at least for a period of time are unable to go through further cell division. Apoptosis occurs as the radiation injured neoplastic cells attempt delayed cell division. Other cells
may undergo sufficient genetic repair to begin again the cell division
process. The tumor progresses, or more ominously, devolves to a more
aggressive cell with higher mitotic index and more anaplastic features.

Let us assume that a superb surgeon does craniotomy, enhanced by
multiple technological adjuncts, and achieves a 99.9% tumor removal.
At this point, 3–6 $\times 10^7$ cells remain, reduced to 10^5 if radiation therapy is administered thereafter. Actually, this surgical resection is not
even remotely possible except for the most benign glial tumor variants
such as the pilocytic tumor or DNETs. How many cells must remain before the patient is cured? There is no answer to this question, although

TABLE 3.1
The Effect of Surgery and Radiation on Tumor Volume (Goal = 1 × 10⁵ cells?)

Size of Tumor at Presentation (30–60 g)	Extent of Cytoreduction	Log Kill	Cells Remaining	Cells Remaining after XRT (55–60 Gy)
3–6 $\times 10^{10}$	90%	1	3–6 $\times 10^9$	3–6 + 10^7
3–6 $\times 10^{10}$	99%	2	3–6 $\times 10^8$	3–6 $\times 10^6$
3–6 $\times 10^{10}$	99.90%	3	3–6 $\times 10^7$	3–6 $\times 10^5$

Legend: XRT = Fractionated radiation therapy
Modified from concepts of W. R. Shapiro: **BNI Quarterly** 3:48–52, 1985.

it is possible that with an optimistic view, perhaps the body can recognize these 10^5 residual abnormal tumor cells and annihilate them itself. From the pessimistic view, one could take the stand that the brain did not recognize the first tumor cell when it began to divide, failed to kill it then, and is unlikely to be successful further down the road. In this pessimistic view of the world, not a single tumor cell must remain after surgical successful treatment in order to accomplish the final result, i.e., long-term cure.

The Role of Stereotactic Biopsy

Between 1975 and 1980 with the advent of CT at our institution, the senior author began to see an increasing number of patients with newly diagnosed or suspected glial tumors. These patients had no neurological deficits, but presented with a single seizure or headache. The tumors were often deep in the white matter, often located in areas of critical brain function. In reviewing the literature at that time, the median survival from large series suggested that 7 years (after craniotomy and radiation therapy) was an expected survival (12). It seemed unreasonable to me to condemn patients to an observational status with such poor statistics, and so we embarked on a prospective trial of early diagnosis and early adjuvant management strategy (13, 14). For those patients who presented with mass effect and focal neurological deficits, cytoreductive surgery by craniotomy was performed first. For patients without signs of increased intracranial pressure or focal neurological deficit, and for those with focal deficits with tumors in critical areas of brain function (such as those spanning the Sylvian fissure), we performed stereotactic biopsy *(Fig. 3.2)*. We were gratified that we could define these lesions histologically with a more than 98% probability. We also found a few patients who were suspected of having glial neoplasms, but who instead had infarcts, cerebritis, or vasculitis. Clearly such patients did not warrant craniotomy and cytoreductive surgery; they certainly didn't require adjuvant radiation therapy either.

We placed our stereotactic CT scanner in the operating room in 1982, beginning an 18-year process of evaluating the role of intraoperative imaging in neurosurgical patients (15). Several thousand stereotactic biopsies were performed during this interval for a wide variety of indications, both diagnostic and therapeutic. We developed this CT imaging suite in order to combine the neurodiagnostic imaging and surgical sites, to facilitate minimally invasive surgery, to allow rapid recognition of potential complications, and hopefully to allow us to do better cytoreductive surgery in carefully selected cases.

Stereotactic biopsy was safe (less than 0.3% risk of morbidity, largely related to the rare development of symptomatic postoperative hemor-

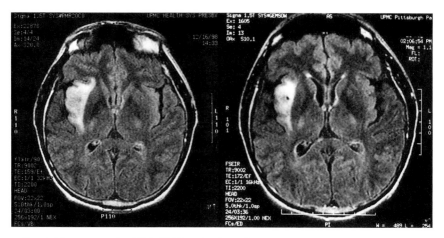

FIG. 3.2 Intraoperative Flair MRI at the time of stereotactic biopsy (left) and two years after fractionated radiation therapy (right). The tumor volume is smaller (right).

rhage requiring craniotomy), effective (a 98% neurodiagnostic rate for glial neoplasms), and facilitated appropriate grading of glial tumors. After a number of years, we noted that both CT and MRI frequently were insufficient tests to be able to accurately grade a glial neoplasm (16). A noncontrast enhancing expansile suspected neoplasm in the brain is not always a fibrillary astrocytoma. Some are not tumors at all. Often these imaging abnormalities proved to be anaplastic glial tumors, for which a much more aggressive treatment strategy was warranted in view of the significantly worse prognosis. We began a prospective biopsy study in 1982, and in 1995 published our long-term assessment of results. For this group of patients with fibrillary astrocytoma, the median survival in a nonrandomized study was 12.3 years after symptom onset and 9.8 years after stereotactic biopsy (13, 14). From a historical standpoint, this statistic alone was significantly better than most studies previously reported. What could not be discerned from this study was the impact of earlier diagnosis. In other words, was this increase in median survival artificial because we elected to perform early biopsy when patients still had minimal signs or symptoms? Most previous studies reported the results of craniotomies on patients with advanced signs and symptoms (17).

The Addition of Technology

Image-guided stereotactic techniques revolutionized our ability to accurately diagnose these tumors earlier and eliminated the misgivings of our neurology colleagues, who recalled mortality rates as high as 30%

by free hand biopsy technique in suspected glioma patients. Mortality is virtually nonexistent in current studies based on using CT or MRI guidance. We use stereotactic techniques for many reasons: (1) precise pre-plotting of probe trajectories; (2) accurate sampling of the abnormal areas at multiple sites; (3) avoidance of pial ependymal structures in which blood vessels reside; (4)avoidance of trajectories through such vascular beds such as the Sylvian fissure; (5) early recognition of potential complications by immediate postoperative neuroimaging; and (6) rigid probe fixation. These techniques in the early years eliminated the apprehension toward stereotactic surgery: two frightened people separated by a needle.

When we began intraoperative stereotactic imaging during craniotomy, we were faced by a number of hurdles: (1) the need to reverse the scanner within the operating room to allow full access to the head, both to the surgeon and to the anesthesiologist; (2) the need to turn the patient's head for optimal position for craniotomy; (3) the need to maintain sterility during repeated imaging during the procedure itself; (4) and the hurdles faced by the crude but anatomically accurate imaging depiction provided by CT. For example, we found out rather early that with the bone flap off, the intraoperative imaging algorithm for CT reconstruction failed to recognize that the bone was removed. This led to a faint white glow in the collapsed cortical tissue at the site of the tumor resection. This could be mistaken for contrast enhancement, but also obscured the potential value of estimating the maximal resection. Faced with the continuing goal of the ever increasing need for higher quality neurodiagnostic imaging, we switched to using MRI biopsy techniques in the mid-1980s for selected cases. This provided us with multiplanar recognition of the tumors and enhanced our trajectory planning. By then, our enthusiasm for intraoperative CT as a guidance technique had waned, because MRI in the same group of patients always showed residual, abnormal signal which was compatible with residual neoplasm. As imaging improved, so did localization techniques and computer programs, and frameless stereotactic intervention was born. Like many other neurosurgeons in academic medical centers, we pursued these techniques with the zeal of any "technogroupie." We evaluated the ISG wand®, Sofmor-Danek Stealth System®, the Brain-Lab Vector Vision®, and eventually the Elekta Robotic Surgical Microscope (Surgiscope®).

The Benefits of Technology Utilization

We were never impressed with the neurodiagnostic resolution of intraoperative ultrasound. We abandoned it because localization of a target required a large craniotomy followed by wheeling in a cumbersome imaging tool with poor resolution. Treatment was always much easier using stereotactic localization techniques, even if it meant following a probe down to the target before cytoreductive surgery. The image-guided frameless stereotactic system revolutionized our approach, allowing us to perform small trephine craniotomies and maximizing our ability to do cytoreductive surgery. We continued our tradition, however, of applying such technologies to those patients who presented with symptomatic mass effect or patients with tumors in lobar locations where the risk of such surgery was limited. We never embraced with enthusiasm the concept of aggressive cytoreductive surgery in areas of the motor strip, the primary sensory cortex, or speech areas. Instead we evaluated the possible usage of radiosurgery as an alternative *(Figs. 3.3, 3.4)*. The addition of image guidance has provided increased safety, eliminated "the hunt for red October," and returned the ultrasound instrument to the Radiology Department where it belongs. Frameless stereotaxy reduced hospital costs, reduced hospital stays (which now

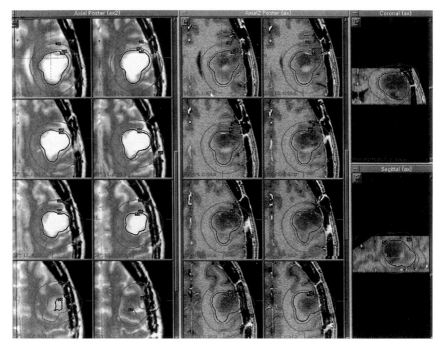

FIG. 3.3: Stereotactic radiosurgery dose plan for biopsy proved grade II fibrillary astrocytoma. Short TR with contrast and long TR images were used for the conformal radiation delivery (15 Gy at 50% isodose).

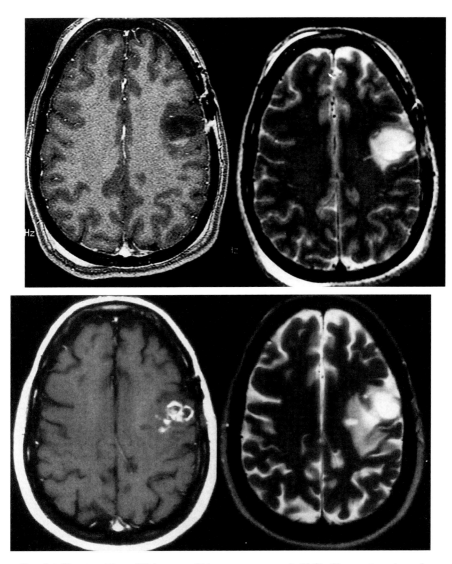

FIG. 3.4 Short and long TR images of biopsy proven grade II fibrillary astrocytoma in the dominant hemisphere (upper). Two years after radiosurgery the tumor volume is stable but contrast enhancement is evident (lower).

average 3.1 for craniotomy for this condition), and reduced postoperative morbidity. We usually perform such operations through a linear incision with a trephine craniotomy accurately located based on intraoperative imaging. All of the technologies (except Surgiscope® which proved to be technologically overpowering) were useful, dependable, and reliable. A dedicated team of neuroimaging personnel with computer skills was needed.

The beauty of these systems is that the surgeon could order the localization technique, have it performed by others, have the data show up in the operating room with the patient, digitize the data of entry points from the patient's head using fiducial or patient landmarks, and be "ready to roll" with no more than an 8 to 10 minutes of additional O.R. time. This additional set up time of 8 to 10 minutes dramatically reduced the average operative time by probably more than an hour. Using a linear incision and trephine craniotomy, the time from scalp incision to tumor debulking can be as little as 20 minutes, the tumor debulking accomplished in another 30 minutes, and the closure completed in 30 minutes. There can be no question as to the benefits of this enhanced technology in terms of patient outcomes and the elimination of morbidity. We have marveled at the success of a number of centers that use sophisticated intraoperative awake craniotomies with speech guidance for removal of such tumors. We await with interest the long-term results of such patients (at 10 to 20 years) to see whether this approach enhances survival. While we continue to use intraoperative stereotactic CT in the resection of some tumors and stereotactic guidance during resection of some skull base tumors, we believe that the overwhelming problems of tumor biology and tumor morphology have not conspired to make image guided craniotomy alone a likely successful venture. We further suspect that the role of intraoperative MRI will prove to be the same, but time will tell. Whether the benefit of a more aggressive resection (90%? 99%? 99.9%?) will enhance long-term survival, especially if no other adjuvant treatments are administered, will require a great deal of experience.

What Do the Current Outcome Studies Show?

To date, there has been little substantive evidence to support aggressive cytoreductive surgery in the glial neoplasms. Several studies in the past have shown that the extent of surgery did not significantly influence survival (12, 18). McCormack et al. retrospectively reviewed 53 cases of adult supratentorial astrocytomas. The median survival was 7 1/4 years with a 5-year survival of 64% (12). Multivariate regression analysis demonstrated that the most important prognosticators for improved survival were young age, absence of contrast enhancement of the original tumor on computed tomography (CT), and the performance status of the patient. Recently Iwabuchi et al. retrospectively evaluated prognostic factors and their effect on survival in 56 adult patients with supratentorial low grade astrocytomas treated between 1967 and 1993 (18a). The median patient age in their study was 42 years and the median survival was 5.0 years. These authors evaluated 15 factors with uni- and multivariate analysis to investigate their importance in predicting the length of survival. Although age group, preoperative Karnofsky scale, and extent of surgery were associated with improved patient survival by univariate analysis, only age group and Karnofsky scale were significant by multivariate analysis. In another recent study Bauman et al. pooled 401 cases of histologically confirmed supratentorial fibrillary astrocytomas (WHO Grade II) from three institutions and analyzed several pretreatment factors (age at diagnosis, gender, seizures at presentation, presence of enhancement on CT or MRI, Karnofsky Performance Status (KPS) at diagnosis, histology, extent of surgical resection, timing of radiotherapy, and treating institution). Median survival for the entire group was 95 months/7.9 years (10). On univariate analysis, ages 18 to40, presence of seizures at presentation, KPS > or = 70, treating institution, and absence of contrast enhancement were associated with improved overall survival. On multivariate analysis, these factors remained independent predictors of improved overall survival. Using recursive partitioning analysis they found that age, KPS, and contrast enhancement on CT/MRI defined distinct prognostic subgroups in a pooled database of patients with fibrillary astrocytoma. Extent of surgery was not a significant predictor for overall survival within this analysis (10).

Most studies show median survivals ranging from 5 to 12.7 years, depending upon the year of publication, the type of patient in the study, and the influence of early versus late surgery (12, 14). These studies are all Phase I or at most Phase II studies, are usually single institution, and are longitudinal in nature. None of these features, however, should lead us to dismiss the relevance of such studies. For example, two recent reports have cast the first glimmer of doubt on the overall value of performing Phase III multi-institution randomized prospective double blinded studies for most of the clinical conditions that are relevant (19, 20). These reports indicate that relatively few studies have actually shown a different outcome than those studies predicted by earlier generation Phase I or II studies. This heretical assessment should give us pause as we embark upon the possibility of future studies under the aegis of our professional societies. For example, the American College of Surgeons Oncology Group (ACOSOG) has advocated the development of a multicenter trial for assessment of the role of cytoreductive surgery versus observation (Z0330). To some surgical oncologists, this relegation to observational status has serious ethical concerns. The recommendation for such a study suggests that we seriously question whether doing anything improves upon the natural history of this disorder. Such a study has got many ambiguities about it, and would require an enor-

mous number of patients even to detect a 20% increase in survival
(Table 3.2). Patients would need to be properly stratified because of the
variables that clearly affect outcomes regardless of treatment modality:
volume, location, presence or absence of neurological symptoms or signs,
presence of increased intracranial pressure, relationship to critical
structures that influence our ability to do cytoreductive surgery, the importance of adjuvant treatment strategies such as radiation therapy, the
need for multimodality treatment in many patients serially over the
course of time, the possibility of missed diagnosis to begin with (unless
all patients are biopsied), the variability in tumor morphology and biology (proliferation indices and chromosome deletions, etc.).

The Need for Additional Management

Previously published studies have clearly defined the benefit of fractionated external beam radiation therapy as an adjuvant in the management of patients who underwent either biopsy or cytoreductive
surgery for their fibrillary astrocytoma (17, 21–31). Median survivals
are extended significantly in published studies, and we have seen a
number of patients with a dramatic imaging response to radiation therapy. The dosage and fractionation scheme as well as tumor volume to
be treated have been much more carefully worked out over the last 10
to 15 years, again dramatically supplemented by the availability of enhanced neurodiagnostic imaging. Radiation therapy is administered in
a coned down version treating the T_2 signal abnormality plus a margin
of 2 cm. The dose per fraction should be 1.8 Gy in a total dose of ap-

TABLE 3.2
Hypothetical Fibrillary Astrocytoma Study to Detect a 20% Increased
Survival Time After Image-Guided Resection

Median Survival of Historical Controls*	Follow-Up Duration Needed	Image-Guided Resection, No. of Patients Needed
7.5 years	7.5 years	587
	10 years	484
	12 years	434
	15 years	385
10.5 years	10.5 years	587
	14 years	484
	16.8 years	434
	21 years	385

*Assumptions
The no. of historical control is very large compared to image guided resection group, level
of 0.05 log-rank test with 90% power used, survival fraction is exponential (Courtesy:
Douglas Potter, MS, Ph.D.)

proximately 55 to 59 Gy to provide the therapeutic benefit desired including the tumor margin, the brain adjacent to the tumor, and the larger infiltrated area of tumor and normal brain. The latter area, of course, cannot be seen on the current imaging studies. The potential of a two log cell kill effect of radiation therapy has the benefit of a direct cell mitosis inhibition, and may secondarily reduce the chances of cell division in those cells which have received sublethal radiation effect. Some will have delayed cellular apoptosis. It is likely that the reason for ultimate failure of radiation therapy lies in the development of resistance or repair of sublethal injury by cell mechanisms that develop or are augmented after exposure to radiation. Nonetheless, it seems likely that the two log kill provided by radiation on top of a single log surgical kill (achieved by a 90% surgical resection) may provide a significant benefit and at least delay the number of cells which may ultimately undergo malignant transformation. The evidence for this hypothesis as yet eludes us. In selected cases stereotactic radiosurgery may be an option *(see Fig. 3.4)*.

Is There a Price to Pay with Radiation Therapy?

Almost certainly, for patients who have long-term survival to fractionated brain radiation therapy develop an increasingly more distressful syndrome of cognitive deterioration affecting memory at first and progressing to a more severe cognitive disorder (32, 33). Coned down irradiation, which significantly restricts the volume of brain irradiated based on current treatment planning techniques (as opposed to the older studies which used AP and lateral ports), will likely improve the outcomes. Very little is known about the long-term price that glioma patients pay in order to reach a 10- to 12- to 15-year survival. Prospective neuropsychological studies need to be performed, and their importance needs to be emphasized in the overall work-up of such patients well in advance of either their surgery or their subsequent radiation therapy. We cannot condone withholding radiation therapy in patients who have had biopsies or incomplete resection of their tumors. We realize that even guidelines for management of this tumor, 125 years later, are still ephemeral.

CONCLUSIONS

The controversy over the rationale, role, extent, and outcomes of radical resection versus stereotactic diagnosis of grade II fibrillary astrocytomas remains. Neurosurgeons love to perform surgery. We would like to believe that a surgical extirpation is a rational and achievable goal. In order to continue to strive for this goal, we are sometimes willing to suspend our understanding of the tumor biology and morphology of fibrillary astrocytoma. The argument for cytoreductive surgery in patients with mass effect is cogent. It is far less compelling in patients with multilobar tumors or in patients with tumors located in areas of critical brain function. Cytoreductive surgery is necessary in some, benefits some, unnecessary in many, hurts a few, helps a few, but it is never enough. We need innovative investigators who will master new imaging techniques and translate emerging molecular biology knowledge into effective therapies.

There are a number of exciting molecular-based conceptual therapies under evaluation. In the year 2000 grants funded by the American Brain Tumor Association included gene vector trials, tumor sensitizer trials, chemosensitivity enhancing agents, and tumor vaccine agents. The clarification of natural history with cytological and molecular biological analysis will eventually establish the optimum management strategy for fibrillary astrocytomas (34–39).

Real advances in the outcome management for fibrillary astrocytoma are likely over the next 10 to 20 years. Providing that funding remains strong, a meaningful management strategy or even cure lies over the horizon. Over the next 20 years, we will forget or forego the argument about cytoreducive surgery versus biopsy. The future generation of neurosurgeons and neuro-oncologists will laugh at our adoption of rigid postures about the role of surgery for fibrillary astrocytomas. They will probably come to realize that in some patients you need it and in some patients you don't. They will understand that whether you need it or you don't, some other potent management strategy (yet to be discovered) is the real answer. We should concentrate our attention on the search for this strategy.

REFERENCES

1. Afra, D, Osztie E: Histologically confirmed changes on CT of reoperated low-grade astrocytomas. **Neuroradiology** 39:804–810, 1997.
2. Afra D, Osztie E, Sipos L, Vitanovics D: Preoperative history and postoperative survival of supratentorial low-grade astrocytomas. **Br J Neurosurg** 13:299–305, 1999.
3. Dropcho EJ, Soong SJ: The prognostic impact of prior low grade histology in patients with anaplastic gliomas: A case-control study. **Neurology** 47: 684–690, 1996.
4. Hirano H, Asakura T, Yokoyama S: The prognostic factors in astrocytic tumors: Analysis by the Kaplan- Meier method and the Weibull log-linear model. **No Shinkei Geka** 24: 809–815, 1996.
5. Janny P, Cure H, Mohr M: Low grade supratentorial astrocytomas. Management and prognostic factors. **Cancer** 73: 1937–1945, 1994.
6. Laws ER Jr, Taylor WF, Bergstralh EJ, Okazaki H, Clifton MB: Neurosurgical management of low-grade astrocytoma of the cerebral hemispheres. **J Neurosurg** 61: 665–673, 1984.

7. Matsumoto K, Abe T, Terada K, et al.: Clinical results of supratentorial astrocytoma grade II. **No Shinkei Geka—Neurological Surgery** 27:139–145, 1999.
8. Peraud A, Ansari H, Bise K, Reulen HJ: Clinical outcome of supratentorial astrocytoma WHO grade II. **Acta Neurochirurgica** 140:1213–1222. 1998.
9. Berger MS, Deliganis AV, Dobbins J, Keles GE: The effect of extent of resection on recurrence in patients with low grade cerebral hemisphere gliomas. **Cancer** 74: 1784–1791, 1994.
10. Bauman G, Lote K, Larson D, et al.: Pretreatment factors predict overall survival for patients with low-grade glioma: A recursive partitioning analysis. **Int J Radiat Oncol Biol Phy** 45:923–929, 1999.
11. Shapiro WR: Multimodality therapy of malignant glioma. **BNI Quarterly** 3:48–52, 1985.
12. McCormack BM, Miller DC, Budzilovich GN, Voorhees GJ, Ransohoff J: Treatment and survival of low-grade astrocytoma in adults-1977–1988. **Neurosurgery** 31: 636–642, 1992.
13. Lunsford LD, Somaza S, Kondziolka D, Flickinger JC: Brain astrocytomas: Biopsy, then irradiation. **Clin Neurosurg** 42:464–479, 1995.
14. Lunsford LD, Somaza S, Kondziolka D, Flickinger JC: Survival after stereotactic biopsy and irradiation of cerebral nonanaplastic, nonpilocytic astrocytoma. **J Neurosurg** 82:523–529, 1995.
15. Lunsford LD, Kondziolka D, Bissonette DJ: Intraoperative imaging of the brain. **Stereo Funct Neurosurg** 66:58–64, 1996.
16. Kondziolka D, Lunsford LD, Martinez AJ: Unreliability of contemporary neurodiagnostic imaging in evaluating suspected adult supratentorail (low-grade) astrocytoma. **J Neurosurg** 79:533–536, 1993.
17. Shaw EG: The low-grade glioma debate: Evidence defending the position of early radiation therapy. **Clin Neurosurg** 42:488–494. 1995.
18. Boyages J, Tiver KW: Cerebral hemisphere astrocytoma: Treatment results. **Radiother Oncol** 8: 209–216, 1987.
18a. Iwabuchi S, Bishara S, Herbison P, Erasmus A, Samejima H: Prognostic factors for supratentorial low grade astrocytomas in adults. **Neurologia Medico-Chirurgica** 39:273–281, 1999.
19. Benson K, Hartz AJ: A comparison of observational and randomized controlled trials. **N Engl J Med** 342;1878–1886, 2000.
20. Concato J, Shah N, Horwitz R: Randomized, controlled trials, and observational studies, and the hierarchy of research designs. **N Engl J Med** 342:1887–1892, 2000.
21. Akyol FH, Atahan IL, Zorlu F, Gurkaynak M, Alanyali H, Ozyar E: Results of postoperative or exclusive radiotherapy in grade I and grade II cerebellar astrocytoma patients. **Radiother Oncol** 23: 245–248, 1992.
22. Bauman G, Pahapill P, Macdonald D, Fisher B, Leighton C, Cairncross G: Low grade glioma: Measuring radiographic response to radiotherapy. **Can J Neurol Sci** 26: 18–22, 1999.
23. Chassard JL, Dutou L, Gerard JP, Papillon J: Postoperative radiotherapy of hemispheric glioma in the adult. A propos of 134 cases. **Neuro-Chirurgie** 21:377–389, 1975.
24. Grabenbauer GG, Roedel, CM, Paulus W, et al: Supratentorial low-grade glioma: Results and prognostic factors following postoperative radiotherapy. **Strahlenther Onkol** 176: 259–264, 2000.
25. Landy HJ, Schwade JG, Houdek PV, Markoe AM, Feun L: Long-term follow-up of gliomas treated with fractionated stereotactic irradiation. **Acta Neurochir Suppl** 62: 67–71, 1994.

26. Leibel SA, Sheline GE, Wara WM, Boldrey EB, Nielsen SL: The role of radiation therapy in the treatment of astrocytomas. **Cancer** 35:1551–1557. 1975.

27. Nakamura M, Konishi N, Tsunoda S, et al.: Analysis of prognostic and survival factors related to treatment of low-grade astrocytomas in adults. **Oncology** 58:108–116, 2000.

28. Salazar OM, Rubin P, McDonald JV, Feldstein ML: Patterns of failure in intracranial astrocytomas after irradiation: analysis of dose and field factors. **Am J Roentgenol** 126: 279–292, 1976.

29. Scanlon PW, Taylor WF: Radiotherapy of intracranial astrocytomas: Analysis of 417 cases treated from 1960 through 1969. **Neurosurgery** 5:301–308. 1979

30. Shibamoto Y, Kitakabu Y, Takahashi M, et al.: Supratentorial low-grade astrocytoma. Correlation of computed tomography findings with effect of radiation therapy and prognostic variables. **Cancer** 72:190–195, 1993.

31. Trautmann TG, Shaw EG: Supratentorial low-grade glioma: Is there a role for radiation therapy? **Ann Acad Med Singapore** 25: 392–396. 1996.

32. Mulhern RK, Ochs J, Kun LE: Changes in intellect associated with cranial radiation therapy, in Gutin PH, Leibel SA, Sheline GE, (eds): *Radiation Injury to the Nervous System*. New York, Raven Press,1991, pp325–340.

33. Taphoorn MJ, Schiphorst AK, Snoek FJ, et al.: Cognitive functions and quality of life in patients with low-grade gliomas: The impact of radiotherapy. **Ann Neurol** 36.48–54, 1994.

34. Coons SW, Davis JR, Way DL: Correlation of DNA content and histology in prognosis of astrocytomas. **Am J Clin Path** 90:289–293, 1998.

35. Ellison DW, Steart PV, Bateman AC, Pickering RM, Palmer JD, Weller RO: Prognostic indicators in a range of astrocytic tumours: An immunohistochemical study with Ki-67 and p53 antibodies. **J Neurol Neurosurg Psychiat** 59:413–419, 1995.

36. Iuzzolino P, Ghimenton C, Nicolato A, et al.: p53 protein in low-grade astrocytomas: a study with long-term follow-up. **Br J Cancer** 69:586–591, 1994.

37. McKeever PE, Strawderman MS, Yamini B, Mikhail AA, Blaivas M: MIB-1 proliferation index predicts survival among patients with grade II astrocytoma. **J Neuropath Exp Neurol** 57:931–936, 1998.

38. Raghavan R, Steart PV, Weller RO: Cell proliferation patterns in the diagnosis of astrocytomas, anaplastic astrocytomas and glioblastoma multiforme: A Ki-67 study. **Neuropath Appl Neurobiol** 16:123–133, 1990.

39. Schiffer D, Cavalla P, Chio A, Richiardi P, Giordana MT: Proliferative activity and prognosis of low-grade astrocytomas. **J Neuro-Oncol** 34:31–35. 1997.

4

SURGICAL MANAGEMENT OF INTRACRANIAL GLIOMAS—BIOPSY, RESECTION, OR WATCHFUL WAITING

EDWARD R. LAWS, M.D., AND MARK E. SHAFFREY, M.D.

Brain tumors continue to represent one of the most dramatic forms of human illness. Gliomas can quickly alter an individual's intellectual capabilities and abilities to function independently. However, this is not the case in all instances. The diagnosis of "glioma" describes a heterogeneous group of neoplasms that can vary widely in their prognosis. There is not one clear pathway or approach that will encompass the treatment of all types of gliomas. When considering the options for surgical management of gliomas of the brain, there are a number of issues that must be carefully assessed and balanced before a final recommendation is in order.

BIOLOGICAL ASPECTS OF GLIOMAS

First of all, one must consider the likelihood that the lesion the surgeon is dealing with is benign or malignant. The biology of malignant gliomas is such that at present very little in the way of significant benefit can be achieved by adjunctive therapies beyond the traditional treatment of surgical removal followed by conventional radiation therapy. Anaplastic oligodendrogliomas remain one of the few malignant gliomas for which survival may be significantly extended with combination chemotherapy. For benign gliomas the situation is entirely different. A significant proportion of benign gliomas are either curable or associated with excellent long-term outcomes depending upon capacity for growth, infiltration, and genomic instability. Reflecting the inherent biology of gliomas is a classification system that illustrates a continuum from low-grade to high-grade lesions, with low-grade tumors having a significantly more favorable prognosis, and in some cases a better response to therapy.

ANATOMICAL AND NEUROIMAGING FEATURES OF GLIOMAS

The basis for preoperative evaluation of many gliomas of the brain is the neuroimaging. The details identified by high resolution MRI scanning with the use of intravenous contrast agents provide a superb assessment of the anatomic, and to some extent the pathologic, features of the lesion. These include whether the tumor is circumscribed in nature or diffuse, whether it is localized to one area of the brain or is multifocal, or whether it is primarily solid, infiltrative, or cystic. Enhancement with intravenous contrast agents provides some indication regarding the metabolic activity of the tumor and its effect on the blood-brain barrier, with nonenhancing tumors tending to be much more benign than tumors that have either diffuse or focal enhancement. One must be mindful, however, that gadolinium enhancement is only a surrogate indicator for both biologic activity and invasion. A small but concerning proportion of malignant gliomas may not show contrast enhancement. Despite the fact that many malignant gliomas have clearly enhancing borders on MRI, biopsy distal to the margins of tumor enhancement usually reveals infiltrating tumor cells (3).

Another factor important for surgical management is tumor vascularity (relatively avascular or hypervascular). Occasionally one can make these determinations on the basis of MR imaging, but often an angiogram can assist in the demonstration of tumor vessels. Angiograms of patients with low-grade astrocytomas may be interpreted as normal in approximately 50% of cases, but abnormalities are present in over 90% of anaplastic astrocytomas and glioblastomas(9).

From the standpoint of surgical approach, whether a lesion is superficial or deep makes a profound difference, as does the location of the lesion in either eloquent or noneloquent areas of the brain. Cortical mapping of patients with superficial gliomas has led to the understanding that infiltrative lesions may contain functional neural tissue within the substance of the tumor(7). The abnormal appearance of brain tissue is not always the most reliable guide for resection without new postoperative deficits(6).

Patient Condition

Because of the enormous impact of age on the outcome of patients with gliomas of the brain, the age of the patient makes a significant difference in therapeutic decisions, for it is known that young patients respond in a much more favorable fashion than older ones. The patient's preoperative functional status, usually measured by the Karnofsky Performance Score, and the duration of symptoms have also been directly correlated to survival for patients with malignant gliomas.

The aforementioned factors are summarized in *Table 4.1.*

TABLE 4.1
Biological and Morphological Aspects of Gliomas

Benign vs. malignant
Low grade vs. high grade
Superficial vs. deep
Circumscribed vs. diffuse
Localized vs. multifocal
Noneloquent vs. eloquent
Cystic vs. solid vs. infiltrative
Nonenhancing vs. enhancing
Homogeneous enhancement vs. nodular enhancement
Edema and mass effect vs. lack of brain reaction
Avascular vs. hypervascular
Young patient vs. old patient
Healthy patient vs. debilitated patient

ARGUMENTS AGAINST RESECTION

Although resection of gliomas has been the standard for neurosurgical management, there are powerful arguments that lead to a conclusion that resection alone may have very little impact on the outcome of patients with gliomas, particularly those with malignant gliomas. It is evident that the vast majority of malignant gliomas and a significant proportion of the "benign" gliomas are basically infiltrative in nature. Even tumors that appear to be circumscribed and very focal may have infiltrative tumor cells around the border, and these tumor cells may extend as far as 4 or 5 cm from the epicenter of the lesion(3, 8). It had been demonstrated as early as the 1930s that even a hemispherectomy on the side of a malignant glioma would not result in a cure in most cases. At autopsy, a substantial proportion of patients with malignant gliomas have tumor cells present in both hemispheres. Elegant whole mount sections of the brain and brain tumors and careful autopsies of patients who died as a result of cerebral gliomas confirm this concept, and show the basic infiltrative nature of most of these lesions(5).

One could contend that in all but a minor number of glioma patients a curative resection is not possible, and that residual tumor will continue to be a problem and will eventually result in the death of the patient. Resective surgery can now be accomplished with relatively low rates of morbidity and mortality, and its accuracy can be significantly enhanced by computer guided methods of resection and functional mapping. Despite this, radical resection of gliomas of the brain may still result in a decline in functional status, which can occur in as many as 12% of carefully examined postoperative patients (1). Clearly, there is a category of tumors that infiltrate vital structures of the brain such as the medulla, pons, midbrain, and hypothalamus where resective surgery is not a valid option. A few studies have suggested the possibility that surgical intervention may destabilize a benign tumor and accelerate its transformation to a malignant lesion.

These arguments are summarized in *Table 4.2*.

ARGUMENTS FOR RADICAL RESECTION

There are many powerful arguments in favor of attempting a radical resection of all gliomas of the brain, including both the "malignant" and "benign" varieties. A basic principle of oncology is one of reducing the tumor burden. This becomes particularly important in the brain, especially when patients are suffering from mass effects related to the tumor, either from the tumor directly or from its effect on surrounding brain in the form of edema and shift of intracranial structures (2, 4). It is clear that patients with increased intracranial pressure from brain tumors and those with progressing disabling neurological deficits can have their clinical symptomatology significantly improved by resection of the underlying glioma. There is a theoretical argument that cytoreduction will allow the body's inherent defenses to deal with smaller numbers of tumor cells that may be left behind. Furthermore, cytoreduction may, by chance, remove cells that are more likely to undergo malignant degeneration or are resistant to adjuvant therapies. A further argument in favor of radical resection is the fact that practically every retrospective study of surgical management of gliomas has shown a survival advantage to those patients who undergo radical resection. Unfortunately, virtually all of these retrospective studies are flawed by significant selection bias wherein the multifocal tumors and those in older patients are less likely to be treated with radical surgery than are the well circumscribed noneloquent superficial cystic tumors in younger individuals. We have yet to see a truly effective prospective study that would be necessary to clarify the controversy with regard to extent of resection.

Another argument in favor of resection, particularly for low-grade gliomas, is the fact that some gliomas can be cured by surgical removal

TABLE 4.2
Arguments Against Resection

Infiltrative nature of most gliomas
Multifocal gliomas—field effect
Potential deficits and complications related to surgery
Tumors may involve eloquent areas of brain
Intervention may provoke progression

alone. These unusual lesions share some characteristics with the more typical and more difficult gliomas of the brain that characteristically recur.

A great advantage of surgical resection is the ability to obtain significant amounts of tissue. This may eliminate a major degree of the sampling error that can occur with stereotactic biopsies. Surgical resection also provides tissue that can be utilized for studies to guide adjunctive therapy and for material that may be utilized for making vaccines and producing natural killer cells and other forms of immunologicallybased adjunctive therapy.

Many patients who present with seizures, particularly those with lower grade gliomas, may have the seizure disorder significantly benefited by resection of the lesion. Resection of the tumor alone may result in postoperative reduction of the patient's seizures but the use of electrocorticography to define extratumoral epileptic foci may further improve postoperative control.

Finally, for low-grade gliomas, the effect of radiation therapy has not been proven and is marginal at best. Thus, in these cases, surgical resection may be the most effective treatment currently available.

Table 4.3 summarizes the arguments in favor of radical resection.

WHEN TO BIOPSY

The following are some general guidelines as to when biopsy is a logical form of management of an intracranial glioma (see *Table 4.4*).

1. To establish a diagnosis when the diagnosis is in doubt. Although imaging studies are highly accurate and most helpful in suggesting a presumptive diagnosis, there is really no substitute for having histology available.
2. To establish a diagnosis that will support or guide therapy. The utilization of adjunctive therapy (or clinical trials) often is quite dependent upon the details of the histology of the lesion being treated.

TABLE 4.3
Arguments for Radical Resection

Decrease the tumor burden—cytoreduction
Reverse neurological deficits
Relieve increased intracranial pressure
Eliminate seizures
Reduce sampling error
Obtain tissue for study and therapy (vaccines, etc.)
Some gliomas are curable by surgery alone
Uncertain/limited effect of radiation therapy on low-grade gliomas

TABLE 4.4
When to Biopsy

To establish a diagnosis when diagnosis is in doubt
To establish a diagnosis that will support or guide therapy
To confirm a presumptive diagnosis for prognosis
To detect molecular features of the tumor
To empty an associated cyst

Obtaining a representative histologic sample is often the only way to do this with accuracy and, therefore, biopsy becomes a highly important aspect of the overall management and decision making.

3. To confirm a presumptive diagnosis for purposes of prognosis. Even though one can assume that a given patient has either a malignant or relatively benign glioma based on the clinical presentation and the imaging studies, many patients will require an assessment that is accurate enough to allow for a prognosis —something that may be important to the patient and his or her family.
4. To empty an associated cystic component of the lesion.
5. To detect and analyze molecular features of the tumor. Progress in our understanding of the biology and management of gliomas of the brain depends upon careful assessment of the molecular biology of the lesion. Essential data regarding the genetic and molecular features of these tumors can only be obtained by the study of tissue obtained from a living patient.

There are a number of specific situations where this neurosurgeon would recommend biopsy only, and these include:

I. Diffuse glioma such as is seen in gliomatosis cerebri.
II. A presumed malignant glioma in a vital or eloquent area of the brain where resection would cause unacceptable neurological consequences.
III. A presumed low-grade glioma located directly in vital or eloquent areas of the brain.
IV. An asymptomatic diffuse nonenhancing glioma that presents with a seizure disorder and no evidence of increased intracranial pressure or shift of intracranial structures. This is a controversial area, but particularly in younger patients, one may argue that it is perfectly reasonable to follow such a patient without planning adjunctive therapy with and without biopsy. For many patients, however, secure knowledge of the nature of the tumor will be desirable.

V. Some ring-enhancing lesions, for example when the differential diagnosis might include metastasis, brain abscess, or a focal area of demyelinating or inflammatory disease.
VI. Some multifocal lesions, particularly if the differential diagnosis includes cerebral lymphoma.
VII. Some hypointense infiltrative lesions of the brain where the diagnosis may not be secure and where the differential diagnosis might include problems such as PML.
VIII. When adjunctive therapy is clearly dependent upon a tissue diagnosis. This will be true for virtually any patient who is being considered for radiation therapy and most patients who are being considered for adjunctive chemotherapy or immunotherapy.

WHEN TO RESECT

There are some reasonably clear indications for radical resection of presumed gliomas of the brain, and they include the following (see *Table 4.5*).

1. When mass effect produces progressive symptoms or impairs the quality of life.
2. When the glioma may be a variety that is surgically curable.
3. To reduce tumor burden by radical resection thereby enhancing the efficacy of adjunctive therapy.
4. To obtain tissue for the production of a vaccine, cytotoxic lymphocytes, natural killer cells, or specific immunologically based adjunctive therapy.

We are prepared to recommend radical resection in the following circumstances.

I. Well-circumscribed lesions that are surgically accessible whether they are presumed to be either high-grade or low-grade gliomas.
II. Suspected pilocytic astrocytomas and other curable gliomas (PXA, DNET, SEGA, central neurocytoma, etc.).
III. Ring enhancing and cystic gliomas when the location permits radical resection.

TABLE 4.5
When to Resect

When mass effect produces symptoms or impairs quality of life
When the glioma may be curable
To reduce tumor burden, enhancing adjunctive therapy
To obtain tissue for production of vaccine, CTL, NK cells, etc.

IV. When adjunctive therapy depends upon a decrease in the tumor burden.

WHEN TO RECOMMEND WATCHFUL WAITING

The initial symptoms of cerebral glioma often occur in otherwise healthy vigorous and productive individuals. Some will wish to move rapidly to a complete diagnostic evaluation and an aggressive treatment plan; others will wish to control symptoms and to maintain an excellent quality of life and continued productivity. Until more secure knowledge is acquired and more truly effective treatment strategies are developed, these desires on the part of the patient should be respected.

The young patient with a homogeneously hypointense infiltrative lesion, without mass effect or increased intracranial pressure can safely be followed. Noninvasive studies such as 2-deoxy-glucose PET can help confirm hypometabolism is a low-grade glioma, and serial PET studies can be used as a guide for the timing of subsequent therapeutic interventions.

There are few studies that argue against a strategy of watchful delay even in potentially resectable, curable gliomas when symptoms and signs are minor in nature and not progressive.

General guidelines and specific recommendations for watchful waiting include the following.

1. Young, otherwise healthy patient with minimal symptoms, no mass effect, no increased intracranial pressure, and a homogeneous infiltrative hypointense cerebral lesion.
2. An asymptomatic or well-controlled similar patient with evidence from imaging studies of a static benign glioma such as a presumed DNET, PXA, ganglioglioma, hamartoma, chiasmal or pilocytic astrocytoma.
3. An older patient, clinically stable, without significant deficit or increased intracranial pressure, with a static lesion on serial imaging studies.

CONCLUSION

These basic principles are excellent guidelines for the management of difficult clinical problems associated with gliomas of the brain *(Table 4.6)*. Each patient must be considered individually, and quality of life should be a guiding principle; one that on balance is more important than simple survival. Hopefully, sophisticated and carefully designed scientific studies will help to clarify and direct our management of intracranial gliomas in the future.

TABLE 4.6
Glioma Management

Biopsy only
- Diffuse tumor — e.g., gliomatosis
- Presumed malignant glioma involving vital or eloquent area
- Presumed low-grade glioma involving vital or eloquent area
- Asymptomatic glioma (seizure only), no ↑ ICP or shift
- Some ring-enhancing lesions (ddx: met., abscess, demyelinating disease)
- Some multifocal lesions (e.g., lymphoma)
- Some hypointense infiltrative lesions (e.g., PML)
- When adjunctive therapy is dependent on tissue diagnosis

Resect
- Well-circumscribed lesions, accessible-malignant or low grade
- Suspected pilocytic astrocytomas and other curable gliomas (PXA, DNET, central neurocytoma)
- Ring-enhancing gliomas (when possible)
- When adjunctive therapy depends on decreased tumor burden

Watchful waiting
- Productive asymptomatic patient with stable disease and characteristic imaging studies

ACKNOWLEDGMENT

The author is grateful to Barbara Behnke for her expert assistance in the preparation of this manuscript.

REFERENCES

1. Ciric I, Ammirati M, Vick N, Mikhael M: Supratentorial gliomas: Surgical considerations and immediate postoperative results. **Neurosurgery** 21:21–26, 1987.
2. Curran WJ Jr., Scott CB, Horton J, Nelson JS, Weinstein AS, Fischbach AJ, Chang CH, Rothman M, Asbell SO, Krisch RE, etal.: Recursive partitioning analysis of prognostic factors in three Radiation Therapy Oncology Group malignant glioma trials. **J Natl Cancer Inst** 85:704–710, 1993.
3. Kelly PJ, Daumas-Duport C, Kispert DB, Kall BA, Scheithauer BW, Illig JJ: Imaging-based stereotactic serial biopsies in untreated intracranial glial neoplasms. **J Neurosurg** 66:865–874, 1987.
4. Kreth FW, Berlis A, Spiropoulou V, Faist M, Scheremet R, Rossner R, Volk B, Ostertag CB: **Cancer** 86:2117–2123, 1999.
5. Laws ER, Goldberg WJ, Bernstein JJ: Migration of human malignant astrocytoma cells in the mammalian brain: Scherer revisted. **Int J Devl Neuroscience** 11:691–697, 1993.
6. Laws ER, Shaffrey ME: The inherent invasiveness of cerebral gliomas: Implications for clinical management. **Int J Devl Neuroscience** 17:413–420, 1999.
7. Ojemann JG, Miller JW, Silbergeld DL: Preserved function in brain invaded by tumor. **Neurosurgery** 39:253–259, 1996.
8. Silbergeld DL, Chicone MR: Isolation of human malignant glioma cells from histologically normal brain. **J Neurosurg** 86:525–531, 1997.
9. Weisberg LA: Cerebral computed tomography in the diagnosis of supratentorial astrocytoma. **Comput Tomogr** 4:87–105, 1980.

CHAPTER

5

An Appraisal of Chemotherapy: In the Blood or in the Brain?

MEIC H. SCHMIDT, M.D., SUSAN M. CHANG, M.D., AND MITCHEL S. BERGER, M.D.

INTRODUCTION

Every year 29,000 new cases of primary brain tumors are diagnosed. About 50% of these are tumors derived from glial cells (46). The incidence rate of primary malignant brain tumors is 6 to 7 per 100,000. Overall the incidence and mortality of malignant brain tumors is increasing, in particular in the elderly population over the age of 75 (34).

Malignant gliomas are a heterogeneous group of neoplasms derived from neuroepithelial tissue. The vast majority of malignant gliomas consist of anaplastic astrocytomas and glioblastoma multiforme. In addition, mixed anaplastic tumors like oligoastrocytoma, oligodendroglioma, and ependymoma are increasingly recognized.

Despite major advances in surgical techniques and radiation strategies, the prognosis for these tumors remains poor. Median survival expectations remain below 1 year despite mulimodality treatment for glioblastoma multiforme. Other anaplastic tumors have longer median survivals ranging from 3 to 5 years. Nontreatment variables such as age at diagnosis, performance status, and glioma histology remain the most important prognostic factors (15). Therapeutic strategies that potentially increase survival are extent of surgical resection, radiation dose, and chemotherapy. Median survival after surgical resection alone is 17 weeks and when combined with postoperative radiation is extended to 37 weeks for glioblastoma multiforme. The majority of treatment failures are due to local progression of tumor (37). This is most likely due to microscopic, infiltrating tumor cells not treatable with surgery and radiation. In addition, microscopic glioma cells have been cultured from histological normal brain tissue away from the primary site (40). Chemotherapy strategies have been developed to treat these malignant cells, but increases in survival with the addition of single or combination chemotherapy to surgery and radiation have not been forthcoming.

This article will review systemic (in the blood) and local (in the brain) strategies that have been evaluated to increase the efficacy of chemotherapeutic agents in the treatment of malignant gliomas.

IN THE BLOOD: THE ROLE OF SYSTEMIC CHEMOTHERAPY

The effectiveness of chemotherapy for malignant gliomas depends on many factors. The antineoplastic agent must be cytotoxic to the glioma cell. The cytotoxic effect should be selective in order to minimize side effects. In addition, cytotoxicity must be efficient so that drug resistance can be minimized or overcome by the agent. For a chemotherapeutic agent to exert its effect it must reach the target cell in high enough concentration. For the treatment of gliomas the blood brain barrier (BBB) is an additional consideration for drug delivery. Systemic drug delivery is most commonly done by the intravenous route. The drug must pass through the circulation and be transferred from the blood to the tumor cell. Many forces determine the uptake and distribution of systemic drugs. These can influence drug concentration in the target tissue and have consequences in nontarget tissues (systemic side effects). Transcapillary drug transfer in particular with intact BBB is influenced by physiochemical characteristics of the chemotherapeutic agent. Lipid solubility, molecular charge, and weight influence drug transfer to gliomas. In general , smaller, lipophilic agents without molecular charge cross the blood brain barrier more readily.

Systemic and intracerebral drug metabolism may activate drugs or decrease the concentration of drugs. It is important to characterize the pharmacological interaction of the chemotherapeutic agent with drugs that are commonly used in the brain tumor population. Steroids and anticonvulsants can significantly alter metabolism and pharmacokinetics of chemotherapeutic agents (12). Steroids may stabilize the blood brain barrier and alter drug uptake in the brain. Many anticonvulsants can cause hepatic enzyme induction and decrease the effective concentration of drug in the plasma. Once the drug reaches the glioma cells it might be deactivated by drug resistance molecules and mechanisms. All these factors make the actual drug concentration in the tumor tissue difficult to predict and may influence the effect of the drug on tumor cells.

Single Agent Chemotherapy

BCNU and related nitrosoureas are most frequently used chemotherapeutic agent in the treatment of malignant gliomas *(Table 5.1)*. They are alkylating agents that cause cross-linking of DNA leading to cell death. BCNU was selected for chemotherapy trials of malignant

TABLE 5.1
Common Chemotherapeutic Agents used in the Treatment of Malignant Gliomas

Class	Agent
Alkylating agents	
Nitrosoureas	BCNU
	CCNU
Metal salts	Cisplatin
	Carboplatin
Nitrogen mustard	Cyclophosphamide
	Ifosfamide
Imidazotetrazine	Temozolomide
Antimetabolites	
Folic acid anolog	Methotrexate
Pyrimidine analog	5-Fluorouracil
	Cytarabine
Purine analogues	Thioguanine
Natural products	
Vinca alkaloids	Vincristine
Podophyllotoxins	Etoposide (VP-16)
Antibiotics	Bleomycin
	Mitomycin C
Taxanes	Paclitaxel
Miscellaneous	
Methylhydrazines	Procarbazine
PKC modulator	Tamoxifen (high dose)

gliomas because of good lipid solubility, which increases the ability to effectively cross the blood brain barrier. It also demonstrated good efficacy with low toxicity in preclinical studies.

The initial phase III trial by the Brain Tumor Study Group (BTSG) showed that BCNU in addition to radiation and surgery increased the proportion of patients surviving at 12 and 18 months as compared to postoperative radiation alone (44). At 12 months 32 % of patients receiving BCNU in addition to surgery and radiation survived compared to 24 % in the surgery postoperative radiation group. This difference persisted at 18 months where 19 % of BCNU patients and 4 % of radiation alone patients survived. However, the addition of BCNU did not significantly increase overall survival (40 to 45 weeks). This result suggests that a subgroup of patients with malignant gliomas may be chemoresponsive.

In addition to therapeutic effectiveness, the recommendation for a chemotherapeutic agent are influenced by local and systemic side effects. BCNU is commonly administered in 6 cycles at 150 to 200 mg/m^2 every 6 to 8 weeks by intravenous infusion on an outpatient basis. Toxicities are in general mild to moderate. Nausea and vomiting are usually controlled with antiemetics. Hematological abnormalities include mild to moderate depression of platelets and white blood cells. White blood cell counts of less than $2000/mm^3$ and platelets of less than $50,000/mm^3$ are rare. Treatment with blood transfusion and growth factors is seldom required and hematological abnormalities improve when BCNU is discontinued. Renal, hepatic, and pulmonary side effects are limited with pulmonary fibrosis being the most significant. The risk of serious complications is limited if the cumulative dose does not exceed 1200 mg/m^2, approximately 6 cycles of BCNU.

Many additional clinical trials were conducted with BCNU or other nitrosoureas. A recent meta-analysis combined the data of 16 studies with more than 3000 patients with malignant gliomas (19). They concluded that there is a proportionate increase in survival for patients treated with radiation and chemotherapy. Specifically, the estimated increase in survival was 10.1 % at 1 year and 8.6 % at 2 years for patients treated with chemotherapy after radiation. But there was only a subgroup of GBM or AA patients that benefited from chemotherapy. In summary, the modest increase in a subgroup of patients with GBM and the tolerable side effect profile make single agent BCNU the chemotherapeutic agent of choice to which other strategies and agents are compared.

Temozolomide is a promising new agent in the treatment of malignant glioma (48). It is a second-generation alkylating agent that can be orally administered. Temozolomide it converted to 5-(3-methyltriazen-1-yl)imidazole-4-carboximide, the active alkylating agent. This conversion occurs spontaneously and does not require metabolic activation. Several preclinical studies indicated temozolomide's antineoplastic activity, with good penetration of the blood brain barrier and cerebrospinal fluid. Temozolomide has been tested with good responses for recurrent malignant gliomas. A multicenter phase II study for patients with anaplastic astrocytoma or oligoastrocytoma at first relapse demonstrated a median overall survival of 13.6 months (48). The 6- and 12-month survival rates were 75 % and 56 %, respectively. Objective response rates as determined by gadolinium-enhanced MRI scans were good. 8% of patients had a complete response, 27 % partial response, and 26% of patients had stable disease. Side effects were mild to moderate, hematological abnormalities occurred in less than 10% of patients. Another phase II study of temozolomide versus procarbazine with 225 recurrent glioblastoma multiforme patients demonstrated a 6-month progression free survival of 21 % and 8 %, respectively (47). In addition, the good treatment response with a low side effect profile was associated with health related quality-of-life benefit (36, 47).

Combination (Multi-agent) Chemotherapy

One strategy to increase the effectiveness of nitrosourea chemotherapy is the use of multiple agents. A study comparing PCV (Procarbazine, CCNU, Vincristine) and single agent BCNU for malignant gliomas was conducted by the Northern California Cooperative Study Group (29, 30). This study demonstrated that combination chemotherapy with PCV was superior to BCNU alone for anaplastic gliomas. Specifically , anaplastic astrocytoma patients treated with radiation and then with either PCV chemotherapy or BCNU only had a median survival of 157 weeks and 82 weeks, respectively. There was no significant difference for the GBM group. Thus, many anaplastic gliomas like anaplastic astrocytomas and oligodendrogliomas constitute a chemosensitive subgroup. As with BCNU, the combination of PCV is usually well tolerated but certainly has more significant side effects. CCNU and Procarbazine are both myelo-suppressive. Procarbazine is a monoamine oxidase inhibitor and requires patients to modify medications and diets. Neuropathy from vincristine can be significant and in 10 % of patients the agents need to be discontinued. In general, PCV is still well tolerated but requires more careful monitoring of patients when compared to BCNU alone. Thus, PCV is recommended for anaplastic gliomas such as anaplastic astrocytomas, anaplastic oligodenrogliomas and anaplastic ependymoma but not for GBM. It is important to know that the less common anaplastic oligoden-droglioma appears to be more chemosensitive than other astrocytomas (10, 11, 33). A phase II study for new and recurrent anaplastic oligoden-drogliomas demonstrated a 71 % objective response rate. Recent studies have also shown a link between anaplastic oligodendrogliomas that had loss of heterozygosity at chromosomes 1p and 19q and their responsive-ness to chemotherapy (9). Specifically, 1p loss was associated with 100% response and 5-year survival of 95 %. When 1p was present there was only a 25 % response and the 5-year survival decreased to 25 %.

In addition to BCNU and PCV many other chemotherapeutic agents have been evaluated for combination chemotherapy and demonstrated activity against malignant gliomas. These are listed in *Table 5.1* and include procarbazine, cisplatin, cyclophosphamide, VP-16, carboplatin, tamoxifen, and crisnatol. None of them has shown to be more effective or less toxic than BCNU for GBM and are reserved for recurrent disease. New combination chemotherapy using anti-angiogenesis drugs and inhibition of chemotherapy resistance mechanisms are being investigated (16, 18, 20).

STRATEGIES TO INCREASE DOSE DELIVERY

In order to increase the therapeutic efficacy and to decrease systemic side effects single and combination chemotherapy has been administered via the carotid and vertebral artery. Nitrosoureas, cisplatin, and methotrexate achieve high intratumoral concentration after intra-arterial (IA) injection (13, 21, 25). In theory this should increase the efficacy of chemotherapy and minimize systemic side effects.

The Brain Tumor Cooperative Group conducted a phase III trial for malignant gliomas comparing intravenous versus intra arterial BCNU with and without 5-Fluorouracil (38). One hundred sixty-seven patients received BCNU intravenously, and 148 patients had intra-arterial administration. There was no significant difference in survival among glioblastoma multiforme patients. Patients with anaplastic gliomas had decreased survival with intra-arterial BCNU. Other studies using intra-arterial cisplatin and carboplatin did not fare better (13, 14, 23). Seizures, weakness, hearing loss, aphasias, and coma have been reported and toxic effects have been reported in many intra-arterial trials (39).

Osmotic blood brain barrier disruption can potentially increase drug transfer into the brain tissue (22). The blood brain barrier may be disrupted iatrogenically via the intra-arterial infusion of hyerosmolar mannitol. This is followed by rapid infusion of chemotherapy. Tumor responses have been reported using blood brain barrier disruption, but there continues to be a high incidence of complications with limited therapeutic success. Thus, there continues to be controversy about this approach and further research is needed to determine the ultimate role of blood brain barrier disruption.

High dose chemotherapy followed by autologous bone marrow rescue has been attempted for malignant gliomas (17, 32). The barrier to increase the systemic dose for many chemotherapeutic agents including BCNU is hematopoietic toxicity. Autologous stem cell or bone marrow rescue can overcome this limitation. It involves the reinfusion of previously harvested stem cells from the peripheral blood or bone marrow after completion of high dose chemotherapy. Hochberg et al treated 11 patients with recurrent glioblastoma multiforme (24). They gave 600 to 1400 mg/m^2 of BCNU followed by autologous bone marrow rescue. At 1400 mg/m^2 of BCNU acute and permanent central nervous system side effects were noted consisting of memory loss and seizure disorders. Survival was not significantly improved. A recent study of myeloablative chemotherapy for recurrent aggressive oligodendroglioma was disappointing (8). 20 patients received high dose thiotepa after induction chemotherapy using PCV or cisplatin with etoposide. Median event-free, progression-free and overall survival times from recurrence were 17, 20, and 49 months, respectively. Fatal treatment toxicity occurred in 20% (4 patients) and consisted of progressive encephalopathy and intratumoral hemorrhage.

Overall, it appears that dose intensification chemotherapy by either intra-arterial infusion, autologous bone marrow rescue, or blood brain barrier disruption did not yield an improvement in survival. In addition, these strategies increase central nervous system toxicity and decrease the quality of life for the patients. One reason why dose intensification might not work is because of the limited intrinsic cytotoxicity of BCNU and BCNU resistance mechanisms.

RESISTANCE MECHANISM TO CHEMOTHERAPY

Tumor cells have several mechanisms to overcome the effect of chemotherapy. Intrinsic and acquired resistance mechanisms include p170 glycoprotein, loss of p53 activity, and DNA repair enzymes. The failure of dose intensification of nitrosourea based chemotherapy indicates that tumor cells have mechanisms to decrease cytotoxicity. Alkylating and methylating agents (BCNU, CCNU, Procarbazine, Temozolomide) cause several forms of DNA damage by a variety of mechanisms. Alkylating agents react with nucleophilic DNA sites. This results in purine and pyrimidine derivatives that can cause DNA-DNA cross links and other damage that can impair DNA replication. The treatment of tumors with nitrosoureas produces a lesion at the O^6 position of guanine. Procarbazine and methyl nitrosourea produces O^6 methyguanine. BCNU and CCNU produces O^6chloroethyl guanine. The tumor cells have mechanisms to repair DNA damage prior to replication. Bodell et al demonstrated that human glioma cell lines that are capable of repairing the O^6 alkyl lesions were more resistant to nitrosoureas.

AGT or O^6 alkylguanine DNA alkyltransferase is part of an inducible repair system for the DNA damage caused by alkylating agents (2–4). High levels of alkyltransferase can repair DNA damage caused by alkylating agents. O^6 BG (benzylguanine) is a new agent that can deplete tumor cells of AGT and thus increase the effectiveness of nitrosourea based chemotherapy. O^6 BG may enhance tumor control when combined with BCNU in vivo and in vitro. Subcutaneous and intracranial glioma xenografts that are resistant to BCNU demonstrate complete or partial responses when BCNU is combined with O^6 BG. No additional toxicity was seen using reduced doses of BCNU. O^6 benzylguanine has been shown to decrease AGT levels in patients with malignant gliomas (20). At 100 mg/m^2 of O^6 benzylguanine the AGT level in tumor specimens were less than 10 fmol/mg protein for 18 hours after treatment. Based on these results the North American Brain Tumor Consortium (NABTC) is currently conducting a phase 1 study to define the dose of O^6 BG that produced total depletion of AGT in patients with anaplastic astrocytomas and glioblastoma multiforme.

Opportunities to increase sensitivity to therapy relate to the p53 gene. This gene and its product are absent in many tumors. The p53 gene product is important in the regulation of apoptosis. New gene therapeutic approaches use vectors that are capable to transfer this gene into tumor cells. Together, with more efficient target delivery, this could result in transduced brain tumor cells more sensitive to chemotherapy (42).

IN THE BRAIN: INTRATUMORAL CHEMOTHERAPY FOR MALIGNANT GLIOMAS

Since the major cause of treatment failure is local recurrence and gliomas rarely metastasize outside the central nervous system, local chemotherapy seems a logical approach. In theory, intratumoral chemotherapy circumvents the blood brain barrier, decreases systemic drug levels, minimizes systemic side effects, and elevates drug levels in tumors. Drug interactions that occur with steroids and anticonvulsants during systemic injection are negligible with local drug delivery. Only agents that do not require systemic metabolism for activation are suitable for this approach. In addition, local delivery implies an invasive procedure with all its associated risks, and as with systemic dose intensification (intra-arterial delivery) the local side effects can dramatically increase. BCNU, methotrexate bleomycin and other agents have been studied. Many of the new systemic agents described above have not yet been used in local, in the brain, delivery.

Direct Injection of Liquid-phase Chemotherapeutic Agents

Injection into the tumor via Ommaya reservoir, infusion pumps, microdialyses probes, and stereotactic delivery have been used to deliver local chemotherapy (45). Preclinical studies have shown that intratumoral chemotherapy is effective and limits systemic toxicity. Intratumoral chemotherapy increased also the effectiveness of systemic therapy when used in combination. Single injection and multiple injection over several days have been used. Several clinical studies using cyclophosphamide, Fluorouracil, methotrexate, Bleomycin, Cisplatin, and BCNU have been reported. Significant increases in median survival were not achieved, but the clinical data confirmed only mild local toxic effects. Treatment failure is most likely due to inadequate drug delivery to the irregular infiltrating brain tumor margin. The data on diffusion distance of local administered chemotherapeutic agent is not available for most agents. The evaluation of new local administered therapy must include quantitative data on diffusion of chemotherapeutic agents into brain tissue. One study that is currently initiated involves the stereotactic injection of DTI-015 prior to tumor resection for recurrent malignant gliomas. DTI-015 is a solution of BCNU and ethanol designed to increase tissue penetration from the injection site. The antitumor effect is mediated though the formation of chemical adducts between BCNU reactive fragments and DNA bases (guanine etc). In this study adduct formation will be assessed at graded distances from the injection site within the tumor. This will yield important information on effective tissue penetration.

Intratumoral Chemotherapy with Polymer Drug Delivery

Direct injection BCNU into tumors has yielded little success. In order to further increase local drug concentrations polymer systems for controlled release have been developed (26, 45). Nonbiodegradable systems using EVAc (Ethylene-vinyl acetate) were used first and has found applications for glaucoma therapy. In addition, 5-fluorouracil with silicone rubber capsules has been used for local glioma therapy. Polyanhidride poly[bis(carboxyphenoxy-propane)-sebacic acid] or PCPP-SA matrix is a biodegradable polymer drug delivery compound that has been investigated for glioma therapy. Drug release occurs at a constant rate and the degradation of the polymer causes only minimal inflammation. Most clinical studies use BCNU wafers despite its limited success by direct injection and systemic administration. The first phase I-II study was completed using BCNU wafers with increasing drug concentration in 21 patients with recurrent anaplastic astrocytomas and glioblastoma multiforme (6). Median survival was 46 weeks at the time of reoperation and BCNU wafers were found to be safe at BCNU concentration of 3.85 %. In 1995, a randomized, prospective, double blind, placebo-controlled study with 222 patients using 3.85% BCNU wafers after surgical resection of recurrent malignant gliomas was published (7). The median survival in BCNU wafer and the placebo wafer were 31 and 23 weeks, respectively. The survival difference was larger for patients with glioblastoma multiforme. Intracranial infection, seizures, and cerebral edema were the most pronounced complications. In a separate study in 1995, 22 patients with newly diagnosed malignant glioma (21 glioblastoma multiforme and 1 anaplastic astrocytoma) received 3.85% BCNU wafers after the initial resection prior to radiation therapy (5). Median survival was 42 weeks and the authors concluded that BCNU wafers could safely be used prior to radiation. A prospective, randomized double blind study with "up front" BCNU wafers in 32 patients with malignant gliomas showed that this approach could be used (43). Median survival was better in the treatment group but there were also a significant number of patients with postoperative complications (21 of 32). The number of patients in each treatment group were small and not balanced by histology. A study published in 1999 used BCNU wafers in 62 patients with recurrent glioblastoma multiforme was unable to demonstrate significant increase in survival (41). Complications were significantly increased in the BCNU wafer group.

Currently it appears that the use of BCNU wafers is a valid option for selected patients and that most complications can be limited. The main factors why increases in survival for BCNU wafers are modest is probably due to intrinsic resistance of tumor cells to BCNU and to limited BCNU penetration into brain/tumor tissue. In addition, no clinical trial has compared systemic BCNU with BCNU wafers. The development of new, more effective chemotherapeutic agents might also increase the usefulness of polymer drug delivery. In addition, the polymer delivery of anti-angiogenesis factors and steroids is being evaluated.

Convection-Enhanced Intratumoral Chemotherapy

A relatively new approach in the intra tumoral delivery of experimental drug therapy for malignant glioma is based on convection enhanced microinfusion. Current methods for intratumoral drug delivery rely on diffusion of the agent. Diffusion is defined as movement of drug along a concentration gradient. In the brain, diffusion of agents result in inhomogeneous distribution of the drug within the parenchyma. The rate of diffusion depends on the concentration gradient and is inversely related to the molecular weight (1). Since the local tissue clearance of drug in the tumor/brain can be faster than the rate of drug diffusion it is possible that most of the intratumoral administered chemotherapy is cleared before it can take effect. In convection delivery, the movement of drug is by bulk solute flow which is dependent on the pressure gradient rather than tissue drug concentration. Chemotherapy administered locally by convective flow can significantly increase the volume and homogeneity of the agent in the target tissue (31). Larger molecules such as monoclonal antibodies and ligand exotoxins can be delivered by convection enhanced microinfusion over larger volumes as compared to systemic or other local delivery.

Preclinical and clinical data from delivery of pseudomonas exotoxin to brain tissue and tumor is improved with bulk flow microinfusion. Studies report distribution of therapeutic molecules up to 4 cm from the point of infusion (1, 27, 28, 35). The results of bulk flow infusion into patients with brain tumors has been reported (28). Eighteen patients received transferrin immunotoxin conjugate by microinfusion. Transient neurologic symptoms were noted during 3 of 44 infusions. Four patients had a seizure during administration. Infusion volume averaged from 5 to 180 ml. No life-threatening complications were noted. This study demonstrated that large volumes of fluid can be delivered to the brain by microinfusion. Further studies to assess the efficacy of this approach are in progress.

CONCLUSION

This review highlights the expanding role of chemotherapy in the treatment of malignant gliomas. Although significant advances in survival have not been achieved yet, it is clear that chemotherapy can affect tumor cells. Research that has evolved from some of the failed chemotherapy agents have yielded significant insight into resistance mechanisms. Molecular analysis and the identification of chemosensitive markers might help to guide therapy in the near future. The delivery of chemotherapy directly into the brain is expanding quickly and the neurosurgeons' role will be significant in selecting and administering chemotherapy in this setting. Chemotherapy in the brain is the ideal and logical approach for local, recurrent disease. Yet new culturing techniques have shown malignant glioma cells in histological normal-appearing brain tissue at distances away from the local recurrence site. The role of systemic chemotherapy in the treatment of these "distant" microscopic tumor nests might not become apparent until local disease is controlled. Therefore, it is clear that the development of new chemotherapy strategies should continue to be in the blood *and* in the brain.

REFERENCES

1. Bobo RH, Laske DW, Akbasak A, Morrison PF, Dedrick RL, Oldfield EH: Convection-enhanced delivery of macromolecules in the brain. **Proc Natl Acad Sci USA** 91(6):2076–2080, 1994.
2. Bobola MS, Berger MS, Silber JR: Contribution of O6-methylguanine-DNA methyltransferase to resistance to 1,3-(2-chloroethyl)-1-nitrosourea in human brain tumor-derived cell lines. **Molecular Carcinogenesis** 13(2):81–88, 1995.
3. Bobola MS, Blank A, Berger MS, Silber JR: Contribution of O6-methylguanine-DNA methyltransferase to monofunctional alkylating-agent resistance in human brain tumor-derived cell lines. **Molecular Carcinogenesis** 13(2):70–80, 1995.
4. Bobola MS, Tseng SH, Blank A, Berger MS, Silber JR: Role of O6-methylguanine-DNA methyltransferase in resistance of human brain tumor cell lines to the clinically relevant methylating agents temozolomide and streptozotocin. **Clin Cancer Res** 2(4):735–741, 1996.
5. Brem H, Ewend MG, Piantadosi S, Greenhoot J, Burger PC, Sisti M: The safety of interstitial chemotherapy with BCNU-loaded polymer followed by radiation therapy in the treatment of newly diagnosed malignant gliomas: phase I trial. **J Neuro-Oncol** 26(2):111–123, 1995.
6. Brem H, Mahaley MS Jr, Vick NA, Black KL, Schold SC Jr, Burger PC, Friedman AH, Ciric IS, Eller TW, Cozzens JW, et al: Interstitial chemotherapy with drug

polymer implants for the treatment of recurrent gliomas. **J Neurosurg** 74(3):441–446, 1991.

7. Brem H, Piantadosi S, Burger PC, Walker M, Selker R, Vick NA, Black K, Sisti M, Brem S, Mohr G, et al: Placebo-controlled trial of safety and efficacy of intraoperative controlled delivery by biodegradable polymers of chemotherapy for recurrent gliomas. The Polymer-brain Tumor Treatment Group. **Lancet** 345(8956):1008–1012, 1995.

8. Cairncross G, Swinnen L, Bayer R, Rosenfeld S: Myeloablative chemotherapy for recurrent aggressive oligodendroglioma. **Neuro-Oncology** 2:114–119, 2000.

9. Cairncross G, Ueki K, Zlatescu M, Lisle D, Finkelstein D, Hammond R: Specific genetic predictors of chemotherapeutic response and survival in patients with anaplastic oligodendrogliomas. **J Natl Cancer Inst** 90:1473–1479, 1998.

10. Cairncross JG, Macdonald DR: Oligodendroglioma: a new chemosensitive tumor. **J Clin Oncol** 8(12):2090–2091, 1990.

11. Cairncross JG, Macdonald DR: Chemotherapy for oligodendroglioma. Progress report. **Arch Neurol** 48(2):225–7, 1991.

12. Chang SM, Kuhn JG, Rizzo J, et al: Phase I study of paclitaxel in patients with recurrent malignant glioma: A North American Brain Tumor Consortium report. **J Clin Oncol** 16(6):2188–2194, 1998.

13. Cloughesy TF, Black KL, Gobin YP, Farahani K, Nelson G, Villablanca P, Kabbinavar F, Viñuela F, Wortel CH: Intra-arterial Cereport (RMP-7) and carboplatin: a dose escalation study for recurrent malignant gliomas. **Neurosurgery** 44(2):270–278; discussion 278–279, 1999.

14. Cloughesy TF, Gobin YP, Black KL, Viñuela F, Taft F, Kadkhoda B, Kabbinavar F: Intra-arterial carboplatin chemotherapy for brain tumors: a dose escalation study based on cerebral blood flow. **J Neuro-Oncol** 35(2):121–131, 1997.

15. Curran WJ Jr, Scott CB, Horton J, Nelson JS, Weinstein AS, Fischbach AJ, Chang CH, Rotman M, Asbell SO, Krisch RE, et al: Recursive partitioning analysis of prognostic factors in three Radiation Therapy Oncology Group malignant glioma trials. **J Natl Cancer Inst** 85(9):704–710, 1993.

16. D'Amato RJ, Loughnan MS, Flynn E, Folkman J: Thalidomide is an inhibitor of angiogenesis. **Proc Natl Acad Sci USA** 91:4082–4085, 1994.

17. Dunkel IJ, JL F: High-dose chemotherapy followed by autologous bone marrow rescue for high grade gliomas, in Berger MS, CB, W., eds: *The Gliomas.* Philadelphia: WB Saunders, 1999, pp549–554.

18. Fine HA, Loeffler JS, Ap K: A phase II trial of the anti-angiogenic agent ,thalidomide, in patients with recurrent high-grade gliomas. **Proc Am Soc** Clin Oncol 16:385a–385a, 1997.

19. Fine HA, Dear KB, Loeffler JS, Black PM, Canellos GP: Meta-analysis of radiation therapy with and without adjuvant chemotherapy for malignant gliomas in adults. **Cancer** 71(8):2585–2597, 1993.

20. Friedman HS, Kokkinakis DM, Pluda J, et al: Phase I trial of O6-benzylguanine for patients undergoing surgery for malignant glioma. **J Clin Oncol** 16(11):3570–3575, 1998.

21. Greenberg HS, Ensminger WD, Seeger JF, Kindt GW, Chandler F, Doan K, Dakhil SR: Intra-arterial BCNU chemotherapy for the treatment of malignant gliomas of the central nervous system: a preliminary report. **Cancer Treatment Reports** 65(9–10):803–810, 1981.

22. Gumerlock MK, Belshe BD, Madsen R, Watts C: Osmotic blood-brain barrier disruption and chemotherapy in the treatment of high grade malignant glioma: patient series and literature review. **J Neuro-Oncol** 12(1):33–46, 1992.

23. Hiesiger EM, Green SB, Shapiro WR, Burger PC, Selker RG, Mahaley MS Jr, Ransohoff J 2nd, VanGilder JC, Mealey J Jr, Robertson JT, et al: Results of a randomized trial comparing intra-arterial cisplatin and intravenous PCNU for the treatment of primary brain tumors in adults: Brain Tumor Cooperative Group trial 8420A. **J Neuro-Oncol** 25(2):143–154, 1995.

24. Hochberg FH, Parker LM, Takvorian T, Canellos GP, Zervas NT: High-dose BCNU with autologous bone marrow rescue for recurrent glioblastoma multiforme. **JNeurosurg** 54(4):455–460, 1981.

25. Hochberg FH, Pruitt AA, Beck DO, DeBrun G, Davis K: The rationale and methodology for intra-arterial chemotherapy with BCNU as treatment for glioblastoma. **J Neurosurg** 63(6):876–880, 1985.

26. Langer R, Folkman J: Polymers for the sustained release of proteins and other macromolecules. **Nature** 263(5580):797–800, 1976.

27. Laske DW, Morrison PF, Lieberman DM, Corthesy ME, Reynolds JC, Stewart-Henney PA, Koong SS, Cummins A, Paik CH, Oldfield EH: Chronic interstitial infusion of protein to primate brain: determination of drug distribution and clearance with single-photon emission computerized tomography imaging. **J Neurosurg** 87(4):586–594, 1997.

28. Laske DW, Youle RJ, Oldfield EH: Tumor regression with regional distribution of the targeted toxin TF-CRM107 in patients with malignant brain tumors. **Nat Med** 3(12):1362–1368, 1997.

29. Levin VA, Edwards MS, Wright DC, Seager ML, Schimberg TP, Townsend JJ, Wilson CB: Modified procarbazine, CCNU, and vincristine (PCV 3) combination chemotherapy in the treatment of malignant brain tumors. **Cancer Treatment** Reports **64(2–3):237–244, 1980.**

30. Levin VA, Silver P, Hannigan J, Wara WM, Gutin PH, Davis RL, Wilson CB: Superiority of post-radiotherapy adjuvant chemotherapy with CCNU, procarbazine, and vincristine (PCV) over BCNU for anaplastic gliomas: NCOG 6G61 final report. **Int J Radiation Oncol Biol Phys** 18(2):321–324, 1990.

31. Lieberman DM, Laske DW, Morrison PF, Bankiewicz KS, Oldfield EH: Convection-enhanced distribution of large molecules in gray matter during interstitial drug infusion. **J Neurosurg** 82(6):1021–1029, 1995.

32. Linassier C, Benboubker L, Velut S, Calais G, Saudeau D, Jan M, Autret A, Berger C, Biron P, Colombat P: High-dose BCNU with ABMT followed by radiation therapy in the treatment of supratentorial glioblastoma multiforme. **Bone Marrow Transplantation** 18 Suppl 1(4):S69–72, 1996.

33. Macdonald DR, Gaspar LE, Cairncross JG: Successful chemotherapy for newly diagnosed aggressive oligodendroglioma. **Ann Neurol** 27(5):573–574, 1990.

34. Mao, Y, Desmeules, M, Semenciw, RM, Hill, G, Gaudette, L, Wigle, DT: Increasing brain cancer rates in Canada. **CMAJ** 145(12):1583–91, 1991.

35. Morrison PF, Laske DW, Bobo H, Oldfield EH, Dedrick RL: High-flow microinfusion: tissue penetration and pharmacodynamics. **Am J Physiol** 266(1 Pt 2):R292–305, 1994.

36. Osoba D, Brada M, Yung WK, Prados M: Health-related quality of life in patients treated with temozolomide versus procarbazine for recurrent glioblastoma multiforme. **J Clin Oncol** 18(7):1481–1491, 2000.

37. Salcman M. Glioblastoma and malignant astrocytoma, in: Kaye AH, Laws ER, eds: *Brain tumors.* Churchill Livingstone, 1995, pp449–477.

38. Shapiro WR, Green SB, Burger PC, Selker RG, VanGilder JC, Robertson JT, Mealey J Jr, Ransohff J, Mahaley MS Jr: A randomized comparison of intra-arterial ver-

sus intravenous BCNU, with or without intravenous 5-fluorouracil, for newly diagnosed patients with malignant glioma. **J Neurosurg** 76(5):772–781, 1992.

39. Shingleton BJ, Bienfang DC, Albert DM, Ensminger WD, Chandler WF, Greenberg HS: Ocular toxicity associated with high-dose carmustine. **Arch Ophthalmol** 100(11):1766–1772, 1982.

40. Silbergeld DL, Chicoine MR: Isolation and characterization of human malignant glioma cells from histologically normal brain. **J Neurosurg** 86(3):525–531, 1997.

41. Subach BR, Witham TF, Kondziolka D, Lunsford LD, Bozik M, Schiff D: Morbidity and survival after 1,3-bis(2-chloroethyl)-1-nitrosourea wafer implantation for recurrent glioblastoma: a retrospective case-matched cohort series. **Neurosurgery** 45(1):17–22; discussion 22–3, 1999.

42. Trepel M, Groscurth P, Malipiero U, Gulbins E, Dichgans J, Weller M: Chemosensitivity of human malignant glioma: modulation by p53 gene transfer. **J Neuro-Oncol** 39(1):19–32, 1998.

43. Valtonen S, Timonen U, Toivanen P, Kalimo H, Kivipelto L, Heiskanen O, Unsgaard G, Kuurne T: Interstitial chemotherapy with carmustine-loaded polymers for high-grade gliomas: a randomized double-blind study. **Neurosurgery** 41(1):44–8; discussion 48–49, 1997.

44. Walker MD, Alexander E Jr, Hunt WE, MacCarty CS, Mahaley MS Jr, Mealey J Jr, Norrell HA, Owens G, Ransohoff J, Wilson CB, Gehan EA, Strike TA: Evaluation of BCNU and/or radiotherapy in the treatment of anaplastic gliomas. A cooperative clinical trial. **J Neurosurg** 49(3):333–343, 1978.

45. Walter KA, Tamargo RJ, Olivi A, Burger PC, Brem H: Intratumoral chemotherapy. **Neurosurgery** 37(6):1128–1145, 1995.

46. Wrench RW, Yuriko M, Bondy ML. Epidemiology, in: Bernstein M, Berger MS, eds. *Neuro-Oncololgy: The Essentials.* New York: Thieme, 1999:

47. Yung WK, Albright RE, Olson J, et al.: A phase II study of temozolomide vs. procarbazine in patients with glioblastoma multiforme at first relapse. **Br J Cancer** 83(5):588–593, 2000.

48. Yung WK, Prados MD, Yaya-Tur R et al.: Multicenter phase II trial of temozolomide in patients with anaplastic astrocytoma or anaplastic oligoastrocytoma at first relapse. Temodal Brain Tumor Group. **J Clin Oncol** 17(9):2762–2771, 1999.

ACKNOWLEDGMENT

This research was supported by NIH grant T32CA09291.

6

New Innovations and Developments for Glioma Treatment

DAVID CROTEAU, M.D., FRCP(C), TOM MIKKELSEN, M.D., FRCP(C),
SANDRA A. REMPEL, PH.D., OLIVER BOGLER, PH.D.,
AND MARK ROSENBLUM, M.D.

INTRODUCTION

There have been tremendous advances over the past few years in understanding the molecular mechanisms underlying glioma behavior and the complex interaction between tumor cells and their environment. Recent discoveries have created new therapeutic avenues for targeting these neoplasms. The concept of using cytostatic agents to restrain tumor progression rather than focusing efforts to induce cytotoxicity has emerged with this progress in molecular biology. The cornerstones of glioma treatment include surgery, radiation therapy, and chemotherapy. These treatment modalities are derived from microbiology therapeutic principles where cancer cells are considered to be different from the host. Conventional wisdom has purported that unless tumor cells are killed and totally eliminated, they will overwhelm the host. In contrast, a regulatory model has recently been proposed in which cancer can be viewed as a dynamic maladaptive process that originates within the host, is constantly in evolution, and is potentially reversible. This model is consistent with the molecular genetic understanding of cancer processes such as clonal evolution that has also been demonstrated in gliomas. One of the implications of such a model is that, by reimposing biological control on a cell population with malignant phenotype, functional control of a tumor may be gained and this may not require complete tumor elimination. Some of these treatment strategies are currently under investigation in clinical trials whereas others are still in preclinical study or in development. We review some of these new therapeutic strategies as well as their underlying molecular bases.

BIOLOGY OF GLIOMAS

When a glial cell becomes neoplastic due to altered gene expression and acquired genetic mutations, it hijacks normal biologic cell processes such as cell growth, cell migration, and neovessel formation for its own proliferation, invasion, and angiogenesis, respectively. These processes are modulated by external influences, such as growth factors, proteases, extracellular matrix (ECM), and associated molecules. By interacting and/or interfering with cell surface molecules, such as receptors and integrins, these external influences regulate a network of complex and integrated signaling pathways that determine whether a tumor will proliferate, invade, and/or create new vessels. Signaling, or signal transduction, refers to a series of events that results in a transfer of information received at the cell surface into the cell that is necessary for the cell to perform the biological processes of cell division, neovessel formation and cell migration *(Fig. 6.1)*.

1. Glial Tumorigenesis

The identification of common genetic alterations in glioma has suggested that there may be a sequence of genetic changes leading to increasingly anaplastic changes and clonal complexity. The initial event triggering the cascade of genetic changes and conferring a growth advantage on that cell is unknown; however, the molecular progression following it has been described for astrocytomas and oligodendrogliomas. There are numerous alterations, and an exhaustive description is beyond the scope of this chapter and has been reviewed elsewhere (1). Rather, the most clinically relevant alterations will be briefly described. Two clonal evolution hypotheses have been proposed to explain the origin of the tumor. In the first hypothesis, the tumor may arise through a process by which a mature glial cell becomes progressively less differentiated *(Fig. 6.2)* (1). Clinical evidence of this progression model comes from patients with low-grade glioma that develop recurrent tumors of a higher grade. Several of these neoplasms appear to be characterized by specific molecular alteration, including alteration on chromosome 17 associated with the tumor suppressor gene TP53 and absence of EGFR gene amplification (2). Since the TP53 gene alteration does not increase significantly in higher-grade tumors, this appears to be an early event in the progression of astrocytoma (2). The recent finding that the chemosensitivity of mature oligodendrocytes resembles that of some oligodendrogliomas suggests that certain cellular characteristics are retained by cells in the course of this dedifferentiation (3). The second hypothesis suggests that multipotent precursor cells (either committed glial progenitors such as oligodendrocyte-type-2 astrocyte progenitor (4) in rat or pluripotent stem cells that have been identified in adult human brain) may give rise to a neoplastic undifferentiated glial cell (5). This occurs through a misdifferentiation process resulting

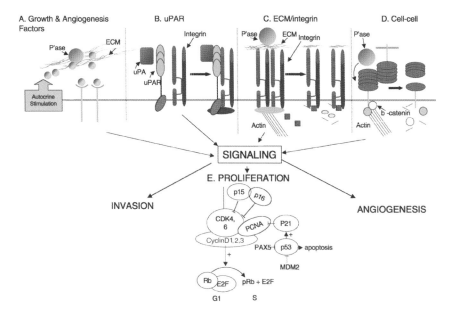

FIG. 6.1 Genetic alterations associated with tumor cell proliferation, adhesion and motility, and angiogenesis. Cell-cell and cell-ECM interactions are important in regulating tumor proliferation, adhesion, motility and angiogenesis. Degradation or activation of cell-surface and ECM proteins and the loss, mutation or amplification of intracellular proteins can mediate rapid and irreversible responses, individually or simultaneously. (*A*) Enhanced expression of growth factors by autocrine secretion or release by degradation of ECM by proteinases, signals cells to proliferate. Positive stimulation induces CDK4,6/CyclinD1,2,3/PCNA complex formation (panel E) which results in the phosphorylation of Rb and dissociation of the Rb/E2F complex. The release of E2F is essential for the cell to cross the restriction point and commit to cell division. p16, p15 and p21 act as negative regulators of this process. P53 acts to negatively regulate tumor growth by positively regulating p21 (cells stay in G1) or by inducing apoptosis under conditions of stress. MDM2 and PAX5 negatively regulate p53. (*B*) uPA binds to uPA-R triggering lateral binding with integrins. The complex binds to caveolin inducing a signaling pathway. (*C*) Proteolysis of ECM proteins alters integrin-mediated anchorage, focal adhesions, cytoskeletal architecture, and signaling molecules. (*D*) Proteolysis of cell-cell adhesion molecules releases their linkage with the cytoskeleton, thereby altering signaling. (*E*) Angiogenic factors may be secreted or released from the ECM by proteinase degradation to stimulate neovessel formation within the tumor or in adjacent normal tissue. [Adapted with permission from Werb Z and the journal, *Cell*. Werb Z: ECM and cell surface proteolysis: Regulating cellular ecology. **Cell** 91:439–442, 1997.]

in a cell with a state of limited or blocked differentiation but accompanied by uncontrolled proliferation *(Fig. 6.3)* (1). The histomorphologic features of such a tumor would reflect the stage at which development was halted. Several of these neoplasms also appear to be characterized by specific ge-

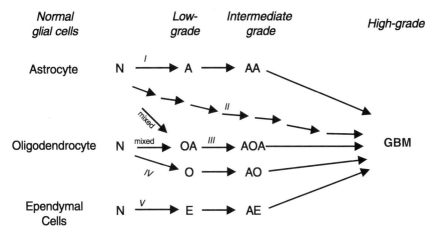

FIG. 6.2 Dedifferentiation hypothesis. Differentiated normal glial cells including astrocytes, oligodendrocytes, and ependymal cells undergoing genetic alterations would allow the formation of low-grade gliomas (A = astrocytoma, OA = oligoastrocytomas, O =
oligodendroglioma, E = ependymoma). Further alterations would permit progression to
an intermediate grade with anaplastic phenotype, AA, AOA, AO and AE, respectively. Finally, further aberrations would permit the progression of all tumors into the highest
grade tumor, glioblastoma multiforme (GBM). Pathways I-II represent alternate routes
for astrocytoma progression based on molecular variants. Pathways III-V represent the
progression of oligodendrogliomas, mixed oligoastrocytomas, and ependymomas, respectively. The accumulation of mutations results in the outgrowth of clonal tumors. Tumor
heterogeneity results as a tumor increases in malignancy, having regions associated with
higher and lower grade. The tumors are graded on their histomorphological appearance
that becomes less differentiated as the tumor increases in malignancy. [Adapted with permission. Dudas SP, Rempel SA: Development, molecular genetics, and genetic therapy of
glial tumors, in Rock JP, Rosenblum M, Shaw E, Cairncross G (eds): *The Practical Management of Low-Grade Primary Brain Tumors.* Philadelphia, Lippincott Williams &
Wilkins, 1999, pp 193–229.]

netic alterations, the most common being EGFR gene amplification without loss or alteration of the TP53 gene (2, 6). Glioblastoma multiforme
(GBM) occurring de novo without antecedent low-grade glioma might
represent an example of misdifferentiation. Another clinically relevant
example of genetic alteration is with oligodendroglioma. The concurrent
loss of 1p and 19q in the absence of TP53 gene alteration early in the onco-
genic transformation appears to be specific to oligodendroglioma and predictors of chemoresponsiveness and survival at least for higher-grade
oligodendroglioma (7). Moreover, the chromosome 1p loss appears to have
a similar significance in high-grade astrocytic tumors (8).

All of these molecular genetic alterations in turn influence the normal cellular biologic processes described below. Replacing these altered

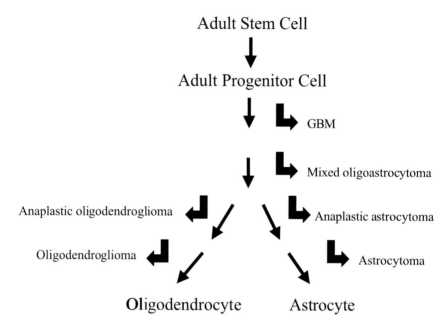

FIG. 6.3: Misdifferentiation hypothesis. Adult multipotential stem cells proliferate, eventually giving rise to adult progenitor cells. A mutation early in the developmental pathway to mature astrocytes or oligodendrocytes would give rise to glioblastoma multiforme (GBM) and mixed oligoastrocytomas. Mutations occurring after the developmental pathway splits giving rise to astrocytes or oligodendrocytes would result in anaplastic astrocytoma or anaplastic oligodendrogliomas. Mutations occurring in cells almost completely differentiated would give rise to the astrocytomas and oligodendrogliomas. Therefore, the further along the differentiation pathway that a mutation occurs in a cell, the more histological resemblance or differentiation there is to the cell it was intended to become. [Adapted with permission. Dudas SP, Rempel SA: Development, molecular genetics, and genetic therapy of glial tumors, in Rock JP, Rosenblum M, Shaw E, Cairncross G (eds): *The Practical Management of Low-Grade Primary Brain Tumors.* Philadelphia, Lippincott Williams & Wilkins, 1999, pp 193–229.]

genes with normal genes to reverse or halt the neoplastic phenotype is one premise upon which gene therapy is based.

2. Proliferation and Apoptosis

One consequence of the acquisition of these genetic molecular alterations is an uncontrolled cell growth through an imbalance between growth-promoting genes, also called proto-oncogenes, and growth-inhibiting or tumor-suppressor genes. Mutations of the former result in a gain of function, whereas alteration of the latter causes a loss of function *(Fig. 6.4)* (1). The control of proliferation involves a series of checks

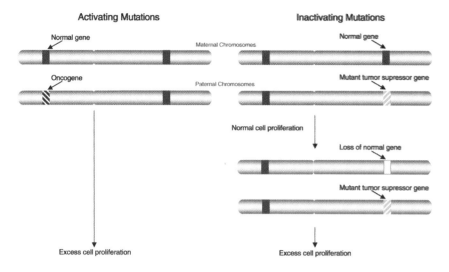

FIG. 6.4 Oncogenes and tumor suppressor genes. Activating mutations result when one allele of an oncogene is mutated and produces too much or abnormal protein. Enhanced expression of an oncogene (which positively regulates cell growth) leads to excess cell proliferation. Inactivating mutations result when one allele of a tumor suppressor gene (which negatively regulates cell growth) is mutant, producing none or abnormal protein and the second normal allele is still functional. Subsequent loss or mutation of the normal allele unmasks the mutant allele. The loss of expression of the normal allele also leads to excess proliferation. [Adapted with permission from Jared Schneidman Design and Scientific American. Cavenee WK, White RL: The genetic basis of cancer. **Sci Am** 272:72–79, 1995.]

and balances, including the interaction of growth factors with their receptors, activation of cytoplasmic signaling, and signal transduction into the nucleus where the decision to divide is regulated by positive effector proteins (e.g., CDK/cyclin, MDM2, PAX5) and negative regulator proteins (e.g., p16, p15, p21, p53, Rb) (9).

Growth factors and their receptors are present in normal glia and are often overexpressed or amplified in glioma. The resultant enhanced mitogenic effect can occur through an autocrine or paracrine mechanism, or through degradation of the ECM and the release of bound growth factors (see *Fig. 6.1*) (1). In addition to the mitogenic effect, growth factors and receptors often have additional angiogenic or immunosuppressive activities. The signaling is achieved through a series of phosphorylation events involving several kinases. The Ras protein appears to be a pivotal component of these proliferation-promoting signaling cascades (*Fig. 6.5*) (10). The signaling cascade ultimately impacts on the expres-

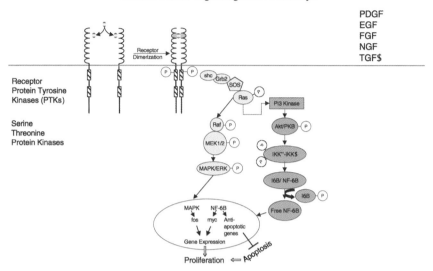

FIG. 6.5 Growth factor signaling: RAS pathways. Growth factors bind to their respective receptors to promote dimerization. This pairing activates the kinase domains of the receptors thereby inducing the transphosphorylation of the partner receptor in several locations and resulting in protein docking sites to recruit the Shc, Grb2, and SOS complex. This complex in turn phosphorylates the ras protein. The activated ras protein induces a phosphorylation cascade starting with RAF kinase followed by MEK and then MAPK/ERK activation. The activated MAPK/ERK translocates into the nucleus where it upregulates the expression of fos and jun that form a transcription factor complex capable of inducing the transcription of proliferation-associated genes. Alternatively, ras can activate PI3 kinase that in turn activates Akt/PKB followed by activation of the IKK complex. This complex phosphorylates the IkB inhibitor of NF-kB, thus freeing the transcription factor to translocate into the nucleus where it promotes proliferation by inducing transcription of myc and inhibits proliferation by inducing transcription of the antiapoptosis genes. [Adapted with permission. Lala P, Provias J, Guha A: Growth factors and nervous system tumors, in Black P, Loeffler JS (eds): *Cancer of the Nervous System*. Oxford: Blackwell Science Ltd, 1997, pp 744–772.]

sion of the cell cycle-control genes coding for the positive and negative effectors mentioned above thus further affecting the level of cellular proliferation.

   There have been tremendous advances in the understanding of apoptosis in recent years. Broadly speaking, there are two major pathways in apoptosis: extrinsic and intrinsic. The former involves ligand-mediated activation of transmembrane death receptors such as Fas, Apo1, and CD95, whereas the latter involves a protein complex called apoptosome as well as proapoptotic and antiapoptotic regulator proteins such as Bax and Bcl-2, respectively. The common final pathway involves the recruitment of enzymes called caspases that dismantle the cell (11–13). P53 protein plays a central role in apoptosis induction especially through genomic damage. An extension of this overall view of apoptosis is the integration of several inputs from a variety of sources both pro- and antiapoptotic in the decision to undergo apoptosis including growth and death signals, cell-cell and cell-matrix contacts, genome, membrane and organelle states, and other direct survival signals. Signal processing appears to be largely based on protein interaction via protein-protein binding motifs. Apoptosis results if the sum of these signals leads to the activation of the cascade of caspases. The ability to undergo death via apoptosis in glioma appears to be suppressed through tumor suppressor gene mutation such as *TP53* and *PTEN/MMAC,* which results in the reduction of proapoptotic signals. Alternately, genes with a proapoptotic effect such as *bax,* are also potential targets for gene therapy (14). Lastly, antiapoptotic molecules such as bcl-2 can be targeted, either with strategies aimed at down-regulation of their expression or by the introduction of dominant-negative proteins (15). The recent implication of a glioma-associated gene, the SH3-domain containing adapter molecule SETA (16) in the regulation of apoptosis of normal and malignant glia (17) suggests that additional targets for these approaches are still being found *(Fig. 6.6).*

3. Invasiveness

The invasive nature of gliomas is the main feature that makes these neoplasms so difficult to cure. It explains tumor persistence beyond therapeutic margins and is the primary reason for tumor recurrence. This invasive behavior is well illustrated by histopathologic correlations with radiologic abnormalities of glial neoplasm, which have demonstrated tumor cells beyond the T2 hyperintensity on MRI (18). Tumor invasiveness is illustrated in *Figure 6.7.* Invasion requires the coordination of several processes. The dissolution of ECM and cell-cell contacts is a critical event in invasion, removing the physical barrier and allowing neoplastic cells to move away from the tumor core. Most major protease classes are involved, including serine proteases such as plasmin, plasminogen activator (PA) and urokinase, and cysteine proteases such as cathepsin B, as well as several matrix metalloproteinases (MMPs) (19).

Cellular adhesion and de-adhesion are also important mechanisms. The adhesion to the surrounding matrix is modulated by glioma cells through substrate adhesion molecules, such as integrins and uPAR (urokinase-type plasminogen activator receptor) as well as antiadhe-

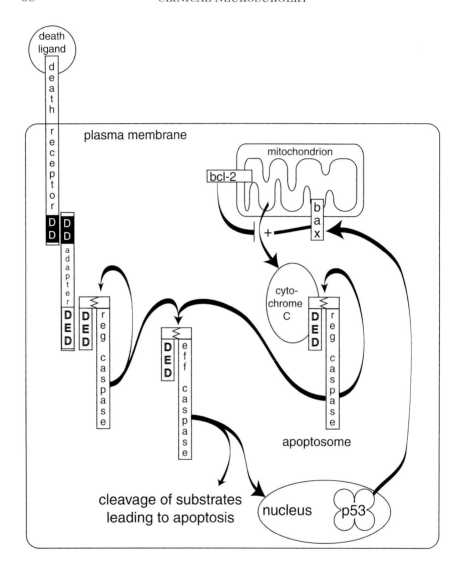

Fig. 6.6 Apoptosis. A diagram showing simplified schemas of the two major apoptosis pathways: the extrinsic and intrinsic. In the extrinsic pathway, binding of a death ligand to its receptor causes receptor clustering and a recruitment of adapter proteins and regulatory caspases via death domains (DD) and death effector domains (DED), respectively. This causes activation of regulatory caspases which cleave their own pro-domains and those of effector caspases, indicated by arrows. The activated effector caspases then dismantle the cell, including the nucleus. In the intrinsic pathway the release of cytochrome C, for example in response to increased bax expression, triggered by DNA damage and p53 activation, causes the formation of the apoptosome. This protein complex also contains apaf1 and regulatory caspases, which become activated, resulting in the activation of effector caspases.

Model of Distant Recurrences in Malignant Glioma

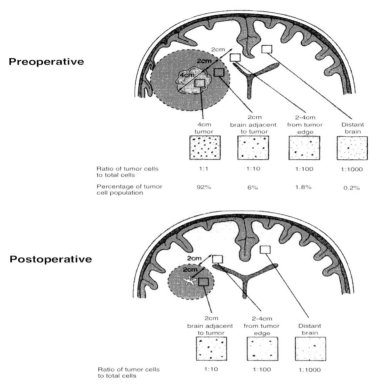

FIG. 6.7 Model of distant recurrences in malignant glioma. The model gives an estimate of the number of tumor cells and its ratio with the normal cells before (upper panel) and after (lower panel) gross total resection of the tumor. [Adapted with permission. Wilson CB: Glioblastoma: The past, the present, and the future, in *Clinical Neurosurgery.* Baltimore, Williams & Wilkins, 1992, p 37.]

sion molecules such as SPARC (secreted protein, acidic and rich in cysteine) (20–23). Integrins are the major membrane-associated molecules involved in modulating invasion, interacting with specific ECM-associated proteins to induce intracellular signaling events necessary to promote cell migration. Focal adhesion kinase (FAK) protein appears to be one of the signaling pathways *(Fig. 6–8)* (24, 25). The motility of glioma cells involves the cytoskeleton, adhesion plaque complexes and membrane extensions (also called invadopodia). Moreover, motility factors with in vitro chemotactic and chemokinetic effects have been described and could play a role in invasiveness (26). Finally, some growth factors seem to have a role in tumor cell shedding and migration in glioma models (27). Invasiveness is the major target for many therapies, including the use of antiprotease, antimotility, and anti-growth factor agents as well as signal transduction inhibitors.

Invasion: Integrin Signaling FAK

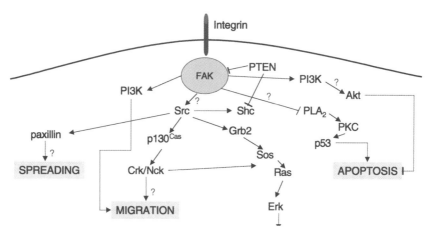

FIG. 6.8 Invasion—integrin/FAK signaling. Integrins interact with ECM-associated proteins to promote migration. Since integrins lack catalytic activity, the recruitment and activation of FAK to focal adhesions is believed to be necessary to transduce the external signal. FAK's catalytic domain becomes activated upon binding to the integrin or through the binding of integrin-associated proteins such as talin or paxillin. FAK then activates P13K protein involved in migration. Alternatively, src can activate FAK-associated p130cas and NCK to promote migration, and src-associated phosphorylation of paxillin participates also in spreading. FAK also activates signaling pathways involved in proliferation and apoptosis.

4. Angiogenesis

To continue growing, a tumor must induce the development of new microvessels from existing ones. The recruitment and proliferation of new vessels, which are dysmorphic and without an intact blood-brain barrier, result in areas of contrast enhancement on imaging. The angiogenic response requires a cascade of biochemical events, including protease secretion, basement membrane remodeling, endothelial cell proliferation, and migration to form capillary sprouts and neovascular tubule formation. The major players include: (1) proteases and protease systems such as MMPs, cysteine and serine proteases, and the extracellular proteosome (EP); (2) basement membrane proteins such as tenascin and fibronectin; (3) endogenous activators such as collagenase activating factor (CAF) and endothelial cell-stimulating angiogenesis factor (ESAF); (4) endogenous inhibitors such as tissue inhibitors of metalloproteinases (TIMPs), angiostatin, endostatin and thrombospondin; and (5) angiogenic growth factors and receptors (e.g., VEGF, bFGF, TGFb).

VEGF appears to be the major growth factor associated with angiogenesis, operating through the activation of several signaling pathways *(Fig. 6.9)* (28–32). Other activators and inhibitors have been described

Angiogenesis: VEGF Signaling

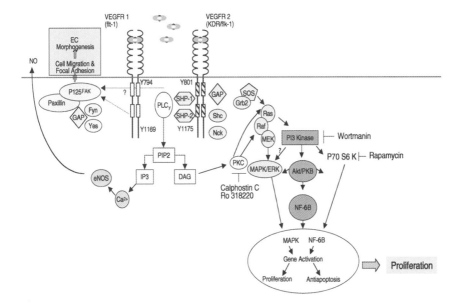

FIG. 6.9 Angiogenesis—VEGF signaling. VEGF appears to be the major growth factor in angiogenesis involving modulation of endothelial cell proliferation and migration. VEGF binding to the KDR/flk-1 receptor is the best-understood mechanism. Activated receptor recruits SHP-1 and SHP-2. The binding of PLC to the receptor via SH-2 binding sites results in the hydrolysis of PIP2 located in the plasma membrane, releasing IP3 and DAG into the intracellular compartment. IP3 immobilizes calcium from the endoplasmic reticulum. DAG and calcium activate protein kinase C that in turn activates the ras/raf pathway. The signaling pathway induced upon VEGF-induced KDR receptor dimerization also activates the ras-mediated proliferation pathway and antiapoptosis pathways elicited by other growth factors. By mechanisms that are still unclear, the activated receptor also induces the phosphorylation of FAK and paxillin promoting the formation of focal adhesions and thereby modulating endothelial cell adhesion and migration.

including some oncogenes, cytokines, and trace elements. An overall view of angiogenesis consists of a tightly regulated balance between oncogenes and tumor suppressor genes, stimulatory and inhibitory peptides, proteases and endogenous inhibitors, and microenvironmental factors such as oxygen or copper ion (33). A major event in initiation is the degradation of ECM and basement membrane by proteases that releases bound growth factors such as VEGF and FGF-2 and makes them available to bind to their receptors. The propagation phase involves upregulation of angiogenic factor receptors and generation of a microenvironment that is conducive to endothelial cell proliferation, migration and tube formation. The termination phase appears to involve TGFb for vessel cannulation and serum protease inhibitors leading to new basement membrane synthesis (34). Since physiologic angiogenesis is limited to wound healing, menses, and trophoblast implantation, tumor angiogenesis has become an excellent specific therapeutic target.

Thus, it is evident that the immediate environment surrounding the tumor plays a pivotal role in modulating the tumor phenotype, including proliferation, invasion, and angiogenesis. Identification of extracellular inducers, their interacting receptors, and characterization of their signal transduction pathways will permit the design of gene-specific or pathway-specific therapies. Although the pathways regulating these biological signals are complex, it is interesting to note that they do share overlapping proteins and other effector molecules. The targeting of such molecules may enable the design of therapeutic treatments that effectively block more than one phenotype (see *Figs. 6.5, 6.7, 6.8, 6.9*) An example discussed below is anti-invasive agents, which often have additional antiangiogenic property.

TREATMENT STRATEGIES

The following molecular strategies are based on glioma biology concepts outlined above and are aimed to selectively target neoplastic cells, with little or no effect on the surrounding normal brain parenchyma. Given the accelerating pace of drug discovery and the limited outcomes with conventional therapy for malignant glioma, significant opportunities exist to translate these new cytostatic agents in this field. Conventional treatment modalities are usually given in conjunction with these new therapeutic strategies in order to evaluate additional benefit and potentially increase the therapeutic index without jeopardizing tumor control. Classification of these new biologic therapies is problematic since several of these compounds have dual mechanisms of action that overlap each other. One approach is to categorize them according to their main mechanism of action or target, such as gene therapy, anti-

invasive agents, anti-angiogenic agents, immunotherapy, antiproliferative signal transduction inhibitors, and differentiating agents.

1. Gene Therapy

Gene therapy refers to the transfer of genetic material into the host's
cells with the aim of eliciting a therapeutic response. The recognition
of specific genetic molecular alterations underlying glial tumorigenesis
and technical advances in molecular biology has provided the necessary
tools for gene therapy. Gliomas are attractive candidates since they
rarely metastasize and are accessible to techniques of direct administration of the therapeutic agent. Gene therapy requires three essential
components: (1) a delivery vehicle, (2) a therapeutic gene, and (3) a delivery method. The delivery vehicles include replication-defective
viruses such as retroviruses with virus-producing cells (VPCs) or adenovirus, cationic liposomes, and plasmids. Therapeutic genes are used
in four applications. The first strategy is to reinsert a gene that has
been lost or mutated during tumorigenesis. Cell cycle control/apoptosis
genes are the most commonly used for this replacement strategy (e.g.,
p53). Derived from this first strategy are replication-conditional
viruses that take advantage of a genetic alteration to promote their
own proliferation and cause selective cytolysis. For example, an E1B-
attenuated adenovirus (E1B is a p53 inhibitor binding protein) that
only replicates in cells without functional p53 protein, is currently being evaluated in phase-I clinical trials (ONYX-015).

The second strategy involves delivery of drug-activating genes followed by administration of a prodrug that is then converted to a cytotoxic drug by the delivered genes. Such a strategy affects mostly transfected tumor cells but also neighboring tumor cells and normal cells
through a bystander effect (e.g., HSV thymidine kinase/ganciclovir, cytosine deaminase/5-fluorocytosine).

The third strategy uses the insertion of genes to promote cellular production of therapeutic peptides, including immune factors such as cytokines, lymphokines, and MHC molecules (immunogene therapy), or
anti-angiogenic molecules such as angiostatin.

Lastly, the fourth strategy inserts antisense cDNA to modify cellular
activity. The antisense oligonucleotide is usually designed to bind to the
mRNA of a protein involved either in cellular proliferation, invasion or
angiogenesis, such as VEGF. A VEGF antisense cDNA construct is still
in preclinical study.

The current delivery methods are either interstitial diffusion or systemic administration combined with blood-brain barrier disruption
agents (35, 36). So far, only a few phase-I/II clinical trials with a small

number of patients have been completed that demonstrate some activity (36). Ongoing gene therapy clinical trials include several drug-activating gene and prodrug strategies, mainly HSVTK/gancyclovir with either adenovirus or retrovirus/VPCs as vehicle. TP53 delivered by adenovirus and a few immunogene therapy trials are also underway.

Gene therapy has not been as successful as anticipated for several reasons. Limited delivery and transduction efficacy of viral vectors, heterogeneity of genetic alterations, and less importantly immune neutralization of vector all appear to affect therapeutic efficacy. Alternative delivery methods, such as interstitial convection-enhanced delivery using hydrostatic pressure to deliver the vector into the brain parenchyma, are currently being assessed in preclinical study.

The efficacy evaluation of gene therapy has been based on clinical and imaging responses. Parameters measured on imaging are similar to those used for cytotoxic agents and include the solid contrast enhancing volume that theoretically represents the pure solid cellular component of the tumor. This instrument is probably adequate for most gene therapy strategies currently used since they either induce apoptosis, cytotoxicity or cytolysis. As gene therapy with cytostatic strategies becomes available, other imaging parameters or methods will be necessary. These alternative methods are discussed under invasion and angiogenesis.

2. Anti-Invasive Agents

Great expectations arise from anti-invasive therapy since control of the invasive phenotype of glioma would represent a major step toward the cure of these neoplasms.

Several proteases involved in the invasive behavior of glioma are potential therapeutic target candidates by specific inhibitors. These protease inhibitors often have dual anti-invasive and anti-angiogenic properties owing to the overlapping role of proteases in both processes. Cysteine protease inhibitors (CPIs) are compounds that down-regulate protease activity such as cathepsin B. Cathepsin B uses laminin and collagen IV as substrates and has been localized in high concentrations at the invasive margin of glioma at both invadopodia and neovascular endothelia. In vitro and in vivo model systems using CPIs have shown interference with cell motility and tumor angiogenesis through inhibition of molecular interactions between the ECM and focal adhesion of glioma cells, and the proteolytic cascade. CPIs are still in preclinical study and no clinical trial is planned at this time.

Among the other protease inhibitors initially designed to overcome invasion but also found to have anti-angiogenic properties, Marimastat was the first MMPI (matrix metalloproteinase inhibitors) tested in humans. A phase-II trial using Marimastat alone in high-grade gliomas has been completed and did not show benefit [unpublished data, British Biotech, internal publication]. Another phase-II study is underway using Marimastat and BCNU in the same patient population. Prinomastat (AG3340), another MMPI without activity on MMP-1 potentially avoiding cartilaginous adverse effect is currently assessed in a comparative phase-II study for newly diagnosed GBM in conjunction with temozolomide. Col-3, a tetracycline analog, appears to inhibit several MMP activities and also down-regulates their expression. A combined phase-I/II study for recurrent high-grade gliomas, within the NABTT consortium is about to be activated.

Carboxyamidoimidazole (CAI) is a novel cytostatic agent that has shown antiproliferative, anti-invasive and anti-metastatic activities in preclinical studies. In vitro glioma models have shown angiogenesis and invasion inhibition at nontoxic concentrations. Moreover, CAI appears to induce apoptosis in glioma and endothelial cells (37). CAI acts as a signal transduction inhibitor possibly by calcium influx interference through voltage-gated and nonvoltage-gated calcium channels. This in turn produces several cellular effects leading to anticancer activity (38). CAI is highly lipophilic leading to a higher concentration in the central nervous system than in the serum. An anti-angiogenic synergistic effect with radiation has also been shown in preclinical studies. This makes CAI an ideal candidate for gliomas, and a phase-II clinical trial is currently underway for newly diagnosed GBM given concurrently and following radiation therapy.

EMD121974, an integrin antagonist discussed under antiangiogenic agents, also has potential anti-invasive properties, since the αvβ3 integrin is also expressed on glioma cells.

As is the case with anti-angiogenic agents, the evaluation of response with conventional imaging parameters such as solid contrast enhancement is not optimal. Potential alternative conventional MR imaging parameter would include FLAIR hypersignal abnormality extent, which theoretically represents the infiltrating component of the tumor. MR diffusion imaging appears to be more sensitive than FLAIR to determine the extent of infiltrating disease and could be more accurate in measuring actual response to anti-invasive agents (39, 40). Finally, MR spectroscopy providing measurement of important cellular metabolites would potentially be another instrument to measure response to cytostatic agents.

3. Anti-Angiogenic Agents

Anti-angiogenic agents can be divided into five categories: protease inhibitors, direct endothelial cell inhibitors, growth factor inhibitors,

inhibitors of endothelial-specific integrin signaling, and drugs with nonspecific or unique mechanisms. Only the most promising drugs currently under investigation for gliomas will be discussed here.

The protease inhibitors with anti-angiogenic properties, Marimastat (BB5416), Prinomastat (AG3340) and Col-3 have been discussed under anti-invasive agents since they have dual properties. TNP-470, a derivative of fumagillin, has been shown to inhibit bFGF- and PDGF-stimulated endothelial proliferation and is currently being evaluated in a phase-II trial for GBM. Thalidomide, developed as a sedative in the 1950s and removed from the market because of its teratogenic effects, has been recently studied in gliomas for its anti-angiogenic property. The drug appears to block angiogenesis growth factors such as bFGF and VEGF. Thalidomide has shown modest activity in recurrent high-grade gliomas (41). A combination of thalidomide with radiation or chemotherapy might better define its usefulness, and several trials are currently underway. Suramin is a polysulfonated molecule interfering with binding of growth factors such as PDGF, bFGF and VEGF to their receptors. It also inhibits induction of uPA. A NABTT phase-I/II trial for recurrent high-grade gliomas revealed marginal short-term activity but few delayed prolonged responses (42). In light of these few cases, a phase-II clinical trial for suramin in conjunction with radiation is currently underway for newly diagnosed high-grade glioma patients.

Other promising angiogenic growth factor antagonists include VEGF receptor signaling antagonists such as SU5416, SU6668 and PTK787/ZK22584. EMD121974 is a synthetic peptide that binds to vitronectin integrin receptors $\alpha v\beta 3$ and $\alpha v\beta 5$ and thereby inhibits their function in endothelial cell proliferation and attachment to ECM. A NABTT phase-I/II study has recently been opened for recurrent high-grade gliomas. Penicillamine appears to be a direct inhibitor of endothelial cell proliferation and migration and has several mechanisms of action in addition to copper chelation, including protease inhibition of uPA, tPA, and gelatinase B, and TIMP stabilization. The inhibition was markedly enhanced when combined with copper depletion. Copper acts as an obligatory cofactor for angiogenic activity of several growth factors, but also has independent effects on proliferation and directional migration of endothelial cells. A NABTT phase-II study has been recently completed for newly diagnosed GBM (43). As discussed above, CAI also has antiangiogenic activity through several mechanisms.

The advent of antiangiogenic agents has brought new challenges in evaluating the radiologic response to these agents. Imaging criteria for tumor response to cytotoxic agents do not seem appropriate for this class of agents. These cytostatic agents may not affect the contrast-enhancing volume and thus other noninvasive imaging techniques appear necessary to monitor antiangiogenesis. Several methods are being developed and include MR spectroscopy and MR perfusion imaging (44–46). Recent advances in brain imaging techniques such as MR perfusion imaging appear more suitable than conventional MR imaging for tumor vascularity evaluation. Several hemodynamic parameters can be measured by MR perfusion imaging. Relative cerebral blood volume (rCBV), including blood flow and volume, as well as vascular permeability can be measured using a dynamic susceptibility T2-weighted contrast technique with CBV- and permeability-weighted images, respectively. rCBV seems to correlate with capillary density and tumor grade, whereas permeability reflects the degree of blood-brain disruption typically associated with neovessels. These parameters would be expected to correlate with the degree of vascular density and they appear to be abnormal well beyond the contrast-enhancing region. The degree of vascular reactivity is another parameter that can be measured using vasodilators and blood oxygenation level-dependent (BOLD) contrast technique. Vascular reactivity relates to the degree of vascular maturation. Immature vessels, which are devoid of pericytes and smooth muscle cells, are highly dependent on VEGF for survival and are poorly reactive (47). Therefore, the degree of vascular reactivity might help to predict susceptibility to anti-angiogenic agents especially those acting through VEGF or its receptor. MR perfusion is a promising tool in evaluating the response to cytostatic agents with antiangiogenic properties.

4. Other Novel Approaches

Immunomodulation is a very diversified and exciting area of cancer treatment. Immunotherapy in glioma consists of four types of strategy: (1) cytokines including interleukin-2, interferon-β and TNF-α; (2) active immunotherapy with methods to prime the host immune system against the tumor; (3) adoptive immunotherapy with actual transfer of activated autologous immune cells; and (4) passive immunotherapy including monoclonal antibody and ligand-target combined with an effector molecule. Immunotherapy has shown modest activity in glioma, although only small series have been reported; however, the combination of active and adoptive immunotherapy appears promising (48, 49). Passive immunotherapy is also promising and involves the use of either a monoclonal antibody reacting to a glioma-specific antigen (e.g., tenascin, gp240, EGFR) or another molecule such as transferrin or IL-13 with chemoaffinity for a receptor overexpressed in gliomas. These are combined with an effector molecule such as a radioisotope (ex: [131]I), a cytotoxin (ex: pseudomonas exotoxin, diptheria toxin), or a drug. A study of IL-13 combined with pseudomonas exotoxin delivered by convection will be activated shortly within the NABTT consortium. Iodine

131 anti-tenascin and anti-gp240 monoclonal antibodies have been used in phase-I/II trials for recurrent malignant gliomas and promising results will prompt a phase-III trial in the near future (50, 51).

Other antiproliferative signal transduction inhibitors include protein kinase C (PKC) inhibitors. PKC is highly expressed in glioma and seems to correlate with the proliferation rate. PKC is involved in the transduction of mitogenic growth factor signals from the cell membrane to the nucleus. Tamoxifen has been found to inhibit PKC and to have activity against high-grade gliomas with a dose-dependent effect on survival (52, 53). Tamoxifen has also been evaluated in combination with other agents and is used in a few ongoing trials. Antisense oligonucleotides have been found ineffective in phase-II studies (54). Other kinase inhibitors include receptor antagonists such as SU101, which is a PDGF-R antagonist, SU5416 and SU6668, which block VEGF-R, and Iressa-blocking EGF-R are currently in clinical trials. Other potential signal transduction inhibitors include inhibitors of Src, a signaling protein, and inhibitors of farnesyl transferase, an enzymatic activity necessary for Ras protein to be inserted into the cytoplasmic membrane.

Tumor differentiating agents are used to revert the anaplastic or malignant phenotype of gliomas. 13-cis-retinoic acid (CRA), which also has antiproliferative activity, has shown activity against high-grade gliomas and is currently being evaluated in combination with other agents (55, 56). Lastly, the short chain fatty acid compound phenylbutyrate has shown good tolerability in phase-I studies for recurrent high-grade astrocytoma conducted in the NABTT consortium and will be evaluated in combination with radiation in newly diagnosed high-grade gliomas (57).

CONCLUSION

The understanding of molecular mechanisms of glioma biology has led to the identification of several potential therapeutic targets. The development of novel agents directed at these targets has resulted in numerous preclinical studies. Many of these promising compounds are currently being assessed in clinical trials, whereas a few others are already available. The treatment of glioma remains based on conventional modalities while we await the results of these trials and the design of further novel agents. It is unlikely that surgery, radiation therapy and chemotherapy will be replaced by these novel therapies in the near future, but it is hoped that gliomas will eventually be treated as chronic nonprogressive conditions.

REFERENCES

1. Dudas SP, Rempel SA: Development, molecular genetics, and gene therapy of glial tumors, in: Rock JP, Rosenblum ML, Shaw E, Cairncross G (eds): *The Practical*

Management of Low-Grade Primary Brain Tumors. Baltimore, Lippincott Williams & Wilkins, 1999, pp193–229.
2. Von Deimling A, Louis DN, Wiestler OD: Molecular pathways in the formation of gliomas. **Glia** 15:328–338, 1995.
3. Nutt CL, Noble M, Chambers AF, Cairncross JG: Differential expression of drug resistance genes and chemosensitivity in glial cell-lineages correlate with differential response of oligodendrogliomas and astrocytomas to chemotherapy. **Cancer Res** 60(17):4812–4818, 2000.
4. Noble M, Gutowski N, Bevan K, Engel U, Linskey M, Urenjak J, Bhakoo K, Williams S: From rodent glial precursor cell to human glial neoplasia in the oligodendrocyte-type-2 astrocyte lineage. **Glia** 15(3):333–340, 1995.
5. Armstrong RC, Dorn HH, Kufta CV, Friedman E, Dubois-Dalq ME: Pre-oligodendrocytes from adult human CNS. **J Neurosci** 12:1538–1547, 1992.
6. Reifenberger J, Ring GU, Gies U, et al.: Analysis of p53 mutation and epidermal growth factor receptor amplification in recurrent gliomas with malignant progression. **J Neuropathol Exp Neurol** 55:822–831, 1996
7. Cairncross JG, Ueki K, Zlatescu MC, et al.: Specific genetic predictors of chemotherapeutic response and survival in patients with anaplastic oligodendrogliomas. **J Natl Cancer Inst** 90:1473–1479, 1998.
8. Ino Y, Zlatescu MC, Sasaki H, et al.: Long survival and therapeutic responses in patients with histologically disparate high-grade gliomas demonstrating chromosome 1p loss. **J Neurosurg** 92:983–990, 2000.
9. Scherr CJ: Cancer cell cycles. **Science** 274:1672–1677, 1996.
10. Lala P, Provias J, Guha A: Growth factors and nervous system tumors, in Black P, Loeffler JS (eds): *Cancer of the Nervous System.* Cambridge, Blackwell Science, 1997, pp744–772.
11. Thornberry NA, Lazebnik Y: Caspases: Enemies within. **Science** 281:1312–1316, 1998.
12. Adams JM, Cory S: The Bcl-2 protein family: arbiters of cell survival. **Science** 281:1322–1326, 1998.
13. Ashkenazi A, Dixit VM: Death receptors: signaling and modulation. **Science** 281:1305–1308, 1998.
14. Vogelbaum MA, Tong JX, Perugu RP, Gutmann DH, Rich KM: Overexpression of bax in human glioma cell lines. **J Neurosurg** 91:483–489, 1999.
15. Ealovega MW, McGinnis PK, Sumantran VN, Clarke MF, Wicha MS: bcl-xs gene therapy induces apoptosis of human mammary tumors in nude mice. **Cancer Res** 56:1965–1969, 1996.
16. Bogler O, Furnari FB, Kindler-Roehrborn A, et al.: SETA: A novel SH_3 domain-containing adapter molecule associated with malignancy in astrocytes. **Neuro-onco!** 2:6–15., 2000.
17. Chen B, Borinstein SC, Gillis J, Sykes VW, Bogler O: The glioma associated protein SETA interacts with AIP1/Alix and modulates apoptosis in astrocytes. **J Biol Chem** 275:19275–19281, 2000.
18. Kelly PJ, Daumas-Duport C, Scheithauer BW, et al.: Stereotactic histologic correlations of computed tomography and magnetic resonance imaging-defined abnormalities in patients with glial neoplasm. **Mayo Clin Proc** 62:450–459, 1987.
19. Giese A, Westphal M: Glioma invasion in the central nervous system. **Neurosurgery** 39:235–252, 1996.
20. Rempel SA: Molecular biology of central nervous system tumors. **Curr Opin Oncol** 10:179–185, 1998.
21. Rempel SA, Golembieski WA, Ge S, Lemke N, Elisevich K, Mikkelsen T, Gutiérrez JA: SPARC: A signal of astrocytic neoplastic transformation and reactive response in hu-

man primary and xenograft gliomas. **J Neuropathol Exp Neurol** 57:1112–1121, 1998.

22. Rempel SA, Ge S, Gutiérrez JA: Characterization of SPARC overexpression in meningiomas, a candidate diagnostic marker of invasive meningiomas. **Clin Cancer Res** 5:237–241, 1999.

23. Golembieski WA, Ge S, Nelson K, Mikkelsen T, Rempel SA: Increased SPARC expression promotes U87 glioblastoma invasion *in vitro*. **Int J Dev Neurosci** 17:463–472, 1999.

24. Cary LA, Guan JL: Focal adhesion kinase in integrin-mediated signaling. **Front Biosci** 4:d102–113, 1999.

25. Howe A, Aplin AE, Alahari SK, Juliano RL: Integrin signaling and cell growth control. **Curr Opin Cell Biol** 10:220–231, 1998.

26. Ohnishi T, Arita N, Hayakawa T, et al.: Purification of motility factor (GMF) from human malignant glioma cells and its biological significance in tumor invasion. **Biochem Biophys Res Commun** 193:518–525, 1993.

27. Lund-Johanson M: Interaction between human glioma cells and fetal rat brain aggregate studied in chemically defined medium. **Invasion Metastasis** 10:113–128, 1990.

28. Zachary I: Vascular endothelial growth factor: How it transmits its signal. **Exp Nephrol** 6:480–487, 1997.

29. Wellner M, Maasch C, Kupprion C, et al.: The proliferation effect of vascular endothelial growth factor requires protein kinase C-α and protein kinase C-δ. **Arterioscler Thromb Vasc Biol** 19:178–184, 1999.

30. Thakker GD, Hajjar DP, Muller WA, Rosengart TK: The role of phosphatidylinositol 3-kinase in vascular endothelial factor signaling. **J Biol Chem** 274:10002–10007, 1999.

31. Ortega N, Hutchings H, Plouet J: Signal relays in the VEGF system. **Front Biosci** 4:d141–152, 1999.

32. Takahashi N, Seko Y, Noiri E, et al.: Vascular endothelial growth factor induces activation and subcellular translocation of focal adhesion kinase (p125[FAK]) in cultured rat cardiac myocytes. **Circ Res** 84:1194–1202. 1999.

33. Brem S: Angiogenesis and cancer control: From concept to therapeutic trial. **Cancer Control** 6:436–457, 1999.

34. Del Maestro RF: Angiogenesis, in Berger MS, Wilson CB (eds): *The Gliomas*. Philadelphia, WB Saunders Company, 1999.

35. Weyerbrock A, Oldfield EH: Gene transfer technologies for malignant gliomas. **Curr Opin Oncol** 11:168–173, 1999.

36. Sasaki M, Plate KH: Gene therapy of malignant glioma: Recent advance in experimental and clinical studies. **Ann Oncol** 9:1155–1166, 1998.

37. Shugang G, Rempel SA, Divine G, Mikkelsen T: Carboxyamido-triazole induces apoptosis in bovine aortic endothelial and human glioma cells. **Clin Cancer Res** 6:1248–1254, 2000.

38. Berlin J, Tutsch KD, Cleary J, et al.: Phase I clinical and pharmacokinetic study of oral carboxyamidotriazole, a signal transduction inhibitor. **J Clin Oncol** 15:781–789, 1997.

39. Gupta RK, Sinha U, Cloughesy TF, Alger JR: Inverse correlation between choline magnetic resonance spectroscopy signal intensity and the apparent diffusion coefficient in human glioma. **Magn Reson Med** 41:2–7, 1999.

40. Krabbe, Gideon P, Wagn P, et al.: MR diffusion imaging of human intracranial tumors. **Neuroradiology** 39:483–489, 1997.

41. Fine HA, Figg WD, Jaeckle K, et al.: Phase II trial of the antiangiogenic agent thalidomide in patients with recurrent high-grade gliomas. **J Clin Oncol** 18:708–715, 2000.

42. Grossman SA, Phuphanich S, Lesser G, et al.: Efficacy, toxicity and pharmacology of suramin in adult with recurrent high-grade astrocytomas [Abstract]. **Proc Am Soc Clin Oncol** 18:142a, 1999.
43. Brem S, Grossman SA, New P, et al.: Phase II study of penicillamine and reduction of copper, for angiosuppressive therapy of glioblastoma: Preliminary safety and feasibility study [Abstract]. **Proc Am Soc Clin Oncol** 19:172a, 2000.
44. Dennie J, Mandeville JB, Boxerman JL, et al.: NMR imaging of changes in vascular morphology due to tumor angiogenesis. **Magn Reson Med** 40:793–799, 1998.
45. Lev MH, Hochberg F: Perfusion magnetic resonance imaging to assess brain tumor responses to new therapies. **Cancer Control** 5:115–123, 1998.
46. Cha S, Knopp EA, Johnson G, et al.: Dynamic contrast-enhanced T2-weighted MR imaging of recurrent malignant gliomas treated with thalidomide and carboplatin. **Am J Neuroradiol** 21:81–89, 2000.
47. Abramovitch R, Dafni H, Smouha E, Benjamin LE, Neeman M: In vivo prediction of vascular susceptibility to vascular susceptibility endothelial growth factor withdrawal: Magnetic resonance imaging of C6 rat glioma in nude mice. **Cancer Res** 59:5012–5016, 1999.
48. Holladay FP, Heitz-Turner T, Bayer WL, Wood GW: Autologous tumor cell vaccination with adoptive cellular immunotherapy in patients with grade III/IV astrocytoma. **J Neurooncol** 27:179–189, 1996.
49. Plautz GE, Barnett GH, Miller DW, et al.: Systemic T cell adoptive of malignant gliomas. **J Neurosurg** 89:42–51, 1998.
50. Cokgor I, Akabani G, Friedman A, et al.: Results of a phase II trial in the treatment of recurrent patients with brain tumor treated with iodine 131 anti-tenascin monoclonal antibody 81C6 via surgically created resection cavities [Abstract]. **Proc Am Soc Clin Oncol** 19:162a, 2000.
51. Bigner DD, Brown M, Coleman RE, et al.: Phase I studies of treatment of malignant glioma and neoplastic meningitis with ^{131}I-radiolabeled monoclonal antibodies anti-tenascin 81C6 and anti-chondroitin proteoglycan sulfate Mel-14 F(ab')2: A preliminary report. **J Neurooncol** 24:109–122, 1995.
52. Couldwell WT, Hinton DR, Surnock AA, et al.: Treatment of recurrent malignant gliomas with chronic oral high-dose tamoxifen. **Clin Cancer Res** 2:619–622, 1996.
53. Vertosick FT, Selker RG, Arena V: A dose escalation study of tamoxifen therapy in patients with recurrent glioblastoma multiforme [Abstract]. **J Neurosurg** 80:385A, 1994.
54. Alavi JB, Grossman SA, Supko J, et al.: Efficacy, toxicity, and pharmacology of an antisense oligonucleotide directed against protein kinase C-a (ISIS 3521) delivered as a 21-day continuous intravenous infusion in patients with recurrent high-grade astrocytomas (HGA) [Abstract]. **Proc Am Soc Clin Oncol** 19:167a, 2000.
55. Yung WA, Kyritsis AP, Gleason MJ, Levin V: Treatment of recurrent malignant gliomas with high-dose 13-cis-retinoic acid. **Clin Cancer Res** 2:1931–1935, 1996.
56. Jaeckle KA, Yung WA, Prados M, et al.: Phase II evaluation of temozolomide and 13-cis-retinoic acid (Isotretinoin; CRA) for the treatment of recurrent ANC progressive malignant gliomas (NABTC 98-03) [Abstract]. **Proc Am Soc Clin Oncol** 19:162a, 2000.
57. Fisher JD, Carducci MA, Baker SD, et al.: Dose escalation study of oral phenylbutyrate (PB) in patients with refractory high grade astrocytomas: Maximum tolerated dose (MTD), toxicity profile, pharmacology, and survival [Abstract]. **Proc Am Soc Clin Oncol** 19:166a, 2000.

CHAPTER

7

Joint Replacement in Neurosurgery

VINCENT C. TRAYNELIS, M.D.

The intervertebral disc constitutes a major component of the functional spinal unit. Aging results in deterioration of the biological and mechanical integrity of the intervertebral discs. Disc degeneration may produce pain directly or perturb the functional spinal unit in such a way as to produce a number of painful entities. Whether through direct or indirect pathways, intervertebral disc degeneration is a leading cause of pain and disability in adults (1). Approximately 80% of Americans experience at least a single episode of significant back pain in their lifetime, and for many individuals, spinal disorders become a lifelong malady. The morbidity associated with disc degeneration and its spectrum of associated spinal disorders is responsible for significant economic and social costs. The treatment of this disease entity in the United States is estimated to exceed $60 billion annually in health care costs (2). The indirect economic losses associated with lost wages and decreased productivity are staggering.

Age-related disc changes occur early and are progressive. Almost all individuals experience diminished nuclear water content and increased collagen content by the 4th decade. This desiccation and fibrosis of the disc blur the nuclear/annular boundary (3).

These senescent changes allow repeated minor rotational trauma to produce circumferential tears between annular layers. These defects, usually in the posterior or posterolateral portions of the annulus, may enlarge and combine to form one or more radial tears through which nuclear material may herniate (4). Pain and dysfunction due to compression of neural structures by herniated disc fragments are widely recognized phenomena. It should be noted, however, that annular injuries may be responsible for axial pain with or without the presence of a frank disc herniation (5, 6). Progression of the degenerative process alters intradiscal pressures, causing a relative shift of axial load-bearing to the peripheral regions of the endplates and facets. This transfer of biomechanical loads appears to be associated with the development of both facet and ligament hypertrophy (7, 8). There is a direct relation between disc degeneration and osteophyte formation (9). In particular, deterioration of the intervertebral disc leads to increased traction on the attachment of the outermost annular fibers, thereby predisposing to the growth of laterally situated osteophytes (10). Disc degeneration also results in a significant shift of the instantaneous axis of rotation of the functional spinal unit (11). The exact long-term consequences of such a perturbation of spinal biomechanics are unknown, but it has been postulated that this change promotes abnormal loading of adjacent segments and an alteration in spinal balance.

Nonoperative therapeutic options for individuals with neck and back pain include rest, heat, analgesics, physical therapy, and manipulation. These treatments fail in a significant number of patients. Current surgical management options for spinal disease include decompressive surgery, decompression with fusion, and arthrodesis alone.

Greater that 200,000 discectomies are performed annually in the United States (12). Although discectomy is exceptionally effective in promptly relieving significant radicular pain, the overall success rates for these procedures range from 48% to 89% (13–15). In general, the return of pain increases with the length of time from surgery. Ten years following lumbar discectomy, 50 to 60% of patients will experience significant back pain and 20 to 30% will suffer from recurrent sciatica (16). In general, the reasons for these less than optimal results are probably related to continued degenerative processes, recurrent disc rupture, instability, and spinal stenosis (17, 18).

There are several specific reasons for failure of surgical discectomy. The actual disc herniation may not have been the primary pain generator in some patients. A number of relapses are due to disc space collapse. Although the disc height is often decreased in the preoperative patient with a herniated nucleus pulposus, it is an exceedingly common occurrence following surgical discectomy (14). Disc space narrowing is very important in terms of decreasing the size of the neural foramina and altering facet loading and function. Disc space narrowing increases intra-articular pressure, and abnormal loading patterns have been shown to produce biochemical changes in the intra-articular cartilage at both the level of the affected disc and the adjacent level (19, 20). The entire process predisposes to the development of hypertrophic changes of the articular processes (21). Disc space narrowing also allows for rostral and anterior displacement of the superior facet. This displacement of the superior facet becomes significant when it impinges upon the exiting nerve root which is traversing an already compromised foramen (4).

Destabilization of the functional spinal unit is another potential source of continued pain. A partial disc excision is associated with significant increases in flexion, rotation, lateral bending, and extension across the affected segment. As the amount of nuclear material which is removed increases, stiffness across the level decreases accordingly (22). Disc excision has also been demonstrated to lead to instability at the level above the injured segment in cadaver studies. This situation has been documented to occur clinically as well (23–25).

Arthrodesis, with or without decompression, is another means of surgically treating symptomatic spondylosis in all regions of the mobile spine. Fusion has the capability of eliminating segmental instability, maintaining normal disc space height, preserving sagittal balance, and halting further degeneration at the operated level. Discectomy with fusion has been the major surgical treatment for symptomatic cervical spondylosis for over 40 years (26–28). A report in 1986 estimated that over 70,000 lumbar fusions were performed annually in the United States (29). Given the explosive development of the instrumentation and interbody device technology, the current annual number of patients treated with a lumbar fusion is even higher. The major rationale for spinal arthrodesis is that pain can be relieved by eliminating motion across a destabilized or degenerated segment (30). Good to excellent results have been reported in 52 to 100% of anterior lumbar interbody fusions and 50 to 95% of posterior lumbar interbody fusions (31–35).

Spinal fusion is not, however, a benign procedure. In numerous patients, recurrent symptoms develop years after the original procedure. Fusion perturbs the biomechanics of adjacent levels. Hypertrophic facet arthropathy, spinal stenosis, disc degeneration, and osteophyte formation have all been reported to occur at levels adjacent to a fusion, and these pathological processes are responsible for pain in many patients (17, 18, 36–41). The long-term results of lumbar fusions have been reported by Lehman et al. These investigators described a series of patients who were treated with uninstrumented fusions and followed for 21 to 33 years. Roughly half the patients had lumbar pain requiring medication at last follow-up, and about 15% had been treated with further surgery over the study period (38). Finally, there are a number of other drawbacks to fusion as a treatment for spinal pain, including loss of spinal mobility, graft collapse resulting in alterations of sagittal balance, autograft harvest site pain, and the possibility of alteration of muscular synergy.

Sir John Charnley revolutionized modern orthopedics with his development of total hip replacement (42). Today, hip and knee arthroplasties are two of the most highly rated surgical procedures in terms of patient satisfaction. It is possible that the development of an artificial disc may impact the treatment of degenerative disc disease in a similar fashion. Although the challenges associated with developing a prosthetic disc are great, the potential to improve the lives of many individuals suffering from symptoms of spinal spondylosis is tremendous.

The idea of spinal disc replacement is not new. One of the first attempts to perform disc arthroplasty was undertaken by Nachemson 40 years ago (43). Fernstrom attempted to reconstruct intervertebral discs by implanting stainless steel balls in the disc space (44). 1966 he published a report on 191 implanted prostheses in 125 patients. Subsidence occurred in 88% of patients over a 4- to 7-year period of follow-up. These pioneering efforts were followed by more than a decade of research on the degenerative processes of the spine, spinal biomechanics, and biomaterials before serious efforts to produce a prosthetic disc resumed.

There are a number of factors which must be considered in the design and implantation of an effective disc prosthesis. The device must maintain the proper intervertebral spacing, allow for motion, and provide stability. Natural discs also act as shock absorbers, and this may be an important quality to incorporate into prosthetic disc design, particularly when considered for multilevel lumbar reconstruction. The artificial disc must not shift significant axial load to the facets. Placement of the artificial disc must be done in such a way as to avoid the destruction of important spinal elements such as the facets and ligaments. The importance of these structures cannot be overemphasized. Facets not only contribute strength and stability to the spine, but they could be a source of pain. This may be especially important to determine prior to disc arthroplasty because it is currently believed that disc replacement will probably be ineffective as a treatment for facet pain. Excessive ligamentous laxity may adversely affect disc prosthesis outcome by predisposing to implant migration or spinal instability.

An artificial disc must exhibit tremendous endurance. The average age of a patient needing a lumbar disc replacement has been estimated to be 35 years. This means that to avoid the need for revision surgery, the prosthesis must last 50 years. It has been estimated that an individual will take 2 million strides per year and perform 125,000 significant bends; therefore, over the 50-year life expectancy of the artificial disc, there would be over 106 million cycles. This estimate discounts the subtle disc motion which may occur with the 6 million breaths taken per year (45).

A number of factors in addition to endurance must be considered when choosing the materials with which to construct an intervertebral disc prosthesis. The materials must be biocompatible and display no corrosion. They must not incite any significant inflammatory response.

The fatigue strength must be high and the wear debris minimal. Finally, it would be ideal if the implant were imaging "friendly."

All currently proposed intervertebral disc prostheses are contained within the disc space; therefore, allowance must be made for variations in patient size, level, and height. There may be a need for instrumentation to restore collapsed disc space height prior to placement of the prosthesis.

The intervertebral disc prosthesis ideally would replicate normal range of motion in all planes. At the same time it must constrain motion. A disc prosthesis must reproduce physiologic stiffness in all planes of motion plus axial compression. Furthermore, it must accurately transmit physiologic stress. For example, if the global stiffness of a device is physiologic but a significant nonphysiologic mismatch is present at the bone–implant interface, there may be bone resorption, abnormal bone deposition, endplate or implant failure. The disc prosthesis must have immediate and long-term fixation to bone. Immediate fixation may be accomplished with screws, staples, or "teeth" which are integral to the implant. While these techniques may offer long-term stability, other options include porous or macrotexture surfaces which allow for bone ingrowth. Regardless of how fixation is achieved, there must also be the capability for revision.

Finally, the implant must be designed and constructed such that failure of any individual component will not result in a catastrophic event. Furthermore, neural, vascular, and spinal structures must be protected and spinal stability maintained in the event of an accident or unexpected loading.

Prosthetic discs have been constructed based on the utilization of one of the following primary properties: hydraulic, elastic, mechanical, and composite. Hydrogel disc replacements primarily have hydraulic properties. Hydrogel prostheses are used to replace the nucleus while retaining the annulus fibrosis. One potential advantage is that such a prosthesis may have the capability of percutaneous placement. The PDN implant is a nucleus replacement which consists of a hydrogel core constrained in a woven polyethylene jacket (Raymedica, Inc., Bloomington, MN) *(Fig. 7.1)* (46, 47). The pellet-shaped hydrogel core is compressed and dehydrated to minimize its size prior to placement. Upon implantation, the hydrogel immediately begins to absorb fluid and expand. The tightly woven ultrahigh molecular weight polyethylene (UHMWPE) allows fluid to pass through to the hydrogel. This flexible but inelastic jacket permits the hydrogel core to deform and reform in response to changes in compressive forces yet constrains horizontal and vertical expansion upon hydration. Although most hydration takes place in the first 24 hours after implant, it takes approximately 4 to 5

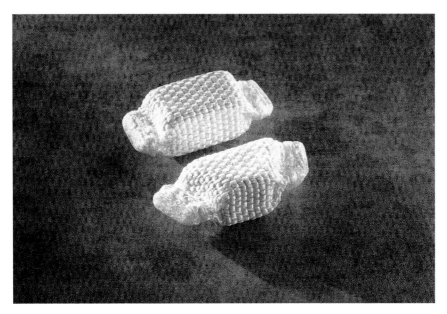

FIG. 7.1 PDN Prosthetic Disc Nucleus

days for the hydrogel to reach maximum expansion. Placement of two PDN implants within the disc space provides the lift that is necessary to restore and maintain disc space height. This device has been extensively assessed with mechanical and *in vitro* testing, and the results have been good (46, 47). Schönmayr et al. reported on 10 patients treated with the PDN with a minimum of 2 years follow-up (47). Significant improvement was seen in both the Prolo and Oswestry scores, and segmental motion was preserved. Overall, 8 patients were considered to have an excellent result. Migration of the implant was noted in 3 patients, but only 1 required reoperation. One patient, a professional golfer, responded favorably for 4 months until his pain returned. He had marked degeneration of his facets, and his pain was relieved by facet injections. He underwent a fusion procedure and since has done well. The devices have been primarily inserted via a posterior route. Bertagnoli recently reported placing the PDN via an anterolateral transpsoatic route (48). The PDN is undergoing clinical evaluation in Europe, South Africa, and the United States.

Two elastic type disc prostheses are the Acroflex prosthesis proposed by Steffee and the thermoplastic composite of Lee (49, 50). The first Acroflex disc consisted of a hexene-based polyolefin rubber core vulcanized to two titanium endplates. The endplates had 7 mm posts for immediate fixation and were coated with sintered 250 micron titanium beads on each surface to provide an increased surface area for bony ingrowth and adhesion of the rubber. The disc was manufactured in several sizes and underwent extensive fatigue testing prior to implantation. Only 6 patients were implanted before the clinical trial was stopped due to a report that 2-mercaptobenzothiazole, a chemical used in the vulcanization process of the rubber core, was possibly carcinogenic in rats (51). The 6 patients were evaluated after a minimum of 3 years, at which time the results were graded as follows: 2 excellent, 1 good, 1 fair, and 2 poor (49). One of the protheses in a patient with a poor result developed a tear in the rubber at the junction of vulcanization. The second generation Acroflex-100 consists of an HP-100 silicone elastomer core bonded to two titanium endplates (DePuy Acromed, Raynham, MA) *(Fig. 7.2)*. In 1993 the FDA approved 13 additional patients for implantation (52). The results of this study have not yet been published.

Lee et al. have published a report on the development of two different disc prostheses created in a manner to simulate the anisotropic properties of the normal intervertebral disc (50). I am not aware of any publications describing the implantation of these devices in humans.

Several articulating pivot or ball type disc prostheses have been developed for the lumbar spine. Hedman and Kostuik developed a set of

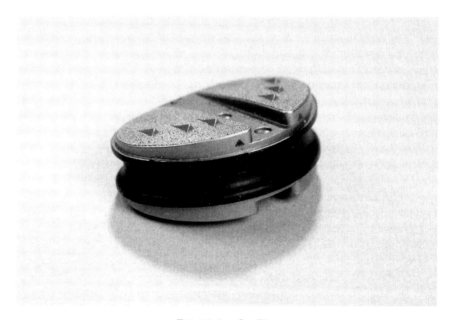

FIG. 7.2 Acroflex Disc

cobalt-chromium-molybdenum alloy hinged plates with an interposed spring (53). These devices have been tested in sheep. At 3 and 6 months post-implantation there was no inflammatory reaction noted and none of the prostheses migrated. Two of the three 6-month implants had significant bony ingrowth. It is not clear whether motion was preserved across the operated segments (45). I am not aware of any publications describing the implantation of these devices in humans.

Dr. Thierry Marnay of France developed an articulating disc prosthesis with a polyethylene core (Aesculap AG & Co. KG., Tuttlingen, Germany). The metal endplates have two vertical wings and the surfaces which contact the endplates are plasma-sprayed with titanium. Good to excellent results were reported in the majority of patients receiving this implant (54).

The most widely implanted disc to date is the Link SB Charité disc (Waldemar Link GmbH & Co, Hamburg, Germany). Currently more than 2000 of these lumbar intervertebral prostheses have been implanted worldwide (35). The Charité III consists of a biconvex ultra high molecular weight polyethylene (UHMWPE) spacer. There is a radiopaque ring around the spacer for x-ray localization. The spacers are available in different sizes. This core spacer interfaces with two separate endplates. The endplates are made of casted cobalt-chromium-molybdenum alloy, each with three ventral and dorsal teeth. The endplates are coated with titanium and hydroxyapatite to promote bone bonding *(Fig. 7.3)*. Although there is great concern regarding wear debris in hip prostheses in which UHMWPE articulates with metal, this does not appear to occur in the Charité III (55). This prosthesis has been implanted in over a thousand European patients with relatively good results.

In 1994 Griffith et al. reported the results in 93 patients with 1-year follow-up (56). Significant improvements in pain, walking distance, and mobility were noted. 6.5% of patients experienced a device failure, dislocation, or migration. There were 3 ring deformations, and 3 patients required reoperation. Lemaire et al. described the results of implantation of the SB Charité III disc in 105 patients with a mean of 51 months of follow-up (57). There was no displacement of any of the implants, but 3 settled. The failures were felt to be secondary to facet pain. David described a cohort of 85 patients reviewed after a minimum of at least 5 years post-implantation of the Charité prosthesis (58). 97% of the patients were available for follow-up. 68% had good or better results. 14 patients reported the result as poor. Eleven of these patients underwent secondary arthrodesis at the prosthesis level. Despite the concern of many other investigators, it is interesting to note that David treated 20 patients with spondylolisthesis or retrolisthesis with an outcome identical to that of the entire group. Clinical trials using the Charité III

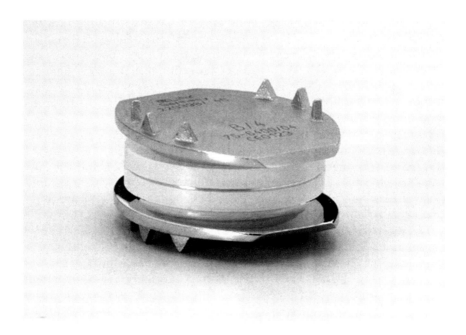

FIG. 7.3 Link SB Charité Disc

prosthesis are ongoing in Europe, the United States, Argentina, China, Korea, and Australia.

There have been several reports on results from a cervical disc prosthesis which was originally developed in Bristol, England. This device was designed by Cummins (59). The original design has been modified. The second generation of the Cummins disc is a ball and socket type device constructed of stainless steel. It is secured to the vertebral bodies with screws. Cummins et al. described 20 patients who were followed for an average of 2.4 years. Patients with radiculopathy improved, and those with myelopathy either improved or were stabilized. Of this group, only 3 experienced continued axial pain. Two screws broke, and there were two partial screw back-outs. These did not require removal of the implant. One joint was removed because it was "loose." The failure was due to a manufacturing error. At the time of removal, the joint was firmly imbedded in the bone and was covered by a smooth scar anteriorly. Detailed examination revealed that the ball and socket fit was asymmetric. It is important to note that the surrounding tissues did not contain any significant wear debris. Joint motion was preserved in all but 2 patients *(Fig. 7.4)*. Both of these patient had implants at the C6–7 level which were so large that the facets were completely separated.

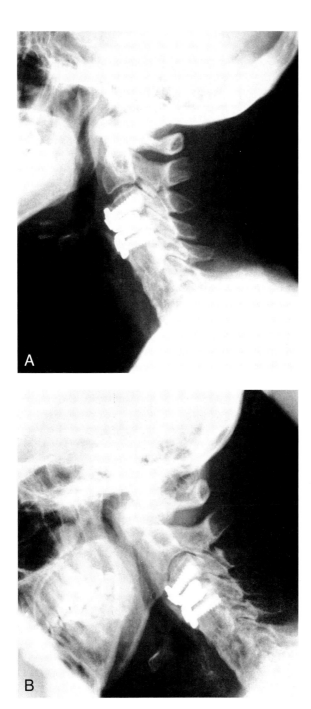

FIG. 7.4 The Bristol Disc. (*A*) Lateral cervical radiograph in extension. (*B*) Lateral cervical radiograph in flexion.

This size mismatch was felt to be the reason motion was not maintained. Subsidence did not occur. This disc prosthesis is currently being evaluated in additional clinical studies in Europe and Australia.

The Bryan Cervical Disc System (Spinal Dynamics Corporation, Seattle) is designed based on a proprietary, low friction, wear resistant, elastic nucleus. This nucleus is located between and articulates with anatomically shaped titanium plates (shells) that are fitted to the vertebral body endplates *(Fig. 7.5)*. The shells are covered with a rough porous coating. A flexible membrane that surrounds the articulation forms a sealed space containing a lubricant to reduce friction and prevent migration of any wear debris that may be generated. It also serves to prevent the intrusion of connective tissue. The implant allows for normal range of motion in flexion/extension, lateral bending, axial rotation, and translation. The implant is manufactured in five sizes ranging from 14 mm to 18 mm in diameter. The initial clinical experience with the Bryan Total Cervical Disc Prosthesis has been promising (Jan Goffin, personal communication, March 2000). Fifty-two devices were implanted in 51 patients by 8 surgeons in 6 centers in Belgium, France, Sweden, Germany, and Italy. There were no serious operative or postoperative complications. Twenty-six of the patients have been followed for 6 months, and complete clinical and radiographic data is available on 23 patients. 92% of the patients were classified as excellent or good outcomes at last follow-up. Flexion/extension motion was preserved in all patients, and there was no significant subsidence or migration of the devices.

In conclusion, spinal disc replacement is not only possible but is an exciting area of clinical investigation which has the potential of revolutionizing the treatment of spinal degeneration. The development of a

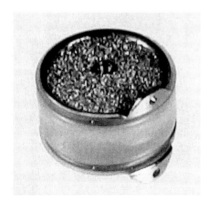

Fig. 7.5 Bryan Cervical Disc Prosthesis

prosthetic disc poses tremendous challenges, but the results from initial efforts have been promising. The future for this field, and our patients, is bright.

REFERENCES

1. Rothman RH, Simeone FA, Bernini PM: Lumbar disc disease, in Rothman RH, Simeone FA, eds: *The spine.* 2nd ed. Philadelphia, WB Saunders, 1982, pp 508–645.
2. Weinstein JN, ed: *Clinical efficacy and outcome in the diagnosis and treatment of low back pain.* New York, Raven Press, 1992.
3. Pearce RH, Grimmer BJ, Adams ME: Degeneration and the chemical composition of the human lumbar intervertebral disc. **J Orthop Res** 5:198–205, 1987.
4. Kirkaldy-Willis WH, Wedge JH, Yong-Hing K, Reilly J: Pathology and pathogenesis of spondylosis and stenosis. **Spine** 3:319–328, 1978.
5. Crock HV: Internal disc disruption: A challenge to disc prolapse 50 years on. **Spine** 11:650–653, 1986.
6. Kääpä E, Holm S, Han X, Takala T, Kovanen V, Vanharanta H: Collagens in the injured porcine intervertebral disc. **J Orthop Res** 12:93–102, 1994.
7. Weinstein PR: Anatomy of the lumbar spine, in Hardy RW, ed: *Lumbar disc disease.* New York, Raven Press, 1982, pp 5–15.
8. Keller TS, Hansson TH, Abram AC, Spengler DM, Panjabi MM: Regional variations in the compressive properties of lumbar vertebral trabeculae. Effects of disc degeneration. **Spine** 14:1012–1019, 1989.
9. Vernon-Roberts B, Pirie CJ: Degenerative changes in the intervertebral discs of the lumbar spine and their sequelae. **Rheumatol Rehab** 16:13–21, 1977.
10. Macnab I: The traction spur: an indicator of segmental instability. **J Bone Joint Surg** 53A:663–670, 1971.
11. Pennal GF, Conn GS, McDonald G, Dale G, Garside H: Motion studies of the lumbar spine: A preliminary report. **J Bone Joint Surg** 54B:442–452, 1972.
12. LaRocca H: Failed lumbar surgery: principles of management, in Weinstein JN, Wiesel SW, eds: *The lumbar spine.* Philadelphia, W.B. Saunders, 1990, pp 872–881.
13. Crawshaw C, Frazer AM, Merriam WF, Mulholland RC, Webb JK: A comparison of surgery and chemonucleolysis in the treatment of sciatica: a propsective randomized trial. **Spine** 9:195–198, 1984.
14. Hanley EN, Shapiro DE: The development of low-back pain after excision of a lumbar disc. **J Bone Joint Surg** 71A:719–721, 1989.
15. Nordby EJ: A comparison of discectomy and chemonucleolysis. **Clin Orthop** 200:279–283, 1985.
16. Hutter CG: Spinal stenosis and posterior lumbar interbody fusion. **Clin Orthop** 193:103–114, 1985.
17. Hsu KY, Zucherman J, White A, Reynolds J, Goldwaite N: Deterioration of motion segments adjacent to lumbar spine fusions. Transactions of the North American Spine Society, 1988.
18. Vaughan PA, Malcolm BW, Maistrelli GL: Results of L4-L5 disc excision alone versus disc excision and fusion. **Spine** 13:690–695, 1988.
19. Dunlop RB, Adams MA, Hutton WC: Disc space narrowing and the lumbar facet joints. **J Bone Joint Surg** 66B:706–710, 1984.
20. Gotfried Y, Bradford DS, Oegema TR Jr: Facet joint changes after chemonucleolysis-induced disc space narrowing. **Spine** 11:944–950, 1986.
21. Schneck CD: The anatomy of lumbar spondylosis. **Clin Orthop** 193:20–37, 1985.

22. Goel VK, Goyal S, Clark C, Nishiyama K, Nye T: Kinematics of the whole lumbar spine: effect of discectomy. **Spine** 10:543–554, 1985.
23. Goel VK, Nishiyama K, Weinstein JN, Liu YK: Mechanical properties of lumbar spinal motion segments as affected by partial disc removal. **Spine** 11:1008–1012, 1986.
24. Tibrewal SB, Pearcy MJ, Portek I, Spivey J: A prospective study of lumbar spinal movements before and after discectomy using biplanar radiography: Correlation of clinical and radiographic findings. **Spine** 10:455–460, 1985.
25. Stokes IAF, Wilder DG, Frymoyer JW, Pope MH: Assessment of patients with low-back pain by biplanar radiographic measurement of intervertebral motion. **Spine** 6:233–240, 1981.
26. Cloward RB: The anterior approach for removal of ruptured cervical disks. **J Neurosurg** 15:602–617, 1958.
27. Cloward RB: Treatment of acute fractures and fracture-dislocations of the cervical spine by vertebral-body fusion. **J Neurosurg** 18:201–209, 1961.
28. Smith GW, Robinson RA: The treatment of certain cervical-spine disorders by anterior removal of the intervertebral disc and interbody fusion. **J Bone Joint Surg** 40A:607–624, 1958.
29. Rutkow IM: Orthopaedic operations in the United States, 1979 through 1983. **J Bone Joint Surg** 68A:716–719, 1986.
30. White AA, Panjabi MM: *Clinical biomechanics of the spine.* 2nd ed. Philadelphia, JB Lippincott, 1990.
31. Watkins RG: Results of anterior interbody fusion, in White AH, Rothman RH, Ray CD, eds: *Lumbar spine surgery: techniques and complications.* St. Louis, CV Mosby, 1987, pp 408–432.
32. Zucherman JF, Selby D, DeLong WB: Failed posterior lumbar interbody fusion, in White AH, Rothman RH, Ray CD, eds: *Lumbar spine surgery: techniques and complications.* St. Louis, CV Mosby, 1987, pp 296–305.
33. Yuan HA, Garfin SR, Dickman CA, Mardjetko SM: A historical cohort study of pedicle screw fixation in thoracic, lumbar, and sacral spine fusions. **Spine** 19 (Suppl 20):2279S–2296S, 1994.
34. Ray CD: Threaded titanium cages for lumber interbody fusions. **Spine** 22:667–680, 1997.
35. Kuslich SD, Ulstrom CL, Griffith SL, Ahern JW, Dowdle JD: The Bagby and Kuslich method of lumbar interbody fusion. History, techniques, and 2-year follow-up results of a United States prospective, multicenter trial. **Spine** 23:1267–1279, 1998.
36. Lee CK: Accelerated degeneration of the segment adjacent to a lumbar fusion. **Spine** 13:375–377, 1988.
37. Frymoyer JW, Hanley EN Jr, Howe J, Kuhlmann D, Matteri RE: A comparison of radiographic findings in fusion and nonfusion patients 10 or more years following lumbar discd surgery. **Spine** 4:435–440, 1979.
38. Lehman TR, Spratt KF, Tozzi JE, et al: Long-term follow-up of lower lumbar fusion patients. **Spine** 12:97–104, 1987.
39. Anderson CE: Spondyloschisis following spine fusion. **J Bone Joint Surg** 38A:1142–1146, 1956.
40. Harris RI, Wiley JJ: Acquired spondylolysis as a sequel to spine fusion. **J Bone Joint Surg** 45A:1159–1170, 1963.
41. Leong JCY, Chun SY, Grange WJ, Fang D: Long-term results of lumbar intervertebral disc prolapse. **Spine** 8:793–799, 1983.
42. Charnley J: Total hip replacement. **JAMA** 230:1025–1028, 1974.

43. Nachemson AL: Challenge of the artificial disc, in Weinstein JN, ed: *Clinical efficacy and outcome in the diagnosis and treatment of low back pain.* New York: Raven Press, 1992.

44. Fernstrom U: Arthroplasty with intercorporal endoprothesis in herniated disc and in painful disc. **Acta Chir Scand** (Suppl)357:154–159, 1966.

45. Kostuik JP: Intervertebral disc replacement, in Bridwell KH, DeWald RL, eds: *The textbook of spinal surgery.* 2nd ed. Philadelphia: Lippincott-Raven, 1997, pp 2257–2266.

46. Ray CD, Schönmayr R, Kavanagh SA, Assell R: Prosthetic disc nucleus implants. **Riv Neuroradiol** 12 (Suppl 1):157–162, 1999.

47. Schönmayr R, Busch C, Lotz C, Lotz-Metz G: Prosthetic disc nucleus implants: the Wiesbaden feasibility study. 2 years follow-up in ten patients. **Riv Neuroradiol** 12 (Suppl 1):163–170, 1999.

48. Bertagnoli R: Anterior mini-open approach for nucleus prosthesis: a new application technique for the PDN. Presented at the 13th annual meeting of the International Intradiscal Therapy Society. June 8–10, 2000. Williamsburg, VA.

49. Enker P, Steffee A, Mcmillan C, Keppler L, Biscup R, Miller S: Artificial disc replacement. Preliminary report with a 3-year minimum follow-up. **Spine** 18:1061–1070, 1993.

50. Lee CK, Langrana NA, Parsons JR, Zimmerman MC: Development of a prosthetic intervertebral disc. **Spine** 16 (Suppl 6):S253–S255, 1991.

51. Deiter MP: Toxicology and carcinogenesis studies of 2-mercaptobenzothiazole in F344/n rats and B6C3F mice. NIH Pub. No. 88–8, National Toxicology Program, Technical Report Series No. 322. Washington DC: US Department of Health and Human Services, 1988.

52. Enker P, Steffee AD: Total disc replacement, in Bridwell KH, DeWald RL, eds: *The textbook of spinal surgery.* 2nd ed. Philadelphia, Lippincott-Raven, 1997, pp 2275–2288.

53. Hedman TP, Kostuik JP, Fernie GR, Hellier WG: Design of an intervertebral disc prosthesis. **Spine** 16 (Suppl 6):S256–S260, 1991.

54. Marnay T: L'arthroplastie intervertébrale lombaire. **Med Orthop** 25:48–55, 1991.

55. Link HD: LINK SB Charité III intervertebral dynamic disc spacer. **Rachis Revue de Pathologie Vertebrale** 11, 1999.

56. Griffith SL, Shelokov AP, Büttner-Janz K, LeMaire J-P, Zeegers WS: A multicenter retrospective study of the clinical results of the LINK® SB Charité intervertebral prosthesis. The initial European experience. **Spine** 19:1842–1849, 1994.

57. Lemaire JP, Skalli W, Lavaste F, et al: Intervertebral disc prosthesis. Results and prospects for the year 2000. **Clin Orthop** 337:64–76, 1997.

58. David TH: Lumbar disc prosthesis: a study of 85 patients reviewed after a minimum follow-up period of five years. **Rachis Revue de Pathologie Vertebrale** 11(No. 4-5), 1999.

59. Cummins BH, Robertson JT, Gill SG: Surgical experience with an implanted artificial cervical joint. **J Neurosurg** 88:943–948, 1998.

8

The Case For and Against
AVM Radiosurgery*

DOUGLAS KONDZIOLKA, M.D., M.SC. FRCS(C),
AND L. DADE LUNSFORD, M.D., F.A.C.S.

INTRODUCTION

Successful arteriorvenous malformation (AVM) radiosurgery is dependent upon achievement of the outcome of complete AVM nidus obliteration that leads to elimination of the future hemorrhage risk (12, 23, 26). While this goal is being achieved, there should be no morbidity or mortality from hemorrhage or radiation-induced brain injury. When these outcomes can be achieved with a high likelihood, a strong case can be made *for* radiosurgery. If clinical or angiographic factors argue *against* the achievement of these goals, then other strategies should more strongly be considered. Physicians who make an argument for radiosurgery cite one or more of the following: (1) that radiosurgery is an effective therapy required for the management of deep-brain AVMs; (2) that radiosurgery is an effective therapy for residual AVMs after subtotal resection; (3) that radiosurgery is worthwhile in an attempt to lower management risks for AVMs in functional brain locations; (4) since embolization does not cure most AVMs, additional therapy such as radiosurgery may be required; (5) microsurgical resection may not be the best choice for some patients depending on their general health; and (6) reduced cost. Since radiosurgery is the first and only biologic AVM therapy, it represents the beginnings of future cellular approaches to vascular malformation diseases. For this reason, the future of radiosurgery may be impacted positively by the development of other biologic strategies such as brain protection or endothelial sensitization.

Those who make an argument against the use of radiosurgery argue the following points: (1) that radiosurgery does not always work especially when only partial AVM obliteration is achieved (25); (2) that brain hemorrhage may occur during the time it takes for radiosurgery to work; (3) that radiation-related morbidity may cause functional neuro-

---

*This paper was presented at the 1999 CNS meeting.

logic deficits; (4) that there may exist "long-term" problems after brain irradiation (36); and (5) that resection may be a more cost-effective treatment over the long term (30). Though all these points can be argued, most neurosurgeons agree that the role of radiosurgery is greatest for patients with small-volume, deep-brain AVMs (1, 2, 23, 37).

It has a lesser role for patients with larger and surgically accessible AVMs. In between these two extremes there exists much debate. The role of radiosurgery for patients with small and yet accessible AVMs is growing steadily (29). For patients with large-volume yet deeply located AVMs, multimodality management often is required. Thus, whether radiosurgery should be considered in the management of an individual patient depends upon the factors of AVM volume, brain location, prior hemorrhage history, patient age, and surgical resectability. These factors have been studied in detail by different groups towards predicting successful AVM outcomes or reasons for radiosurgery failure (7, 8, 11, 19, 26).

CASE ILLUSTRATIONS

Case 1

This 30-year-old man sustained his first seizure and was found to have an ateriovenous malformation within motor cortex. *(Fig. 8.1)*. The argument for the use of radiosurgery would be the location of the AVM within a critical brain area, that its overall size is suitable for radiosurgery, and that the patient had not sustained a prior hemorrhage. If the patient had sustained a hemorrhage that caused neurologic deficits, then resection might more strongly be considered since any potential deficits already would be present. Arguments against the role of radiosurgery would be the chance for hemorrhage during the latency to obliteration, as well as the unknown outcome for seizures. Current reports note a 50 to 80% seizure cessation rate in patients who have AVM radiosurgery, regardless of the obliteration response (14, 16, 33).

Case 2

This 45-year-old man presented with headaches and was found to have a temporal lobe arteriovenous malformation supplied by the middle cerebral artery. An aneurysm just proximal to the arteriovenous malformation was also identified *(Fig. 8.2)*. Arguments for the use of radiosurgery include the small AVM volume, allowing radiosurgery to be used as an alternative to resection or embolization. Arguments against the role of radiosurgery include the resectability of the AVM in this location (with relatively low risk) and the sustained hemorrhage risk during the radiosurgery latency interval. Management of the proximal aneurysm via intraoperative clipping would be a strong argument for

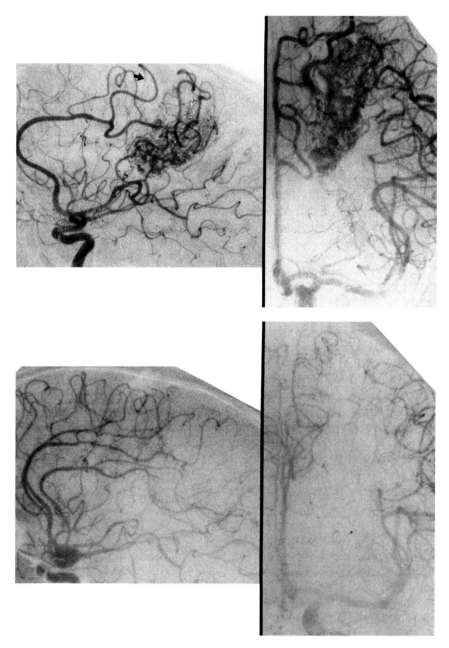

FIG. 8.1 Angiograms before radiosurgery in a young man with a left frontal-parietal AVM that had caused a seizure (*top*). Two years later, repeat angiography showed complete obliteration (*bottom*).

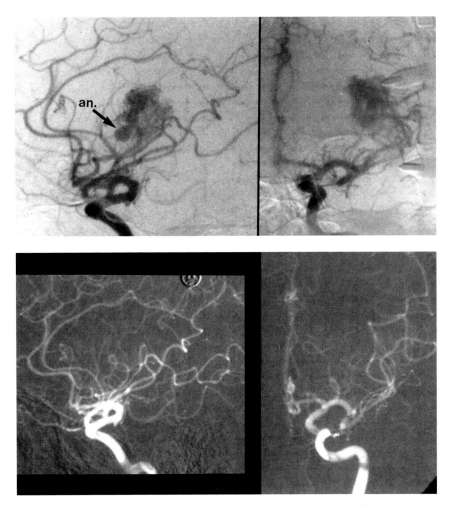

FIG. 8.2 Angiograms before radiosurgery showing a left temporal lobe AVM with a proximal aneurysm (*top*). His 2-year angiogram showed obliteration of the AVM and the aneurysm (*bottom*).

resection. This patient underwent radiosurgery, and his 2-year angiogram showed complete AVM obliteration and eliminination of the aneurysm.

Case 3

This 22-year-old woman suffered an intracerebral hemorrhage from an AVM located in the posterior limb of the left internal capsule. The hemorrhage caused hemiparesis, which had improved to a level of only mild arm weakness *(Fig. 8.3)*. She underwent radiosurgery because of the critical brain location of the malformation, its small and suitable size for radiosurgery, and the belief that this approach represented the lowest overall management risk. An argument could be made against radiosurgery since the patient had already sustained one hemorrhage and remained at a higher risk for a second bleed. However, the potential morbidity of resection appeared to outweigh this risk. Two years after radiosurgery, complete obliteration of the malformation was documented.

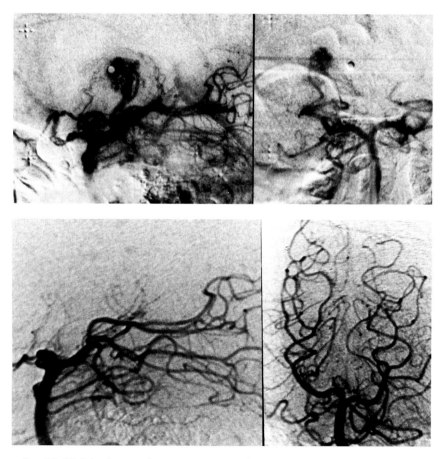

FIG. 8.3 *(Top)* Angiograms in a young woman who sustained a hemorrhage from an internal capsule AVM *(middle)*. Complete obliteration was confirmed on angiography after 2 years with no new neurological deficits *(bottom)*.

Case 4

This 45-year-old man had sustained two intraventricular hemorrhages from a thalamic arteriovenous malformation. He initially presented in 1976 and at that time a conservative approach was recommended. At the time of his second hemorrhage over 15 years later, radiosurgery was advocated. Symptoms from his intraventricular hemorrhage had resolved. The case for radiosurgery included the critical brain location of the malformation and its suitable size. The argument against radiosurgery was that their remained a continued risk of rebleeding prior to nidus obliteration, and that the nidus appeared diffuse on angiography and might present problems for targeting. However, the good functional status of the patient and the critical brain location were stronger arguments for radiosurgery *(Fig. 8.4)*. Three years following radiosurgery complete obliteration of the malformation had been confirmed. However, 1 year after irradiation, he developed sensory dysfunction of the right arm and leg associated with imaging changes in the surrounding thalamus. The symptoms and imaging changes largely resolved over 1 year. He remains active with no major motor deficits.

WHY DOES RADIOSURGERY WORK?

Radiosurgery is effective because the power of single-fraction irradiation causes significant injury to the blood vessels that compose the AVM (6, 2, 31, 35). Stereotactic definition of the AVM target ensures that these radiobiologic effects are limited to the malformation. Conformal radiosurgery allows irradiation of only a small volume of surrounding normal tissue in the region of dose fall-off (20, 23). Dose-prescription formulae are used to help select an appropriate radiation dose depending on imaging and clinical factors (5, 9).

The immediate effect of radiosurgery is to damage the endothelial cells of the AVM vessels. Release of tissue-specific cytokines common to other forms of radiation-induced injury are likely to mediate such acute effects. Inflammatory cells mediate tissue repair in response to irradiation. Later, chronic inflammation consists of the ingrowth of granulation tissue that contains fibroblasts and new capillaries. These events may explain the delayed imaging changes sometimes observed after radiosurgery (as in Case 4 above). Szeifert et al. identified the presence of actin-producing fibroblasts, so-called myofibroblasts, that are hypothesized to exert contractile properties and facilitate AVM obliteration (34). It is common that contrast-enhanced MRI studies at this late stage after obliteration show enhancement of the obliterated AVM. This finding does not indicate a "patent" AVM, but we believe, a marker for the newly formed capillary network within the scarred AVM tissue rem-

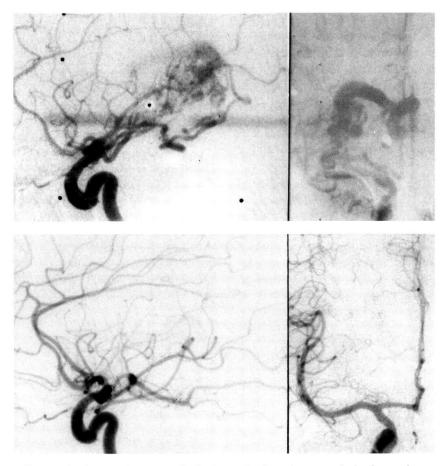

FIG. 8.4 Angiograms in a man who had sustained two intraventricular hemorrhages from a thalamic AVM (*top*). Note that the AVM nidus is non-compact and difficult to define (*arrows*). After 3 years, complete obliteration was documented (*bottom*).

nant. Several reports have noted the rare, late finding of cyst formation at the AVM site, which probably represent expansion of the extracellular fluid space within the fibrosis (15, 36).

CLINICAL EXPERIENCE

At the University of Pittsburgh, 694 AVM patients had Gamma knife radiosurgery during an 11-year interval. The mean patient age was 35 years (range 2–82). Prior intracranial hemorrhage was reported in 51% of patients, headaches in 44%, and seizures in 31%. The wide variety of different clinical presentations ensures discussion of the different treatment options in all patients. All referred vascular malformation cases are discussed at a weekly conference attended by neurosurgeons, neuroradiologists, and radiation oncologists. Intravascular embolization was performed in 114 patients (16%) before radiosurgery. Eighty-five patients (12%) had already undergone one or more surgical procedures prior to radiosurgery. For some of these patients, the goal of surgery had been AVM resection, while in others the goal of surgery was hematoma removal. The mean AVM volume was 3.4 ml (range .03–24 ml.). The 50% isodose was used as the margin isodose in 71% of patients. Only 0.7% of patients were treated below the 50% isodose.

The Spetzler-Martin grading system was used to classify all AVMs according to size, critical location, and venous drainage. As noted above, the most commonly referred patient was one with a small-volume, deeply located AVM (Grade III, n=267, 40%). The most infrequent patient had and AVM (n=23, 3.5%) that was small, superficial and non-critical in location (Grade 1). Sixteen percent of patients (n=104) had a Grade VI AVM. The AVM was located totally within the parenchyma of the brainstem or thalamus. The mean dose delivered to the AVM margin was 20 Gy and the mean maximum dose 37 Gy. The primary brain locations of AVMs in this series are listed in *Table 8.1*.

When radiosurgery did not lead to complete AVM obliteration, further discussion occurred over the merits of repeat radiosurgery or resection. Fifty-two patients underwent repeat radiosurgery for persistent AVM nidus after at least 3 years had elapsed since the first procedure. If after 3 to 4 years, a residual AVM nidus *with* early venous drainage remains, then a second radiosurgical procedure should be per-

TABLE 8.1
Brain Locations of AVMs for Stereotactic Radiosurgery (n=682)

Location	Number of Patients	Percent
Frontal lobe	109	15.7
Parietal lobe	136	19.6
Temporal lobe	117	16.8
Occipital lobe	71	10.2
Intraventricular	16	2.3
Basal ganglia	47	6.7
Thalamus	63	9.1
Cerebellum	52	7.4
Pons/midbrain	41	5.9
Corpus callosum	22	3.1
Medulla	3	0.4
Other	5	0.7

formed (28). We do not recommend additional management for patients who harbor only an early draining vein as this feature resolves over an additional observation interval (18). In addition we know of no patient who sustained a later hemorrhage when only an early draining vein was present. Some patients will have an angiogram that shows some abnormal appearing vessels in the region of the irradiated AVM, without early venous drainage. This fine vascular blush may indicate the neocapillary network within the scarred malformation. Such findings also require no additional therapy.

Retreatment is associated with a 70% probability of obliteration (17). At the second procedure, only the small remnant need be irradiated, usually at a dose lower than the first dose delivered (although sometimes greater if the initial AVM was large and the remnant is small, depending on location) *(Fig. 8.5).*

HOW AVM OBLITERATION AFFECTS DECISION MAKING

Whether an AVM can be successfully obliterated depends on whether proper stereotactic nidus definition can be performed followed by delivery of an adequate radiosurgery dose (10, 24). A complete analysis of 197 AVM patients with up to 3-year angiographic follow-up showed an overall complete obliteration rate of 72% after a single procedure. These results were stratified by volume. In 20 of 197 patients (10%) the targeted AVM nidus failed to obliterate totally. The most important reason for lack of complete obliteration was improper targeting (28). An additional 35 patients (18%) had a residual AVM that was not included in the original treatment volume. Many of these patients then underwent a second radiosurgery procedure. Important obliteration factors were identified in this study: incomplete imaging-definition of the AVM; reappearance of AVM after initial compression by hematoma; and recanalization of a previously embolized nidus. We and others advocate the use of multimodality imaging (MRI, MRA, and conventional stereotactic angiography) to obtain the best results (13, 21). For the smallest AVM (less than 1.3 ml), 90% of patients had complete obliteration (45 of 50), and 98% had obliteration of the target (49 of 50). For AVMs between 1.4 and 3 ml, 41 of 49 patients had complete obliteration (84%) and 47 of 49 had obliteration of the included target (96%). These data indicate that the radiosurgical dose will achieve our goal with a high likelihood if we can accurately tailor it to the entire lesion margin.

In a separate analysis of our date, we reported a multivariate analysis of AVM obliteration as related to dose and volume (10). A clear dose response up to 25 Gy was identified. We concluded that large AVMs have low obliteration rates because of the combination of lower treatment doses used and the greater problems encountered with target definition. A recent analysis of 95 patients with thalamic or basal ganglia AVMs found similar obliteration rates when stratified by volume; overall, 80% of patients were cured after a single procedure. Thus, AVM volume not only means that more tissue exists to undergo obliteration, but that there may be additional challenges in stereotactic targeting.

Pikus et al. argued that the high rate of complete microsurgical resection in their 72 patient AVM series (99%) with 8% rate of new permanent neurological deficits, substantiated their belief that resection was better than radiosurgery for small AVMs (25). However, only three of their patients (4%) had AVMs in the basal ganglia, thalamus, or brainstem. Porter et al. constructed a decision analysis model based on obliteration estimates and morbidity rates for resection and radiosurgery (30). They concluded that resection conferred a clinical benefit because of early protection from hemorrhage. Radiosurgery became a superior treatment if the surgical morbidity rate exceeded 12%. They did not factor the use of second stage or repeat radiosurgery into their model, choosing to leave patients with subtotally obliterated AVMs "unprotected" for the rest of their expected life. This outcome is rare since most patients achieve complete obliteration but may require more than one procedure. Thus, how obliteration data is used, and from where it is obtained (brain locations), is paramount to construct a proper argument on the use of different techniques.

HOW RADIOSURGERY MORBIDITY AFFECTS DECISION MAKING

Since immediate post-radiosurgery complications are rare, many patients and physicians choose radiosurgery because of rapid return to activities and employment. Post-radiosurgery seizures are rare when we administer therapeutic levels of anticonvulsant medication to patients with supratentorial lobar AVMs. One must consider the chance for delayed morbidity after radiosurgery that corresponds with the time course for AVM obliteration. We found that the rate of developing any post-radiosurgery imaging change between 2 and 7 years after radiosurgery is 30% (8). We believe that the majority of these changes are hemodynamic or inflammatory. Most do not cause neurologic symptoms. Symptomatic imaging changes are found in 10%. These changes resolve in half the patients within 3 years of onset as compared to a 95% resolution rate in patients with asymptomatic imaging findings.

There are several ways to predict in advance the chance for adverse radiation effects. A multivariate analysis of imaging changes with various radiosurgical parameters found that the only significant independent correlation was the total volume of tissue that received $\geq$ to 12 Gy

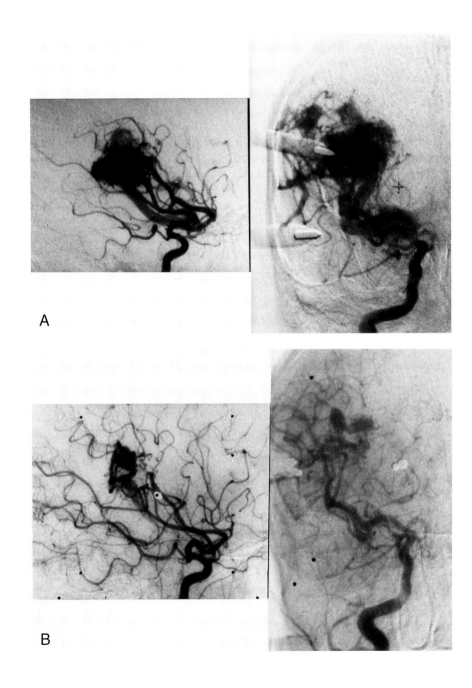

A

B

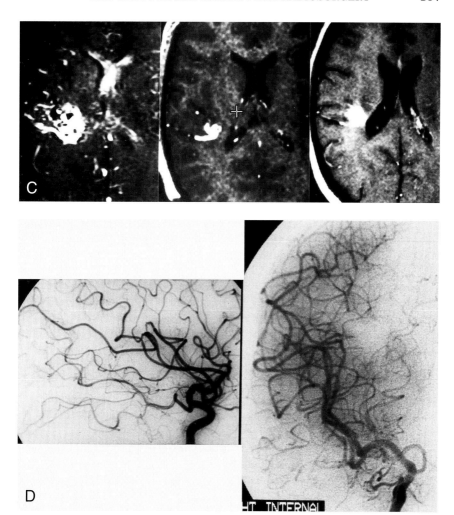

FIG. 8.5 Angiograms at the time of radiosurgery in a woman with a Sylvian fissure AVM (*A*). After 3 years (*B*), a small nidus remained and she underwent repeat radiosurgery. The MR sequence (*C*) showed the patent AVM (*left*), at 3 years (*middle*), and 2 years later (*right*). Persistent contrast enhancement was seen but no more arterial supply or venous drainage. An angiogram (*D*) confirmed complete obliteration after two-stage radiosurgery.

(7). Symptomatic imaging changes were correlated with the volume that received this dose and with location (brainstem versus non-brainstem). Although radiosurgery may seem to be the only viable treatment option for intraparenchymal brainstem AVMs, a higher risk must be expected.

Finally, the persistent risk of hemorrhage during the obliteration latency interval remains one of the strongest arguments against radiosurgery in some cases. Although Karlsson et al. reported protection from re-hemorrhage in the interval prior to complete obliteration, neither the Pittsburgh nor University of Florida series identified such a benefit (11, 19, 27). In our experience the hemorrhage rate after radiosurgery remains the same as the hemorrhage rate before radiosurgery until the AVM obliterates. We have never observed a bleed after obliteration.

THE CASE FOR LARGE AVMs: STAGED VOLUME RADIOSURGERY

We now consider prospective staged radiosurgery for larger AVMs (volume staging) especially for patients who present with hemorrhage and who are not suitable for resection. With this approach, the AVM volume is divided into components to allow radiosurgery of smaller volumes at higher, more effective, and more tolerable doses. Irradiation of an entire large AVM at a low dose (below 15 Gy to the AVM margin) has such a low obliteration rate that it is probably not worthwhile. We separate the AVM radiosurgeries by 4 to 6 months to allow repair of sublethal deoxyribonucleic acid damage in normal brain (4). There is evidence to suggest that even incompletely obliterated AVMs may become easier to resect after a period of several years. Perhaps prophylactic staged radiosurgery may facilitate eventual resection of AVMs previously considered untreatable (32). This approach is a new one and relatively little outcomes data is available to support its widespread use.

SUMMARY

AVM radiosurgery has been in practice for over 30 years and is now a common method to manage properly selected patients with brain AVMs. The techniques have been refined along with our understanding of the expected response. It is this understanding of expected outcomes that should allow a rational discussion of the pertinent issues for management of patients with AVMs. Some patients will require multimodality approaches. All AVM patients should seek to understand whether stereotactic radiosurgery is an appropriate option for their problem.

REFERENCES

1. Betti O, Munari C, Rosler R: Stereotactic radiosurgery with the linear accelerator: Treatment of arteriovenous malformations. **Neurosurgery** 24:311–321, 1989.
2. Colombo F, Benedetti A, Pozza F, et al: Linear accelerator radiosurgery of cerebral ateriovenous malformations. **Neurosurgery** 24:833–840, 1989.
3. Colombo F, Pozza F, Chierego G, et al: Linear accelerator radiosurgery of cerebral arteriovenous malformations: An update. **Neurosurgery** 34:14–21, 1994.

4. Firlik A, Levy E, Kondziolka D, et al: Staged volume radiosurgery and resection: A new treatment for a giant arteriovenous malformation. **Neurosurgery** (in press).

5. Flickinger JC. An integrated logistic formula for prediction of complications from radiosurgery. **Int J Radiat Oncol Biol Phys** 17:879–885, 1989.

6. Flickinger J, Kondziolka D, Kalend AM, et al. Radiosurgery-related imaging changes in surrounding brain: Multivariate analysis and model evaluation. **Radiosurgery** 1:229–236, 1995.

7. Flickinger JC, Kondziolka D, Pollock B, et al: Complications from arteriovenous malformation radiosurgery: Multivariate analysis and risk modeling. **Int J Radiat Oncol Biol Phys** 38:485–490, 1997.

8. Flickinger JC, Kondziolka D, Maitz A, et al: Analysis of neurological sequelae from radiosurgery of arteriovenous malformations: How location affects outcome. **Int J Radiat Oncol Biol Phys** 40:273–278, 1998.

9. Flickinger JC, Lunsford LD, Kondziolka D. Dose prescription and dose volume effects in radiosurgery. **Neurosurg Clin North Am** 3:51–59, 1992.

10. Flickinger JC, Pollock BE, Kondziolka D, et al. A dose-response analysis of arteriovenous malformation obliteration after radiosurgery. **Int J Radiat Oncol Biol Phys** 36:873–879, 1996.

11. Friedman W, Blatt D, Bova F, et al: The risk of hemorrhage after radiosurgery for arteriovenous malformations. **J Neurosurg** 84:912–919, 1996.

12. Friedman W, Bova F: Linear accelerator radiosurgery for arteriovenous malformations. **J Neurosurg** 77:832–841, 1992.

13. Friedman W, Bova F, Mendenhall W: Linear accelerator radiosurgery for arteriovenous malformations: The relationship of size to outcome. **J Neurosurg** 82:180–189, 1995.

14. Gerszten PC, Adelson PD, Kondziolka D, et al: Seizure outcome in children treated for arteriovenous malformation after gamma knife radiosurgery. **Ped Neurosurg** 24:139–144, 1996.

15. Hara M, Nakamura M, Shiokawa Y, et al: Delayed cyst formation after radiosurgery for cerebral arteriovenous malformation: Two case reports. **Minim Invas Neurosurg** 41:40–45, 1998.

16. Huang CF, Somaza S, Lunsford LD, et al: Radiosurgery in the management of epilepsy associated with arteriovenous malformations. **Radiosurgery** 1:195–200, 1996.

17. Karlsson B, Kihlstrom L, Lindquist C, et al: Gamma knife surgery for previously irradiated arteriovenous malformations. **Neurosurgery** 42:1–6, 1998.

18. Karlsson B, Lindquist M, Lindquist C, et al: Long-term angiographic outcome of arteriovenous malformations responding incompletely to gamma knife surgery. **Radiosurgery** 1:188–194, 1996.

19. Karlsson B, Lindquist C, Steiner L: Effect of gamma knife surgery on the risk of rupture prior to AVM obliteration. **Minim Invas Neurosurg** 39:21–27, 1996.

20. Kondziolka D, Lunsford LD: Intraparenchymal brainstem radiosurgery. **Neurosurg Clin North Am** 4:469–479, 1993.

21. Kondziolka D, Lunsford LD, Kanal E, et al: Stereotactic magnetic resonance angiography for targeting in arteriovenous malformation radiosurgery. **Neurosurgery** 35:585–591, 1994.

22. Larsson B, Leksell L, Rexed B, et al: The high-energy proton beam as a neurosurgical tool. **Nature** 182:1222–1223, 1958.

23. Lunsford LD, Kondziolka D, Flickinger J, et al: Stereotactic radiosurgery for arteriovenous malformations of the brain. **J Neurosurg** 75:512–524, 1991.

24. Petereit D, Mehta M, Turski P, et al: Treatment of arteriovenous malformations with stereotactic radiosurgery employing both magnetic resonance angiography and standard angiography as a database. **Int J Radiat Oncol Biol Phys** 25:309–313, 1993.
25. Pikus H, Beach ML, Harbaugh R: Microsurgical treatment of arteriovenous malformations: analysis and comparison to stereotactic radiosurgery. **J Neurosurg** 88:641–646, 1998.
26. Pollock B, Flickinger JC, Lunsford LD, Maitz A, Kondziolka D. Factors associated with successful arteriovenous malformation radiosurgery. **Neurosurgery** 42:1239–1247, 1998.
27. Pollock BE, Flickinger JC, Lunsford LD, et al: Hemorrhage risk after radiosurgery for arteriovenous malformations. **Neurosurgery** 38:652–661, 1996.
28. Pollock BE, Kondziolka D, Lunsford LD, et al: Repeat stereotactic radiosurgery of arteriovenous malformations: Factors associated with incomplete obliteration. **Neurosurgery** 38:318–324, 1996.
29. Pollock BE, Lunsford LD, Kondziolka D, et al: Patient outcomes after stereotactic radiosurgery for "operable" arteriovenous malformations. **Neurosurgery** 35:1–8, 1994.
30. Porter P, Shin A, Detsky A, et al: Surgery versus radiosurgery for small, operable cerebral arteriovenous malformations: a clinical and cost comparison. **Neurosurgery** 41:757–766, 1997.
31. Schneider B, Eberhard D, Steiner L: Histopathology of arteriovenous malformations after gamma knife radiosurgery. **J Neurosurg** 87:352–357, 1997.
32. Steinberg G, Chang S, Levy R, et al: Surgical resection of large incompletely treated intracranial arteriovenous malformations following stereotactic radiosurgery. **J Neurosurg** 84:920–928, 1996.
33. Steiner L, Lindquist C, Adler JR, et al: Clinical outcome of radiosurgery for cerebral arteriovenous malformations. **J Neurosurg** 77:1–8, 1992.
34. Szeifert GT, Kemeny AA, Timperley W, et al: The potential role of myofibroblasts in the obliteration of arteriovenous malformations after radiosurgery. **Neurosurgery** 40: 61–66, 1997.
35. Wu A, Lindner G, Maitz A, et al: Physics of gamma knife approach on convergent beams in stereotactic radiosurgery. **Int J Radiat Oncol Biol Phys** 18:941–949, 1990
36. Yamamoto M, Jimbo M, Hara M, et al: Gamma knife radiosurgery for arteriovenous malformations: Long-term follow-up results focusing oncomplications occurring more than 5 years after irradiation. **Neurosurgery** 38:906–914.
37. Yamamoto Y, Coffey R, Nichols B, et al: Interim report on the radiosurgical treatment of cerebral arteriovenous malformations. **J Neurosurg** 83:832–837, 1995.

II

General Scientific
Session II
Spinal Surgery Outcomes:
The Basis of Practice

9

Neurosurgery for the 21ˢᵗ Century

What Does Neurobiology Justify for Repairing Neurodegenerative Disorders?

PAUL R. SANBERG, PH.D., D. SC., ALISON E. WILLING, PH.D,
AND DAVID W. CAHILL, M.D.

INTRODUCTION

Neurosurgery for the treatment of neurodegenerative disease or brain injury/stroke tends to be a very limited specialty. The predominant view until recently has been that once neurons are destroyed and neural circuitry interrupted, there is little in the way of surgical intervention that can repair the damage. The focus in many cases has been on palliation and to some extent, rehabilitation through the retraining and hence reorganization of the remaining neural circuitry. The exception to this general rule has been in neurosurgical treatments of Parkinson's disease (PD). Neurosurgical approaches to this disease include neural transplantation, deep brain stimulation, pallidotomy, and thalamatomy. Parkinson's disease lends itself to this approach because of the discrete deficit in dopaminergic neurotransmission and the resulting dysregulation of the well-characterized striatal output pathways. Central nervous system diseases with less discrete neuropathologies do not lend themselves as easily to such surgical interventions. However, scientific developments of the last quarter century foreshadow a time when neurosurgical intervention may become more proactive and more widespread, encompassing diseases not formerly within the purview of the neurosurgeon. This revolutionary change will occur through the application of evolving knowledge of developmental and molecular biology to neural transplantation. In the remainder of this discussion, the focus will be on recent developments in neurotransplantation and gene therapy and what these may mean for the treatment of neurological diseases and injury in the coming century.

NEURAL TRANSPLANTATION FOR PARKINSON'S DISEASE

The most extensive investigations of neural transplantation in the last 30 years have been as a treatment for PD. The first published results from animal studies in which fetal ventral mesencephalon (VM) were transplanted into hemiparkinsonian rat appeared in 1979 (1, 2). While early studies in animals demonstrated the utility of the transplant approach, it has taken longer in the clinical setting to establish that transplantation can improve function in the PD patient. In the early clinical studies there was little consistency in the techniques used leading to inconsistencies in the reported benefits of the treatment. However, there are now ample demonstrations that grafts do survive in man and that they can at least partially ameliorate functional deficits observed in this disease (see (3)) for an extensive review). Transplants have been shown to survive, form synaptic connections, and improve motor function in many patients (4). Even while neural transplantation is the only therapeutic strategy that aims to replace lost or diseased cells in the central nervous system (CNS) and its technical feasibility and clinical merit have been demonstrated, it cannot develop into a widely available treatment option for patients with CNS diseases as long as fetal tissue is the cell source of choice. Ethical concerns and difficulties in obtaining enough healthy tissue for transplants, even for a single patient, prevent the widespread use of this treatment strategy. This is even though neural transplantation is now being studied experimentally in many other disease models including Huntington's disease (HD), Alzheimer's disease (AD), spinal cord or brain traumatic injury and stroke.

WHAT MAKES A GOOD ALTERNATIVE CELL FOR TRANSPLANTATION?

With the limited availability of fetal tissue, there are a number of other cell types that have been used in neural transplantation therapies *(Fig. 9.1)*. The utility of the cells depends upon the nature of the defect they are meant to repair *(Table 9.1)*. In some cases, the purpose is to supply a neuroactive substance to a specific site within the CNS. In this case, non-neuronal cells may adequately serve as delivery devices for the desired molecules. For example, providing dopamine to striatal neurons is sufficient to restore function in a PD patient. In addition, the purpose of the grafts may not be to replace lost neurons, but may be to provide support to neuron populations and thereby protect against disease progression or promote plasticity. If, however, the damage is more diffuse, involves more than one type of neuronal population, or repair requires re-establishing the neuronal circuits through synaptic contact, then it is not enough for the transplanted cells to be secre-

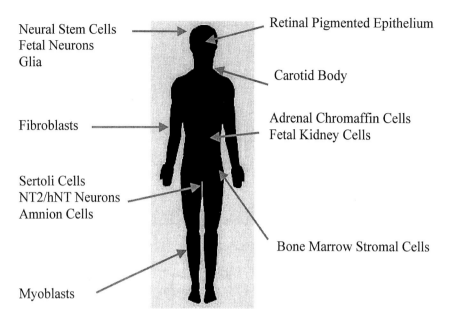

Neural Stem Cells
Fetal Neurons
Glia

Retinal Pigmented Epithelium

Carotid Body

Fibroblasts

Adrenal Chromaffin Cells
Fetal Kidney Cells

Sertoli Cells
NT2/hNT Neurons
Amnion Cells

Bone Marrow Stromal Cells

Myoblasts

FIG. 9.1 Cells used for neural transplantation and the anatomical regions of origin.

tory mini-pumps. The cells must be neuron-like in their ability to develop a particular neuronal phenotype, express specific neurotransmitters, develop appropriate neuritic outgrowth, and form synaptic contacts with host cells in order to achieve regulated delivery of the molecule. While these are very stringent criteria, fetal tissue transplants in PD and HD have been shown to fulfill these requirements.

ALTERNATIVE CELL TRANSPLANTATION STRATEGIES

In this section, we will describe in more detail some of the alternative sources of cells that are being considered for the treatment of neurodegenerative diseases and injuries. This discussion is not exhaustive, however; we have focused on cell sources or therapy approaches that are already being tested for use in humans *(Table 9.2)* or have great potential for clinical treatments in the near future.

Xenografts

With the limited availability of human fetal tissue, a number of groups have begun to examine the feasibility of using tissue from other species, thereby securing an unlimited supply of cells. To date there have been clinical trials on the use of bovine chromaffin cells for the

TABLE 9.1

Strategies for Choosing Cell Sources for Transplantation

Strategy	Cells Used	Model	Purpose
Providing a Neuroactive Substance	Adrenal chromaffin cells	Parkinson's	Dopamine secretion
	Transfected Astrocytes	"	"
	Carotid body cells	"	"
	Retinal Pigmented Epithelium	"	"
	Transfected Myoblasts	"	"
	PC12 cells	"	"
	Adrenal chromaffin cells	Pain	Provide catecholamines and enkephalins/opioids
	Transfected Fibroblasts	Alzheimer's	Trophic Support through NGF delivery
Replacing Lost Neurons and Restoring Neural Circuitry	Embryonic Tissue (human or xenograft)	Parkinson's, Huntington's, Stroke, Injury	Synthesize and secrete lost neurotransmitter at newly formed synapses with the host tissue
	Neural Stem Cells	"	"
	HNT Neurons	"	"
	Bone Marrow Stromal Cells	Stroke	"

treatment of pain, engraftment of hamster cells to treat amyotropic lateral sclerosis (5), and porcine fetal VM for PD (7). However, any time that cross-species transplants are performed there will be a concern about the transmission of new infectious diseases that may be as devastating as AIDS. Currently, a controversy exists over the use of porcine

TABLE 9.2

Alternative Cells Currently Used in a Clinical Setting

Cells	Purpose	Ref.
Xenografts		
Bovine chromaffin cells	Pain Management	(5)
Porcine VM	Parkinson's Disease	(7)
Hamster Kidney Cells	Amyotropic Lateral Sclerosis	(6)
Non-Neural Cells		
Adrenal chromaffin cells	Parkinson's Disease	Reviewed in (58)
Neural Cell Lines		
hNT Neurons	Basal Ganglia Stroke	(30)

tissue since the first report that human cells were infected with an endogenous porcine retrovirus and cells so infected were resistant to lysis (8). While it may not be possible to predict how a specific virus will mutate if it crosses from one species to another, this practice mandates keeping extensive health records and procedural protocols on the donor animals including possible exposures to infectious agents. This would mean that a tissue archive and safety database could be available as tools to identify and/or treat possible disease (9).

A more immediate issue for the use of nonhuman cells is immunogenicity. Without immune suppression, xenografted tissue is rejected. Survival of porcine VM transplanted into striatum of nonimmunosuppressed rats occurred in 7% of animals after 4 months compared to 52% in cyclosporin-treated animals (10). These grafts were infiltrated with lymphocytes, bone marrow derived cells and microglia as determined through immunohistochemistry. In another study in which porcine VM was grafted into rat striatum, rejection occurred in almost two thirds of the animals and the grafts contained natural killer cells, macrophage, CD4 and CD8 positive cells in addition to microglia and extensive scarring (11). Further, Ni et al. (12) showed that intracerebral administration of xeno-antigens resulted in the accumulation of antigen-specific cells in the cervical lymph node and stimulation of a strong CD4 positive T cell response that with time and additional antigenic challenge produced IL-2.

While the brain is relatively immune privileged because of the blood-brain barrier (BBB), which prevents the entry of peripheral immune cells into the brain, during transplantation the BBB is disrupted. This means that MHC antigens in the graft may be recognized and a systemic immune response activated. This may explain why there is unhindered T and B cell infiltration into the graft. But perhaps even more important than this cellular mediated immune response, where T cells may actually have a weaker affinity to the presenting antigens of the nonhuman tissue because they are so dissimilar to those of man, would be the humoral immune response generated by immunoglobulins and complement proteins, which can cross the disturbed BBB (13).

Whether graft rejection occurs through direct cellular interactions or humoral interactions, it becomes imperative to maintain long-term immunosuppression that addresses multiple immune pathways while still trying to minimize the risk of side effects inherent in immunosuppressive treatments. A possible solution to this problem may also lie in an emerging cell-transplantation technology. The Sertoli cells (SCs) of the testes have been shown to provide immune and trophic support to co-transplanted neural tissue. In their natural environment, SCs provide immune protection for developing germ cells in the testes while also providing trophic and nutritional support. This immune support occurs through multiple mechanisms: formation of the blood-testis barrier, production of a paracrine factor that can inhibit interleukin-2 (IL-2) production and T-lymphocyte responsiveness to IL-2, production of CD-95 ligand (FasL), which when bound to the CD-95 receptor (Fas) on activated lymphocytes induces apoptosis and the subsequent down-regulation of the immune response (see 14) for a more extensive review of SCs in neural transplantation). As an adjunct to traditional neural transplantation, the SCs can increase the number of surviving dopaminergic neurons transplanted into the hemiparkinsonian rat striatum (15). Further, these cells decreased microglial infiltration and activation of human hNT neuron xenografts, increased graft survival from 50% in the absence of SCs to 100% with the SCs and increased graft size (16). In another study, microglial infiltration (as demonstrated using lectin histochemistry) of bovine adrenal chromaffin cell grafts in the striatum was reduced when SCs were co-grafted with these DA-producing cells (17). These cells have also been shown to secrete FasL after transplantation in the striatum (18). These data provide a powerful demonstration that the SCs may be able to provide localized, extra-testicular immune suppression capable of protecting xenografted tissue in the CNS from rejection.

Cell Lines

An ideal alternative to the use of fetal tissue would be to have a neural cell line available. This could provide an unlimited supply of neural cells for transplantation. Such cell lines do exist and have been studied in animal models; for example PC12 cells have been studied as a source of dopaminergic cells to treat PD and conditionally immortalized O-2A cells as a source of oligodendrocytes or type II astrocytes to induce myelination in the spinal cord. However, one of the critical issues in the use of cell lines for transplantation is the possibility that the cells will continue to proliferate *in vivo,* generating tumors. One promising cell line is the hNT neuron.

HNT NEURONS

The hNT neurons (or LBS Neurons, Layton BioScience, Inc.) are actually derived from the immortalized human teratocarcinoma cell line, NTera2/D1, which can be induced to differentiate in vitro into post-mitotic neuron-like cells (hNT) that express neurofilaments (19) and a variety of neurotransmitters including dopamine (20), acetylcholine (21), and GABA (22). When the hNT neurons are implanted in the striatum, they develop a morphology and polarity similar to neurons and can survive at least a year without reverting to a tumorigenic phenotype (23). These cells express synaptic proteins in vivo (20) and have been demonstrated to form functional synapses in long-term tissue culture preparations (20).

All of these characteristics make the hNT neurons a very versatile cell for the treatment of neurodegenerative diseases and brain or spinal cord injury. These cells have been tested in models of Huntington's disease (24), PD (25), and spinal cord injury (26, 27). However, the first studies to demonstrate this involved transplanting these cells into the striatum of rats after a middle cerebral artery occlusion, which is a good model of human stroke. Transplanted animals were shown to exhibit less motor asymmetry and improved performance on the passive avoidance test of cognitive function (28). Further, these improvements were dose-dependent (29). These positive results have led to a clinical safety study in 12 patients with basal ganglia stroke and fixed motor deficits (30). At 6 months after transplantation of these cells, there was both a significant improvement in performance on the European Stroke Scale score of 6 patients and improved fluorodeoxyglucose uptake at the implant site.

Gene Therapy

Gene therapy is potentially a very powerful method for treating neurodegenerative diseases. In this method, a delivery vehicle (or vector), which can be viral or non-viral (such as a plasmid or cationic liposome), is used to transfer a gene of interest to a target cell. The efficiency of gene transfer depends on the method of transfer chosen, with viral vectors being more efficient than other methods. However, for transferring genes to the central nervous system (CNS), only the herpes simplex virus (or lentivirus), adenovirus, or adeno-associated virus have been shown to infect post-mitotic cells. There are two basic gene transfer approaches—ex vivo and in vivo.

EX VIVO

In ex vivo gene transfer, a cell is genetically modified prior to transplantation in order to deliver a neurotransmitter, trophic substance, or toxin to the CNS. Cells that have been used include fibroblasts, myoblasts, astrocytes, and neural stem cells. Tuszynski and associates have used autologous fibroblasts transfected with nerve growth factor (NGF) to demonstrate neuroprotection of cholinergic neurons and stimulation of cholinergic fiber ingrowth into these grafts in nonhuman primate models of Alzheimer's disease (31, 32).

Another ex vivo gene application involves transduction of neural stem cells to express agents toxic to glioma cells. The stem cells make a good vehicle for this treatment because they migrate within the CNS using white matter tracts. Aboody and associates (33) have shown that transplanted NSCs migrate into contact with experimental tumor cells. These NSCs were transduced to express a bacterial pro-drug activating enzyme, cytosine deaminase (CD); upon treatment with 5-fluorocytosine, there was a greater than 80% reduction in tumor size. Similarly, Benedetti et al. (34) showed that transferring the gene for interleukin-4 to mouse neural progenitor cells and then injecting the cells into an established glioblastoma resulted in shrinkage of the tumors and mouse survival.

IN VIVO

For in vivo gene transfer, a retrovirus construct that includes the gene of interest is engineered and this construct is then injected into the nervous system. The virus infects nearby cells, thereby transferring the gene to the brain and allowing these cells to make and secrete the gene product. The first demonstration in which long-term transfer of gene expression occurred was in a study in which the herpes simplex type I virus was used as the vehicle to deliver the human tyrosine hydroxylase transgene (35). In this case, behavioral recovery was demonstrated out to 12 months post transplant. Further, immunohistochemistry demonstrated a large number of TH positive cells present in the striatum. These results have now been replicated in a nonhuman primate model (36) with an adeno-associated vector and an initial safety study of the lentivirus vector performed (37). In this latter study, there was long-term expression of the transferred βGal gene and little if any inflammatory response or perivascular cuffing.

Another example of the potential of this treatment approach is for the correction of metabolic diseases of the CNS. In a recent paper, the gene for β-glucoronidase was inserted into an adeno-associated virus and injected at specific sites within the brain of mice deficient in this enzyme (38). The secreted enzyme produced a widespread reversal of pathology, even though the vector was delivered at a limited number of sites.

POTENTIAL PROBLEMS

While the potential of gene transfer is significant, it is not without problems. The less severe problems involve maintaining long-term gene expression in vivo. A more severe example of problems occurred in a recent clinical trial where an adenovirus carrying the gene for ornithine-transcarbamylase, which controls ammonia metabolism, was injected into the liver of patients with an inherited deficiency in this enzyme

(39). One patient died shortly after delivery of the adenovirus and the gene product and traces of the adenovirus were found throughout the body. While the reason for this patient's severe reaction to the treatment is unclear, the incidence of adverse events such as this is rare.

Neural Stem Cells

Perhaps the most exciting development in the field of neural transplantation and science in general is the discovery of neural stem cells (NSCs) in the mammalian brain (see (40) for a recent review). A NSC is a single cell with the ability to proliferate, exhibit self-maintenance or renewal over the lifetime of the organism, and to generate a large number of clonally related progeny. NSCs give rise to neurons, astrocytes, and oligodendrocytes during development and can replace a limited number of neural cells in the adult brain. These cells have been isolated from both embryonic (41, 42) and adult human brain (43, 44).

The new stem cell technologies may provide an unlimited supply of human neural cells for transplantation in the near future. Further, stem cell therapies may increase the number of disease states for which neural transplantation becomes a viable option. As an example, Yandava et al. (45) repaired the genetic deficit in the *shiverer* mouse model, using mouse NSCs to replace myelin basic protein (MBP) expressed by oligodendrocytes and required for myelination. Not only was there an increase in the brain content of MBP and improvement in symptomology, but there was also increased differentiation of the NSCs into oligodendrocytes compared to when these cells were transplanted into a normal brain. This suggests that the cells can read cues within the host environment to direct their development into the appropriate cell type. The implications of this are four-fold. First, it may be possible to effectively treat diseases with more complicated disruptions in neural circuitry, such as Huntington's disease where more than one cell population in more than one region in the brain is affected. Second, it may not be necessary for the cells to be manipulated ex vivo to produce a specific cell population for a specific disease. Another point to consider is that NSCs follow inherent migratory pathways within the host brain and integrate into the host parenchyma (42, 46), making delivery strategies simpler. Finally these cells may provide an ideal vehicle for targeted gene delivery. It may now be possible to cure genetic and metabolic diseases such as Tay Sach's disease, which before were untreatable and led to early death.

AVAILABILITY OF NEURAL STEM CELLS

As with traditional neural transplantation, the major limiting concern is that the best characterized NSCs are still obtained from fetal tissues. It has been recently shown that NSCs can be isolated from the adult brain. This eliminates the ethical objections inherent to fetal tissue; however, until such time as there are fully characterized and immortalized clonal cell lines available this limits the availability of tissue to that obtained post-mortem. The other consideration when using stem cells obtained from the adult is whether the aged stem cell is similar to the stem cell from the younger animal. In studies of hematopoietic stem cells, changes in stem cell function during development occur and correlate with the loss of telomere length, which in turn may decrease the ability of the stem cell to self renew with age (47, 48).

STEM CELLS FROM OUTSIDE THE CNS

Another possibility for obtaining stem cells to differentiate into neural cells is to look outside the CNS to other tissues where these cells are easier to obtain. The recent demonstration that NSCs can produce non-neural hematopoietic cells (49), suggests that the source of stem cells need not be limited to either embryonic or adult NSCs. Adult bone marrow is a good source not only of hematopoietic stem cells but also of nonhematopoietic stem cells (also referred to as bone marrow stromal cells (BMSCs)). These multipotent precursors have the ability to differentiate into osteoblasts, chondroblasts, adipocytes, and myoblasts (50). After systemic infusion of BMSCs into irradiated adult mice, the progeny of the donor precursor cells were found repopulating various nonhematopoietic tissues including the brain (51). Moreover, direct transplantation of human BMSCs into rat striatum or the lateral ventricle of neonatal mice resulted in engraftment, survival, migration, and differentiation into astrocytes (52, 53). We have shown that these BMSCs are capable of differentiating into not only astrocytes, but also neurons (54). When human or mouse BMSCs were cultured in the presence of epidermal growth factor or brain derived neurotrophic factor, a subpopulation of these cells was immuno-labeled with an antibody to neuronal nuclei (NeuN). These results have now been replicated (55); further, clonal cell lines have been established from single cells that produce neuron-like cells. In animal models of neurodegenerative disease or injury, these cells have now been shown to ameliorate behavioral deficits (56) and may promote the proliferation of endogenous stem cells within the subventricular zone (57).

CONCLUSION

In the 20th century, the field of neural transplantation has exploded. At the turn of the century it was almost a biological law that an injured human brain or spinal cord could never be repaired or regenerate. During the last decades, successful proof of principle demonstrations of neural regeneration and transplantation and current theories of CNS plasticity, have fostered high hopes for brain repair in the coming years. The dawn of the 21st century finds us living in a very exciting time with the recent breakthroughs in stem cell biology and human genetics. The challenge in the coming years will be in learning to apply this new knowledge to the treatment and prevention of human disease. We now have the blueprint for the human genome; the Herculean task will be to understand the role each of these genes plays in health and disease. As we delineate these roles, gene therapy will become available for a wider array of neurodegenerative diseases. With the isolation and propagation of neural stem cells or other stem-like cells, we may develop a perfect and widely available delivery vehicle for these therapies. Together these developments will change how we view neurosurgical interventions leading to broader applications of neurotransplantation for repairing the damaged brain and spinal cord.

REFERENCES

1. Bjorklund A, Stenevi U: Reconstruction of the nigrostriatal dopamine pathway by intracerebral transplants. **Brain Res** 177:555–560, 1979.
2. Perlow MJ, Freed WJ, Hoffer BJ, Seiger A, Olson L, Wyatt RJ: Brain grafts reduce motor abnormalities produced by destruction of nigrostriatal dopamine system. **Science** 204:643–647, 1979.
3. Barker RA, Dunnett SB: First clinical trial: Neural grafts in Parkinson's disease, in *Neural Repair, Transplantation, and Rehabilitation.* East Sussex, UK, Psychology Press Lts, 1999, pp 93–132.
4. Kordower JH, Freeman TB, Snow BJ, et al.: Neuropathological evidence of graft survival and striatal reinnervation after the transplantation of fetal mesencephalic tissue in a patient with Parkinson's disease. **N Engl J Med** 332:1118–1124, 1995.
5. Buchser E, Goddard M, Heyd B, et al.: Immunoisolated xenogenic chromaffin cell therapy for chronic pain. Initial clinical experience. **Anesthesiology** 85:1005–1012, 1996.
6. Aebischer P, Schluep M, Deglon N, et al.: Intrathecal delivery of CNTF using encapsulated genetically modified xenogeneic cells in amyotrophic lateral sclerosis patients. **Nat Med** 2:696–699, 1996.
7. Deacon T, Schumacher J, Dinsmore J, et al.: Histological evidence of fetal pig neural cell survival after transplantation into a patient with Parkinson's disease. **Nat Med** 3:350–353, 1997.
8. Patience C, Takeuchi Y, Weiss RA: Infection of human cells by an endogenous retrovirus of pigs [see comments]. **Nat Med** 3(3):282–286, 1997.
9. Barker RA, Kendall AL, Widner H, the Neural Tissue Xenografting Project: Neural tissue xenoplantation: What is needed prior to clinical trials in Parksinon's Disease? **Cell Transplant** 9:235–246, 2000.
10. Pakzaban P, Deacon TW, Burns LH, Dinsmore J, Isacson O: A novel mode of immunoprotection of neural xenotransplants: masking of donor major histocompatibility complex class I enhances transplant survival in the central nervous system

[published erratum appears in **Neuroscience** 66(3):761, 1995]. **Neuroscience** 65(4):983–96, 1995.

11. Larsson LC, Czech KA, Brundin P, Widner H: Intrastriatal ventral mesencephalic xenografts of porcine tissue in rats: Immune responses and functional effect. **Cell Transplant** 9:261–272, 2000.

12. Ni HT, Merica RR, Spellman SR, Wang JM, Low WC: Visualization of antigen-specific T cell activation in vivo in response to intracerebral administration of a xenopeptide. **Exp Neurol** 164(2):362–370, 2000.

13. Iwata H, Ikada Y: Agarose, in Kuhtreiber WM, Lanza RP, Chick WL (eds): *Cell Encapsulation Technology and Therapeutics.* Boston, Birkhauser, 1999 pp 97–107.

14. Willing AE, Cameron DF, Sanberg PR: Sertoli cell transplants: Their use in the treatment of neurodegenerative disease. **Mol Med Today** 4(11):459–504, 1998.

15. Willing AE, Othberg AI, Saporta S, et al.: Sertoli cells enhance the survival of cotransplanted dopamine neurons. **Brain Res** 822:246–250, 1999.

16. Willing AE, Sudberry JJ, Othberg AI: et al.: Sertoli cells decrease microglial response and increase engraftment of human hNT neurons in the hemiparkinsonian rat striatum. **Brain Res Bull** 48:441–444, 1999.

17. Sanberg PR, Borlongan CV, Saporta S, Cameron DF: Testis-derived Sertoli cells survive and provide localized immunoprotection for xenografts in rat brain. **Nature Biotech** 14:1692–1695, 1996.

18. Sanberg PR, Saporta S, Borlongan CV, Othberg AI, Allen RC, Cameron DF: The testis-derived cultured Sertoli cell as a natural Fas-L secreting cell for immuno-suppressive cellular therapy. **Cell Transplant** 6:191–193, 1997.

19. Pleasure SJ, Lee VM-Y: NTera 2 cells: A human cell line which displays characteristics expected of a human committed neuronal progenitor cell. **J Neurosci Res** 35: 585–602, 1993.

20. Miyazono M, Nowell PC, Finan JL, Lee VM-Y, Trojanowski JQ: Long-term integration and neuronal differentiation of human embryonal carcinoma cells (NTera-2) transplanted into the caudoputamen of nude mice. **J Comp Neurol** 376:602–613, 1996.

21. Zeller MS, Strauss WL: Retinoic acid induces cholinergic differentiation of NTera2 human embryonal carcinoma cells. **Int J Dev Neurosci** 13:437–445, 1995.

22. Hartley RS, Margulis M, Lee VM-Y, Tang C.M: Astrocytes are required for the formation of functional synapses between human NT2N neurons in vitro. **J Comp Neurol** 407(1):1–10, 1999.

23. Kleppner SR, Robinson KA, Trojanowski JQ, Lee VM-Y: Transplanted human neurons derived from a teratocarcinoma cell line (NTera-2) mature, integrate, and survive for over 1 year in the nude mouse brain. **J Comp Neurol** 357:618–632, 1995.

24. Hurlbert MS, Gianani RI, Hutt C, Freed CR, Kaddis FG: Neural transplantation of hNT neurons for Huntington's disease. **Cell Transplant** 8(1):143–151, 1999.

25. Baker KA, Hong M, Sadi D, Mendez I: Intrastriatal and intranigral grafing of hNT neurons in the 6-OHDA rat model of Parkinson's disease. **Exp Neurol** 162:350–360, 2000.

26. Makoui AS, Saporta S, Willing AE, et al.: Recovery of motor and sensory evoked potentials after transplantation of hNT neurons in rats with complete spinal cord contusion injury. **Exp Neurol** 164:455, 2000.

27. Velardo MJ, O'Steen BE, McGrogan M, Reier PJ: hNT cells and transplantation repair of rat cervical spinal cord contusions. **Exp Neurol** 164:454, 2000.

28. Borlongan CV, Tajima Y, Trojanowski JQ, Lee VM, Sanberg PR: Transplantation of cryopreserved human embryonal carcinoma-derived neurons (NT2N cells) promotes functional recovery in ischemic rats. **Exp Neurol** 149(2):310–21, 1998.

29. Saporta S, Borlongan CV, Sanberg PR: Neural transplantation of human neurotera-tocarcinoma (hNT) neurons into ischemic rats. A quantitative dose-response analysis of cell survival and behavioral recovery. **Neuroscience** 91(2):519–525, 1999.
30. Kondziolka D, Wechsler L, Goldstein S, et al.: Transplantation of cultured human neuronal cells for patients with stroke. **Neurology** 55:565–569, 2000.
31. Tuszynski MH, Senut M-C, Ray J, Roberts JUH-S, Gage FH: Somatic gene transfer to the adult primate central nervous system: In vitro and in vivo characterization of cells genetically modified to secrete nerve growth factor. **Neurobiol Dis** 1:67–78, 1994.
32. Tuszynski MH, Roberts J, Senut M-C, U HS, Gage FH: Gene therapy in the adult primate brain: Intraparenchymal grafts of cells genetically engineered to produce nerve growth factor prevent cholinergic neuronal degeneration. **Gene Therapy** 3:305–314, 1996.
33. Aboody KS, Brown A, Rainov NG, et al.: Neural stem cells—a new platform for delivery of gene therapy against brain tumors. **Exp Neurol** 164:468, 2000.
34. Benedetti S, Pirola B, Pollo B, et al.: Gene therapy of experimental brain tumors using neural progenitor cells. **Nat Med** 6(4):447–450, 2000.
35. During MJ, Naegele JR, O'Malley KL, Geller AI: Long-term behavioral recovery in parkinsonian rats by an HSV vector expressing tyrosine hydroxylase. **Science** 266:1399–1402, 1994.
36. Bankiewicz KS, Leff SE, Nagy D, et al.: Practical aspects of the development of ex vivo and in vivo gene therapy for Parkinson's disease. **Exp Neurol** 144:147–156, 1997.
37. Kordower JH, Bloch J, Ma SY, et al.: Lentiviral gene transfer to the nonhuman primate brain. **Exp Neurol** 160:1–16, 1999.
38. Skorupa AF, Fisher KJ, Wilson JM, Parente MK, Wolfe JH: Sustained production of ß-glucoronidase from localized sites after AAV vector gene transfer results in widespread distribution of enzyme and reversal of lysosomal storage lesions in a large volume of brain in mucopolysaccharidosis VII mice. **Exp Neurol** 160:17–27, 1999.
39. Marshall E: Gene therapy death prompts review of adenovirus vector. **Science**. 286:2244–2245, 1999.
40. Armstrong RJE, Svendsen CN: Neural stem cells: From cell biology to cell replacement. **Cell Transplant** 9(2):139–152, 2000.
41. Vescovi AL, Parati EA, Gritti A: et al.: Isolation and cloning of multipotential stem cells from the embryonic human CNS and establishment of transplantable human neural stem cell lines by epigenetic stimulation. **Exp Neurol** 156:71–83, 1999.
42. Flax JD, Auroara S, Yang C, et al.: Engraftable human neural stem cells respond to developmental cues, replace neurons, and express foreign genes. **Nat Biotechnol** 16:1033–1039, 1998.
43. Kirschenbaum B, Nedergaard M, Preuss A, Barami K, Fraser R, Goldman S: In vitro neuronal production by precursor cells derived from the adult human brain. **Cerebral Cortex** 4:576–589, 1994.
44. Kukekov VG, Laywell ED, Suslov O, et al.: Multipotent stem/progenitor cells with similar properties arise from two neurogenic regions of adult human brain. **Exp Neurol** 156(2):333–344, 1999.
45. Yandava BD, Billinghurst LL, Snyder EY: "Global" cell replacement is feasible via neural stem cell transplantation: Evidence from the dysmyelinated shiverer mouse brain. Proc Natl Acad Sci USA **96:7029–7034, 1999.**
46. Brustle O, Choudhary K, Karram K, et al.: Chimeric brains generated by intraventricular transplantation of fetal human brain cells into embryonic rats. **Nat Biotechnol** 16:1040–1044, 1998.

47. Lansdorp PM: Self-renewal of stem cells. **Biol Blood Marrow Transplant** 3:171–178, 1997.
48. Globerson A: Hematopoietic stem cells and aging. **Exp Gerontol** 34:137–146, 1999.
49. Bjornson CRR, Rietze R, Reynolds BA, Magli MC, Vescovi AL: Turning brain into blood: A hematopoietic fate adopted by adult neural stem cells in vivo. **Science** 283:534–537, 2000.
50. Prockop DJ: Marrow stromal cells as stem cells for nonhematopoietic tissues. **Science** 276(5309):71–74, 1997.
51. Eglitis MA, Mezey E: Hematopoietic cells differentiate into both microglia and macroglia in the brains of adult mice. **Proc Natl Acad Sci USA** 94(8):4080–4085, 1997.
52. Kopen GC, Prockop DJ, Phinney DG: Marrow stromal cells migrate throughout forebrain and cerebellum, and they differentiate into astrocytes after injection into neonatal mouse brains. **Proc Natl Acad Sci USA** 96(19):10711–10716, 1999.
53. Azizi SA, Stokes D, Augelli BJ, DiGirolamo C, Prockop DJ: Engraftment and migration of human bone marrow stromal cells implanted in the brains of albino rats—similarities to astrocyte grafts. **Proc Natl Acad Sci USA** 95(7):3908–3913, 1998.
54. Sanchez-Ramos J, Song S, Cardozo-Pelaez F, et al.: Adult bone marrow stromal cells differentiate into neural cells in vitro. **Exp Neurol** 164(2):247–256, 2000.
55. Woodbury D, Schwarz EJ, Prockop DJ, Black IB: Adult rat and human bone marrow stromal cells differentiate into neurons. **J Neurosci Res** 61:364–370, 2000.
56. Chen J, Li Y, Chopp M: Intracerebral transplantation of bone marrow with BDNF after MCAo in rat. **Neuropharmacology** 39:711–716, 2000.
57. Li Y, Chen J, Chopp M: Adult bone marrow transplantation after stroke in adult rats. **Cell Transplant** 10(1):31-40, 2001.
58. Quinn NP: The clinical application of cell grafting techniques in patients with Parkinson's disease. **Prog Brain Res** 82:619–625, 1990.

10

Surgical Drug Delivery for Neurodegenerative Diseases

MICHAEL G. KAPLITT, M.D., PH.D.
AND ANDRES M. LOZANO, M.D., PH.D.

With the close of the Decade of the Brain, the explosion in neuroscience research has yielded numerous promising new potential therapies. Immunotherapy, enzyme and growth factor therapy, and cell and gene therapy have all received limited clinical exposure at present. An array of successful experimental studies over the past decade, however, has fostered enthusiasm for expanding applications for patients. When combined with more traditional chemical or drug treatments, these applications are poised to significantly alter future approaches to neurological disorders.

One major impediment to fully realizing the therapeutic potential of these substances is the presence of the blood-brain barrier, which significantly limits brain penetration of even small molecules from the bloodstream following peripheral drug administration. The blood-brain barrier is disrupted in certain disease conditions, such as brain tumors and stroke, permitting increased drug or protein exposure to affected areas. Yet many important neurological disorders, in particular neurodegenerative disorders, are not characterized by a significant blood-brain barrier alteration. Even under those conditions in which blood-brain barrier disruption is seen, the barrier often remains intact in infiltrated or at-risk brain regions, thereby blocking peripheral access to the most desirable targets. Techniques for transiently disrupting the blood-brain barrier have been explored for several years, and they hold great promise for improving intracerebral drug delivery from intravenous sources. At present, however, these approaches have limited utility and even under theoretically optimal conditions, generalized and transient delivery to the whole brain may not be appropriate for many therapies.

Direct surgical infusion of substances into the brain is increasingly viewed as a promising area in the future of neurosurgery. Advances in neurosurgical navigation, electrophysiological monitoring and stereotactic equipment now permit access to previously privileged areas of the brain and brainstem. Brain lesioning and deep brain stimulation allow therapeutic inhibition of hyperactive brain nuclei, however this technique is quite nonspecific and does not readily permit protection or functional alteration of the activity of abnormal brain regions. Infusion of bioactive molecules, cells, or genetic vectors allows selective modulation or protection of specific populations of brain cells within a controllable and targeted brain volume. Here we will consider the known technical factors that may permit maximal surgical safety, efficacy, and control of direct infusion. We will also review the limited clinical experience with infusion of bioactive molecules and gene therapy vectors into the brains of human patients, in order to assess prospects for the future of this field.

TECHNICAL CONSIDERATIONS WITH BRAIN INFUSION

Development of advanced therapeutic molecules is unquestionably important; however, if they do not effectively reach their intended brain targets, even the most ideal treatments will be of no clinical value. In addition to efficiency of delivery, control of the volume of distribution is also necessary to minimize adverse drug effects. Free-hand injection is often uncontrollable and results in fluid backup along the injection tract. In our experience with gene therapy vectors, this can also lead to dissection of brain tissue and creation of a pocket in which fluid settles rather than spreads. Infusion pumps permit longer-term infusion, but without a rational basis for defining parameters such as concentration, volumes, and rates of infusion, they can also suffer from poor control and variable results. Reproducible and predictable methods are necessary for intracerebral infusion to gain wide application and acceptance.

Intraventricular delivery represents the largest human experience to date with intracerebral infusion. For a variety of applications, this is clearly the most appropriate method of drug delivery. Intraventricular chemotherapy via Ommaya reservoirs, for example, can be effective for treatment of leptomeningeal neoplastic disease (1). Similarly, severe ventricular infections can be treated by direct infusion of antibiotics. In these instances, intraventricular chemotherapy is logical because the disease process is in direct contact with ventricular cerebrospinal fluid. Ventricular access is a routine and safe technique that does not require special skills or instrumentation, and extensive clinical experience with this route of drug infusion has lead to an understandable level of comfort with the technique. A desire to circumvent the blood-brain barrier while delivering molecules to wide areas of the brain, in addition to technical familiarity, has led to expansion of this mode of delivery beyond intraventricular diseases *(Table 10.1)*. There is, however, a brain-CSF barrier, and it has long been known that penetration of therapeutic mol-

TABLE 10.1
Human Applications of Intraventricular Infusion

Parkinson's disease
    Dopamine (14–16)
    GDNF
Alzheimer's disease
    Cholinergic agonists (23–25)
    NGF (26–27)
Canavan disease
    Liposome-mediated gene therapy (47)
Brain tumors
    Chemotherapy
    Antibodies
    Immunotoxins, targeted-toxins (35)
    Radiolabelled antibodies
    Cytokines
Infection
    Antibiotics
    Antifungals
Spasticity
    Baclofen

ecules into brain tissue from CSF is at best suboptimal (2). It is not surprising, therefore, that this mode of delivery has met with limited success in treatment of solid tumors, degenerative diseases, and other intraparenchymal pathology. This has resulted in increasing interest in direct infusion of substances into brain parenchyma *(Table 10.2)*.

TABLE 10.2
Human Applications of Intraparenchymal Infusion

Parkinson's disease
    Lidocaine (19, 20)
    Muscimol (22)
    NGF with cell transplantation (17)
Epilepsy
    KCL (21)
Brain tumors
    Chemotherapy (30)
    Antibodies (32)
    Immunotoxins; targeted-toxins (36)
    Cytokines (37, 38)
    Gene therapy (41, 42)
    Oncolytic viruses (45, 46)
Infection
    Antibiotics
    Antifungals
Hemorrhage
    Thrombolytics

Convection-enhanced delivery (CED)is a method of intracerebral infusion that attempts to exploit natural tissue planes and intercellular channels to predictably and reliably deliver controlled fluid volumes to targeted brain regions. Based upon early observations that bulk flow can occur within the brain when pressure gradients are generated, diffusion through the brain extracellular space using CED can be augmented by infusing fluid with sufficient pressure to create such gradients. The resulting active interstitial infusion along natural planes of flow within the brain substantially enhances macromolecular distribution (3). High-flow microinfusion appears to deliver molecules to a far larger area than simple diffusion, with greater control and a mathematically predictable pattern (4, 5). Although it has been suggested that absolute dose may be a more important determinant of distribution volume than convection parameters (6), numerous subsequent studies holding the infusion dose constant have confirmed the validity of convection-enhanced delivery (5, 7–11).

A series of studies has provided insight into some of the factors that may influence drug distribution in convection-enhanced delivery. Both small and very large molecules can be spread over most of the area of an entire deep nucleus (10). This distribution is far more quantitatively uniform than delivery by simple diffusion or low-flow infusion, which results in substantial concentration gradients. Different patterns are also seen in gray and white matter. Although large areas of gray matter can be treated, such as an entire deep brain nucleus, this appears to follow a fairly spherical and somewhat limited distribution pattern (9, 11, 12). By contrast, flow among the interstitium of white matter can yield even larger areas of distribution, and the pattern can often asymmetrically follow preferred axonal tracts (9). In large animals, volumes as high as one-third of the white matter in a cerebral hemisphere have been covered with labeled macromolecules infused from a single site by convection-enhanced delivery (8, 9).

Comparison of different routes of drug administration has confirmed the value of convection infusion for intraparenchymal delivery. Studies with both labeled sucrose (7) and labeled cytosine arabinoside (AraC) (8) have documented widespread distribution but extremely low brain tissue levels following intravenous administration. Intraventricular infusion, as suggested above, resulted in higher brain tissue levels but poor penetration, with most signal concentrated at the ependymal surface and diffusing a small distance into the immediate periventricular tissues. For example, less than 0.4% of the dose of labeled sucrose exposed to the brain via intravenous route entered brain tissue, while delivery efficiency via intraventricular route was 100%. This efficiency dropped to 5% within 2 mm from the ventricular surface (7). Intra-parenchymal infusion of both substances by convection-enhanced delivery also was 100% efficient, but the volume of distribution within the brain was substantially greater than intraventricular delivery. This substantiates the view that neuractive substances are unlikely to significantly improve intraparenchymal disease processes when infused by an intraventricular route, but convection-enhanced delivery can potentially distribute therapeutic molecules to large areas of brain tissue.

Several parameters can predictably modulate the results of convection-enhanced delivery. As expected, flow rate can have both positive and negative effects. Low-flow infusion or passive diffusion yields very focal delivery, while increasing infusion rates resulted in wider areas of drug delivery in several studies (5, 7, 8). Molecules will be cleared by normal flow of interstitial fluid. However, clearance by this route is sufficiently slow that even moderately high flow rates readily overcome this factor. Very rapid infusion can cause significant fluid backup along the injection track, resulting in both poor control of delivery and loss of infusate from the cortical surface (4, 5). Catheter diameter also influences backflow in an inverse relationship to flow rate, so that more rapid infusions can be performed over briefer periods by using catheters with smaller diameters (5). Characteristics of the infused molecule are also important, since differential binding of molecules to cells or internalization by cells can influence delivery volume and clearance. A dual microdialysis study in rodents graphically demonstrated this in real time, since infusion of mannitol, a purely extracellular molecule, reached steady-state levels faster than dopamine, which clears by both extracellular and intracellular paths (13). Distribution characteristics in gray and white matter differ; however, other tissue factors may also be influential. Presence of brain edema can alter delivery (9), and the mere presence of a 6-hydroxy dopamine nigral lesion in rodents can influence the rate of diffusion of both dopamine and mannitol compared with normal controls following infusion into striatum (13). Mathematical models have been created to predict drug distribution and tissue levels based upon idealized models and presumptions (4, 5). However, individual conditions such as drug characteristics and disease states can influence delivery in ways that are not yet fully predictable.

The predictive value of these findings has been tested in experimental models of Parkinson's disease. Thermolesions of the internal pallidum palliate parkinsonian symptoms in MPTP-treated primates. Convection-enhanced infusion of excitotoxins kainic acid and quinolinic acid into GPi resulted in behavioral improvements in these animals (11,

12). The first study used a relatively large volume (75 μl) of kainic acid, with a resulting pallidal distribution of neuronal loss over 180 μl of tissue (12). This represented an 85% efficiency when compared with a predicted distribution of 225 μl of tissue, assuming that the interstitial space represents 35% of the tissue. At this volume, significant neuronal loss was also seen in the GPe and some excitotoxicity was even demonstrated in the hippocampus. The second study used molecular models to determine the volume and concentration of the quinolinic acid solution, as well as the rate of infusion necessary to cover the GPi with a toxic level of drug while sparing surrounding structures (11). The results closely matched predictions, with a near total neuronal loss in GPi but no significant loss in GPe, subthalamic nucleus, thalamus or hippocampus. These provide important preclinical evidence that molecular modeling can provide some guidance to permit planned surgical infusion of substances to a defined brain area.

PARKINSON'S DISEASE

Parkinson's disease (PD) represents a logical target for brain microinfusion, given the long history of stereotactic neurosurgery for movement disorders. A major limitation of drug therapy for PD is the inability to deliver sufficient molecules to brain targets without significant side effects in the periphery or in remote brain regions. One approach to circumvent this is to deliver neurotransmitters or analogs at high levels directly to brain targets. Among the first ventures in this area involved intraventricular infusion of dopamine into PD patients (14, 15). Minimal benefits were observed in these patients, and no larger study was performed to determine if even these effects were truly significant. An interesting consequence of this therapy in one patient was the development of psychotic symptoms with delusions (16). Although the treatment failure could be due to a disease process which was refractory to dopamine therapy, it is more likely that the drug failed to penetrate sufficiently into the depths of the striatum to cause symptomatic improvement. It is possible that the observed psychosis could reflect better drug delivery to periventricular limbic/cognitive structures, including anterior temporal, frontal, and hypothalamic areas.

Growth factors have also been infused into PD patients. An early study employed chronic nerve growth factor (NGF) infusions over 23 days via a subcutaneous pump into the striatum of a woman following adrenal autograft (17). The purpose was to provide support for maintenance of the adrenal graft. Adrenal grafting has largely been abandoned due to poor efficacy, and later studies on nigral trophic factors implicated molecules other than NGF. In particular, glial-derived neurotrophic factor (GDNF) seems to be particularly protective of nigral neurons in tissue culture and in animal models. Based upon this, a phase I dose escalation multicenter clinical study was undertaken to examine the safety of recombinant GDNF in PD patients following intraventricular delivery. At the trial doses used, in 8 patients treated at our center, intraventricular GDNF did not provide significant clinical benefit and was associated with adverse effects including nausea, weight loss, and sensory symptoms. The diffusion of this potent neurotrophic factor throughout the CSF space and within the brain beyond the intended nigral dopaminergic neurons was the likely explanation for the poor therapeutic index observed in this study. Local delivery of recombinant GDNF to the substantia nigra and/or striatum by either infusion pumps or by expression from gene therapy vectors may help to minimize adverse effects while improving efficacy. Recent evidence demonstrating that growth factors may have complicated, and often contradictory, neural modulatory effects distinct from their trophic effects emphasizes the importance of preclinical studies (18).

At the Toronto Western Hospital, we have explored the effects of single infusions of neuroactive substances directly into deep brain nuclei in PD patients. Lidocaine has been shown to block neuronal activity in experimental animals. Early reports of small patient groups suggested that large volume infusion into the globus pallidus could positively influence rigidity and tremor in PD. Using modern imaging and microelectrode-guided stereotactic techniques, 0.5 to 2.0 μl of 2% lidocaine was hand injected into potential thalamic lesion sites (V_{im}) of patients with tremor (19, 20). Infusion was performed only at sites where microstimulation suppressed tremor, and lidocaine also reduced or arrested tremor at nearly 80% of these sites. The drug effect began within 1 minute of injection and lasted for no more than 20 minutes. In one patient, microelectrode recording revealed an absence of spontaneous electrical activity within the target nucleus for approximately 10 minutes (19). All patients then underwent successful thalamic thermocoagulation at these target sites. Chemically induced inhibition of brain electrical activity (manifest as spreading depression on EEG) has also been seen in epilepsy patients following microinjection of potassium chloride into the caudate nucleus or hippocampus (21).

Since lidocaine will inhibit both somatic activity within a nucleus and signal propagation along axonal fibers, we more recently examined the effect of muscimol infusion in deep brain nuclei (22). Muscimol is a selective $GABA_A$ agonist which transiently blocks neuronal firing in cells harboring appropriate receptors but does not influence the activity of fibers of passage. Infusion of up to 5 μl of drug at a rate of 1–2 μl/min resulted in tremor reduction or arrest in all tested essential tremor patients, with time of onset averaging 7 minutes and a mean duration of 9 minutes *(Fig. 10.1)*. No effect on tremor was observed following infusion of equivalent rates and volumes of saline (22). Again, all patients then received successful thalamotomy or thalamic DBS prior. We have subsequently found similar effects following muscimol infusion into GPi and STN of PD patients (A. Lozano, unpublished observations). As with the experimental PD studies using excitotoxin infusions (11, 12), this approach should permit specific modulation of neuronal cell bodies while sparing glial cells and axonal fibers. The ability to selectively influence specific cellular elements within a nucleus may permit more careful dissection of the human pathophysiology of movement disorders. These studies also demonstrate the feasibility of drug infusion as an alternative method for control of movement disorder symptoms. Combination of this approach with advanced, chronic infusion techniques may make direct drug infusion into the brain a viable option for surgical treatment of movement disorders.

ALZHEIMER'S DISEASE

Alzheimer's disease (AD) presents far greater challenges to successful surgical intervention than PD. AD is a more diffuse disease than PD, and currently there is a poor understanding of the relevant dysfunctional anatomical pathways that cause symptoms of AD. Animal models of AD have only recently been developed, and their relevance to human symptoms is still unclear. There is also considerable debate as to the pathophysiology of AD, so there is no consensus as to which molecules might best be employed to treat AD. Such issues of target selection and drug choice are more straightforward in PD, so microinfusion studies in human AD patients have so far been limited to intraventricular infusion of putative therapeutic agents.

Loss of cholinergic tone has long been implicated as one factor that promotes development of memory loss and dementia in AD. Among the few drugs approved for use in AD are oral agents which promote increased cholinergic transmission within the brain. Although the value of such therapy is controversial, any benefit is limited by poor brain penetration and peripheral side effects at higher doses. This was the basis for trials in AD patients examining the efficacy of intraventricular infusion of bethanecol, a muscarinic agonist (23–25). A pilot project documented that chronic infusion with a subcutaneous pump could be performed safely in AD patients, but there was no clear evidence of therapeutic efficacy (24). In some patients, adverse effects were transiently experienced, but these resolved with reduction in flow. After a

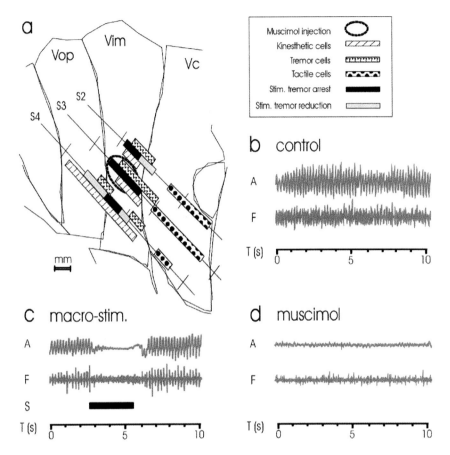

FIG. 10.1 Effects of electrical stimulation and intrathalamic muscimol microinjections in essential tremor patients. (A) Reconstruction of the trajectories of three microelectrode tracks (S2, S3, S4) in a patient with essential tremor on a sagittal map 14.5 mm lateral to the midline. The site of muscimol injection is represented by a dashed ellipse in S3 (i.e., the targeted injection site was V_{im}). The regions where single-unit responses to joint movement (kinesthetic), tremor, and tactile stimuli were recorded are indicated by the patterned bars (see box for code). Regions where microstimulation at 100 µA induced tremor reduction or arrest are indicated by the filled bars. (B) Baseline tremor (control) at 1 min before muscimol microinjection as recorded by accelerometer (A) and wrist flexor EMG (F) over 10 s of time (T) during postural tremor. (C) Macrostimulation blocks tremor (0.5 mm exposed tip, 25 gauge tubing; track S3, 400 µA, 0.1 ms pulses, 300 Hz, 3 s train) performed at the microinjection site. Traces as in (B); period of stimulation (S) indicated by the horizontal bar. (D) The effect of a 5 µL microinjection of muscimol (same site as macrostimulation) on tremor, 8 min after injection. Traces as in (B) Microinjections of muscimol but not saline reduced tremor by approximately 85%. (Modified from Pahapil et al., 1999, *Annals of Neurology*.)

subsequent study found conflicting evidence of improvement (23), a double-blind, multicenter trial was completed. This demonstrated no clear evidence of therapeutic benefit, and cholinergic agonist infusion into the ventricles of AD patients has to date been largely abandoned (25). The failure of this treatment may be at least partially due to over-simplification of the pathophysiology of AD. The intraventricular route would expose the majority of drug to periventricular structures, how-ever, and this might yield unacceptable side effects at doses necessary to permit sufficient therapeutic penetration, if that were even possible.

As with PD, intraventricular growth factor infusion has also been used in an attempt to preserve degenerating neurons in AD patients. Nerve growth factor (NGF) was the first identified neuronal trophic fac-tor. Although numerous growth factors were subsequently found to have greater protective effects on specific neuronal populations, NGF appears to be particularly effective at protecting cholinergic and hip-pocampal neurons in tissue culture and in animal studies. In the ini-tial clinical case report, no significant adverse effects were found fol-lowing a 3-month chronic infusion of NFG (26). An increase in cerebral blood flow was noted on PET scan, but no convincing cognitive changes were seen. Expansion of the trial to include three patients yielded im-provements in selected neuropsychiatric tests but no broad cognitive changes (27). Side effects, including dose-related back pain and weight-loss, were also now noted. Even though this was a small and uncon-trolled study, the suggestion of a benefit and reversible, dose-related side effects again suggests that direct delivery of NGF to parenchymal brain targets may be a viable therapy for AD. Animal studies have ex-plored direct, intraparenchymal infusion of recombinant NGF (28), as well as infusion of cells or gene therapy vectors expressing NGF (29), and these have all yielded positive results. Recently, a clinical protocol was approved and a trial was initiated for infusion of cells engineered to secrete NGF into the basal forebrain. This may hold promise for a new neurosurgical approach to AD therapy.

BRAIN TUMORS

The most widespread use of direct intracerebral infusion in common clinical practice is in neuro-oncology. Intraventricular infusion of chemotherapy through Ommaya reservoirs are frequently used to treat leptomeningeal metastatic disease and CNS lymphoma (1). Although it is important to place the catheter tip properly within a clear CSF space to prevent intraparenchymal toxicity, there are few other technical con-siderations when infusing agents through this route (1). Fairly rapid hand injections are usually performed on an intermittent basis, although implantable pumps with slower, continuous infusion rates have been used. Intraventricular chemotherapy can be quite effective for leptomeningeal disease in some cases. However, use of this technique for treatment intraparenchymal disease has met with poor results (30). This is likely due to the penetration problems outlined in our earlier discussion.

The promise of new technologies that do not penetrate the brain by other routes has led to exploration of direct intratumoral infusion of antineoplastic agents. Intratumoral chemotherapy attempts to massively increase the local drug dose to the tumor while limiting systemic effects. This has largely been popularized by wafer technology, which relies on simple diffusion, however intratumoral catheter-based infusion of chemotherapeutic agents has also been attempted (31). Since tumor resistance to chemotherapy remains a major problem regardless of the method of drug delivery, biological agents with potentially improved efficacy are likely to benefit more from direct intratumoral infusion strategies. Antibodies and immunotoxins are examples of such agents. Unconjugated antibody infusion within tumors attempts to provoke antitumor immune responses following antibody binding to tumor cells. An early use of an antiepidermal growth factor receptor antibody revealed some evidence of necrosis, but it was unclear whether there was a significant treatment effect (32). The infusion rate of 4 ml/hr through four shunt catheters would suggest that there may have been significant backflow of antibody with loss of efficacy, based upon experimental studies. Radioactive conjugates have also been infused into tumors (33), but this is unlikely to improve upon the extensive experience with interstitial radiation therapy in the brain.

Immunotoxins and targeted-toxins represent more promising strategies for brain tumor therapy, and may be applicable to neurodegenerative diseases as well. Immunotoxins are cell-selective antibodies conjugated to modified strong cellular toxins such as ricin A or diphtheria toxin, while targeted-toxins are toxin conjugates that use molecules such as receptor ligands to provide cell-specificity (34–37). The ability to fuse a toxin to any cellular receptor ligand suggests that they may also permit targeted destruction of specific neuronal populations for the treatment of disorders such as Parkinson's disease. Currently, however, these have been considered mostly as brain tumor therapy. A promising study of intraventricular infusion of an immunotoxin for leptomeningeal disease demonstrated mild toxicity at high doses and a possible antitumor effect (35). Most patients received only a single dose, which may have limited efficacy, and assessment of the true value of this treatment awaits publication of more conclusive studies. More relevant to this discussion is a similar study using a mutant diphtheria toxin conjugated to transferrin (36). Transferrin receptors are abundant in most tumor cells but are minimally expressed within normal brain, so the toxin should specifically target tumor cells. This study appears to be the first direct application of convection-enhanced delivery of a molecule into the human brain, and impressive preliminary responses were observed. In similarly preliminary studies, others have also infused cytokines into tumors to provoke immune responses or toxin-conjugated cytokines for direct tumor lysis (37, 38). Further improvements in delivery techniques to tumors may increase the acceptance and efficacy of these therapies. Development of new treatments may, however, be of greater importance to the future of direct infusion in the brain, and among the most exciting of these approaches is gene therapy.

GENE THERAPY

The explosion in genomics has opened previously unimaginable areas of opportunity for new medical diagnostics and therapeutics, and few areas are poised to benefit from this more than neurological disease. As the functions of new genes are discovered at exponential rates, there is great hope for developing a variety of new drugs to mimic or modulate the activity of those genes associated with particular disorders. Cell transplantation can result in local production of therapeutic proteins and potentially replace lost cells. Cells do not significantly diffuse, so strategies to improve delivery to cover a brain region have been developed (39). One of the most direct, logical, and theoretically controllable approaches to therapeutic alteration of gene expression is gene therapy. Most gene therapy strategies use modified viruses as gene delivery vehicles, since viruses have evolved to be highly efficient agents for transfer of genetic material (40). Early issues focused upon improving the safety of vector systems and enhancing the efficiency of gene delivery. These issues have been addressed over recent years (41), and while improvements in vector technology and delivery methods continue, attention has largely turned to choice of gene(s), regulation of expression, and application to human disease.

Until recently, the only clinical experience with gene therapy in the brain has been in the treatment of brain tumors (42). All of the clinical studies can be grouped into two general categories: gene transfer and oncolytic viruses. Gene transfer involves delivery of one or more therapeutic genes into brain tumor cells, and technical issues with this method are not significantly different from other gene transfer strategies for non-neoplastic disorders. Some trials have involved simple transfer of genes, which may cause cell death or correct possible defects in the tumor cell cycle. One such example is a recent trial of the safety of adenovirus-mediated transfer of the p53 tumor suppressor gene in patients with glioblastoma multiforme (GBM)(43). As with other phase I studies, this appears to be safe, but efficacy is unclear. Efficacy may be improved by combining p53 gene therapy with radiation, as p53 is known to sensitize cells to ionizing radiation. Since complete eradication of tumor cells would theoretically require 100% efficiency of gene delivery, others have attempted to transfer genes that would produce diffusible substances (42). For example, transfer of cytokine genes into tumors has yielded mixed results at best, but the consequences of cytokine-induced local inflammation and edema may offset any potential benefits.

The most popular gene transfer agents to date have contained genes for prodrug activating enzymes. When expressed within a cell, these enzymes cleave otherwise inactive agents into active chemotherapeutics with specific antineoplastic activity. The classic example of this is the herpes simplex virus (HSV) thymidine-kinase (TK) gene. TK converts drugs such as ganciclovir into active agents that block DNA synthesis and kill replicating cells. Even if this event occurred in neurons, it should be innocuous since these cells do not divide. The observation that in some situations a "bystander" effect can kill uninfected cells adjacent to those which are infected enhanced enthusiasm for this strategy. Several studies have examined the safety and efficacy of this treatment using infusion of retroviral vectors, retroviral-producer cell lines and adenoviral vectors in both adult and pediatric brain tumors (42). Adenoviral vectors appear to provide much greater tumor distribution than lower titer retroviruses, but trials have thus far failed to document impressive treatment effects with any system (42). Numerous experimental studies are ongoing to develop agents with improved antineoplastic activity.

Oncolytic viruses are modified viruses that selectively replicate in tumor cells while sparing normal tissue. Since they are engineered viruses, which usually do not necessarily transfer a new genetic function to the cell, this may be better called "viral therapy" rather than gene therapy. The first oncolytic virus used in clinical oncology is the ONYX-015 virus, which is an adenovirus deleted for the E1B gene (44). This virus appears to selectively replicate in p53-deficient cells, such as many tumor cells, but replication and toxicity is blocked in normal cells expressing wild-type p53. The exact method of selectivity is still under exploration, since some tumor cells expressing wild-type p53 appear to be sensitive to this virus, but normal cells still appear resistant.

Although a phase I clinical study in patients with brain tumors has recently been initiated, encouraging results from a trial in patients with head and neck cancer suggest that this may be a promising treatment (44). More recently, selectively replicating HSV vectors have been subjected to pilot clinical studies (45, 46). These viruses both harbored deletions in the γ34.5 gene, which has been identified as an HSV neurovirulence gene. One of the studies used a virus with a second deletion in ribonuccleotide reductase gene, which should further disable the virus in nondividing cells that have insufficient pools of nucleotides to support viral replication (45). The double mutant was given at doses up to 3×10^9 pfu (plaque-forming units), and some toxicities were noted which could not be conclusively referred to the virus (45). The single mutant resulted in less toxicity, but it was given at far lower doses (up to 10^5 pfu) (46). Demonstration of the optimal safety profile and the therapeutic value of these agents awaits further studies.

Recently, gene therapy has been applied to the human brain for a non-neoplastic condition (47). Historically, it appeared logical that gene therapy would be initially applied to genetic disorders in which replacement of the defective gene could cure a disease. In practice, however, the damage from a genetic disorder during development often precludes postnatal rescue, and gene replacement likely requires high efficiency, widespread delivery. As a result, even the number of preclinical studies in this area has been limited. Perhaps the most promising targets for gene therapy are neurodegenerative disorders such as Parkinson's disease. This is reflected in the number of preclinical studies that have brought gene therapy to the brink of clinical approval (48–50). Nonetheless, the first gene therapy study for a non-neoplastic disorder has recently been described for the genetic disorder Canavan disease (47).

Canavan disease is an autosomal recessive leukodystrophy which results in spongiform, white matter degeneration secondary to a deficiency in aspartoacylase (ASPA) activity. ASPA deficiency leads to a buildup in N-acetyl-aspartate (NAA), which can be measured in vivo by proton spectroscopy. The ASPA gene in a plasmid was encapsulated into liposomes, since viral vectors did not appear sufficiently advanced when governmental approval was requested. Animal studies suggested that intraventricular infusion would yield widespread delivery, but efficiency was suboptimal. After primate safety studies were completed, a phase I trial was initiated which documented the safety of this technique (47). Although there was some MRI evidence of remyelination *(Fig. 10.2)* and short-term decreases in NAA levels in some brain regions, this was not universally observed and the small number of pa-

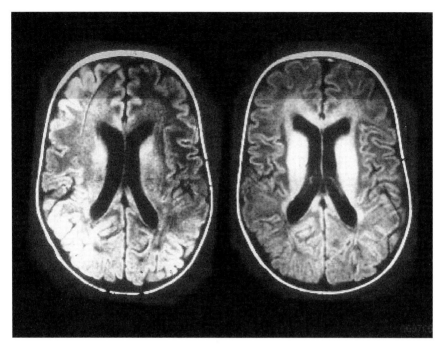

FIG. 10.2 Axial T1 weighted MR image of a patient with Canavan disease before (left) and 12 months after (right) gene therapy. Note the increase in periventricualr myelination after gene therapy.

tients precludes conclusive determination of therapeutic efficacy. Since direct infusion of viral vectors into white matter will likely result in vastly increased gene transfer efficiency, a phase I trial of direct intraparenchymal infusion of an ASPA-containing adeno-associated virus vector is currently under review.

FUTURE DIRECTIONS

The few clinical studies to date using direct microinfusion into the brain reflect the state of a new field in its infancy. Although neuro-oncology will continue to benefit from improvements in this area, potentially revolutionary therapies may result from expansion of direct infusion strategies to non-neoplastic disorders. Drug infusion has already yielded short-term benefits in patients with Parkinson's disease, and chronic infusion technologies may help realize its true clinical potential. Nonviral gene therapy has now been explored in a pediatric neurogenetic disorder, and viral gene therapy will soon follow for both pediatric and adult diseases. Lesioning and deep-brain stimulation are the major modalities currently used in stereotactic procedures, but drug or gene therapy infusion will likely target neuronal populations in a far more specific manner. Also, current surgical procedures only dampen output from hyperactive brain regions. As genomic information expands and we increase knowledge of the biological basis of neurological disorders, the ability to infuse drugs or gene vectors may provide new or improved function specific to neuronal populations. Combined with improvements in delivery technology and predictability, these advances are poised to provide future surgical options for an array of neurological diseases which at present can only be imagined.

REFERENCES

1. Sandberg DI, Bilsky MH, Souweidane MM, Bzdil J, Gutin PH: Ommaya reservoirs for the treatment of leptomeningeal metastases. **Neurosurgery** 47:49–54, 2000.
2. Blasberg RG, Patlak C, Fenstermacher JD: Intrathecal chemotherapy: Brain tissue profiles after ventriculocisternal perfusion. **J Pharmacol Exp Ther** 195:73–83, 1975.
3. Bobo RH, Laske DW, Akbasak A, Morrison PF, Dedrick RL, Oldfield EH: Convection-enhanced delivery of macromolecules in the brain. **Proc Natl Acad Sci USA** 91:2076–2080, 1994.
4. Morrison PF, Laske DW, Bobo H, Oldfield EH, Dedrick RL: High-flow microinfusion: Tissue penetration and pharmacodynamics. **Am J Physiol** 266:R292–305, 1994.
5. Morrison PF, Chen MY, Chadwick RS, Lonser RR, Oldfield EH: Focal delivery during direct infusion to brain: role of flow rate, catheter diameter, and tissue mechanics. **Am J Physiol** 277:R1218–1229, 1999.
6. Kroll RA, Pagel MA, Muldoon LL, Roman-Goldstein S, Neuwelt EA: Increasing volume of distribution to the brain with interstitial infusion: dose, rather than convection, might be the most important factor. **Neurosurgery** 38:746–752, 1996.
7. Groothuis DR, Ward S, Itskovich AC, et al.: Comparison of 14C-sucrose delivery to the brain by intravenous, intraventricular, and convection-enhanced intracerebral infusion. **J Neurosurg** 90:321–331, 1999.
8. Groothuis DR, Benalcazar H, Allen CV, et al.: Comparison of cytosine arabinoside delivery to rat brain by intravenous, intrathecal, intraventricular and intraparenchymal routes of administration. **Brain Res** 856:281–290, 2000.
9. Laske DW, Morrison PF, Lieberman DM, et al.: Chronic interstitial infusion of protein to primate brain: determination of drug distribution and clearance with single-photon emission computerized tomography imaging. **J Neurosurg** 87:586–594, 1997.
10. Lieberman DM, Laske DW, Morrison PF, Bankiewicz KS, Oldfield EH: Convection-enhanced distribution of large molecules in gray matter during interstitial drug infusion. **J Neurosurg** 82:1021–1029, 1995.
11. Lonser RR, Corthesy ME, Morrison PF, Gogate N, Oldfield EH: Convection-enhanced selective excitotoxic ablation of the neurons of the globus pallidus internus for treatment of parkinsonism in nonhuman primates. **J Neurosurg** 91:294–302, 1999.
12. Lieberman DM, Corthesy ME, Cummins A, Oldfield EH: Reversal of experimental parkinsonism by using selective chemical ablation of the medial globus pallidus. **J Neurosurg** 90:928–934, 1999.
13. Hoistad M, Kehr J, Andbjer B, Jansson A, Fuxe K: Intracerebral infusion of H-

dopamine and H-mannitol in the striatum of halothane-anaesthetized male rats. A dual-probe microdialysis study of long-distance diffusion. **Eur J Neurosci** 12:2505–2514, 2000.

14. Venna N, Sabin TD, Ordia JI, Mark VH: Treatment of severe Parkinson's disease by intraventricular injection of dopamine. **Appl Neurophysiol** 47:62–64, 1984.

15. Horne MK, Butler EG, Gilligan BS, Wodak J, Stark RJ, Brazenor GA: Intraventricular infusion of Dopamine in Parkinson's disease. **Ann Neurol** 26:792–794, 1989.

16. Kulkarni J, Horne M, Butler E, Keks N, Copolov D: Psychotic symptoms resulting from intraventricular infusion of dopamine in Parkinson's disease. **Biol Psychiatry** 31:1225–1227, 1992.

17. Olson L, Backlund EO, Ebendal T, et al.: Intraputaminal infusion of nerve growth factor to support adrenal medullary autografts in Parkinson's disease. One-year follow-up of first clinical trial. **Arch Neurol** 48:373–381,1991.

18. Messer CJ, Eisch AJ, Carlezon WA, Jr., et al.: Role for GDNF in biochemical and behavioral adaptations to drugs of abuse. **Neuron** 26:247–257, 2000.

19. Dostrovsky JO, Sher GD, Davis KD, Parrent AG, Hutchison WD, Tasker RR: Microinjection of lidocaine into human thalamus: a useful tool in stereotactic surgery. **Stereotact Funct Neurosurg** 60:168–174, 1993.

20. Parrent AG, Tasker RR, Dostrovsky JO: Tremor reduction by microinjection of lidocaine during stereotactic surgery. **Acta Neurochir Suppl (Wien)** 58:45–47, 1993.

21. Sramka M, Brozek G, Bures J, Nadvornik P: Functional ablation by spreading depression: possible use in human stereotactic Neurosurgery **Appl Neurophysiol** 40:48–61, 1977.

22. Pahapill PA, Levy R, Dostrovsky JO, et al.: Tremor arrest with thalamic microinjections of muscimol in patients with essential tremor. **Ann Neurol** 46:249–252, 1999.

23. Harbaugh RE: Intracerebroventricular cholinergic drug administration in Alzheimer's disease: preliminary results of a double-blind study. **J Neural Transm Suppl** 24:271–277, 1987.

24. Harbaugh RE, Roberts DW, Coombs DW, Saunders RL, Reeder TM: Preliminary report: intracranial cholinergic drug infusion in patients with Alzheimer's disease. **Neurosurgery** 15:514–518, 1984.

25. Harbaugh RE, Reeder TM, Senter HJ, et al.: Intracerebroventricular bethanechol chloride infusion in Alzheimer's disease. Results of a collaborative double-blind study. **J Neurosurg.** 71:481–486, 1989.

26. Seiger A, Nordberg A, von Holst H, et al.: Intracranial infusion of purified nerve growth factor to an Alzheimer patient: the first attempt of a possible future treatment strategy. **Behav Brain Res** 57:255–261, 1993.

27. Eriksdotter Jonhagen M, Nordberg A, Amberla K, et al.: Intracerebroventricular infusion of nerve growth factor in three patients with Alzheimer's disease. **Dement Geriatr Cogn Disord** 9:246–257, 1998.

28. Dekker AJ, Fagan AM, Gage FH, Thal LJ: Effects of brain-derived neurotrophic factor and nerve growth factor on remaining neurons in the lesioned nucleus basalis magnocellularis. **Brain Res** 639:149–155, 1994.

29. Mandel RJ, Gage FH, Clevenger DG, Spratt SK, Snyder RO, Leff SE: Nerve growth factor expressed in the medial septum following in vivo gene delivery using a recombinant adeno-associated viral vector protects cholinergic neurons from fimbria-fornix lesion-induced degeneration. **Exp Neurol** 155:59–164, 1999

30. Kroin JS, Penn RD: Intracerebral chemotherapy: chronic microinfusion of cisplatin. **Neurosurgery** 10:349–354, 1982.

31. Haroun RI, Brem H: Local drug delivery. **Curr Opin Oncol** 12:187–193, 2000.

32. Wersall P, Ohlsson I, Biberfeld P, et al.: Intratumoral infusion of the monoclonal an-

tibody, mAb 425, against the epidermal-growth-factor receptor in patients with advanced malignant glioma. **Cancer Immunol Immunother** 44:157–164, 1997.

33. Lashford LS, Davies AG, Richardson RB, et al.: A pilot study of 131I monoclonal antibodies in the therapy of leptomeningeal tumors. **Cancer** 61:857–868, 1988.

34. Vitetta ES, Fulton RJ, May RD, Till M, Uhr JW: Redesigning nature's poisons to create anti-tumor reagents. **Science** 238:1098–1104, 1987.

35. Laske DW, Muraszko KM, Oldfield EH, et al.: Intraventricular immunotoxin therapy for leptomeningeal neoplasia. **Neurosurgery** 41:1039–1049, 1997.

36. Laske DW, Youle RJ, Oldfield EH: Tumor regression with regional distribution of the targeted toxin TF-CRM107 in patients with malignant brain tumors. **Nat Med** 3:1362–1368, 1997.

37. Rand RW, Kreitman RJ, Patronas N, Varricchio F, Pastan I, Puri RK: Intratumoral administration of recombinant circularly permuted interleukin-4-Pseudomonas exotoxin in patients with high-grade glioma. **Clin Cancer Res** 6:2157–2165, 2000.

38. Martinez R, Vaquero J, Ramiro J, Garcia Salazar F, De Oya S: Intratumoural and intraventricular human lymphoblastoid alpha interferon (HLBI) for treatment of glioblastoma multiforme. **Acta Neurochir (Wien)** 100:46–49, 1989.

39. Qureshi NH, Bankiewicz KS, Louis DN, Hochberg FH, Chiocca EA, Harsh GRt: Multicolumn infusion of gene therapy cells into human brain tumors: technical report. **Neurosurgery** 46:663–668, 2000.

40. Kaplitt MG, Pfaff DW: Viral vectors for gene delivery and expression in the CNS. **Methods** 10:343–350, 1996.

41. Kaplitt MG, Darakchiev B, During MJ: Prospects for gene therapy in pediatric Neurosurgery **Pediatr Neurosurg** 28:3–14, 1998.

42. Qureshi NH, Chiocca EA: A review of gene therapy for the treatment of central nervous system tumors. **Crit Rev Oncog** 10:261–274, 1999.

43. Lang FF, Yung WK, Sawaya R, Tofilon PJ: Adenovirus-mediated p53 gene therapy for human gliomas. **Neurosurgery** 45:1093–1104, 1999.

44. Ganly I, Kirn D, Eckhardt SG, et al.: A phase I study of Onyx-015, an E1B attenuated adenovirus, administered intratumorally to patients with recurrent head and neck cancer. **Clin Cancer Res** 6:798–806, 2000.

45. Markert JM, Medlock MD, Rabkin SD, et al.: Conditionally replicating herpes simplex virus mutant, G207 for the treatment of malignant glioma: results of a phase I trial. **Gene Ther** 7:867–874, 2000.

46. Rampling R, Cruickshank G, Papanastassiou V, et al.: Toxicity evaluation of replication-competent herpes simplex virus (ICP 34.5 null mutant 1716) in patients with recurrent malignant glioma. **Gene Ther** 7:859–866, 2000.

47. Leone P, Janson CG, Bilianuk L, et al.: Aspartoacylase gene transfer to the mammalian central nervous system with therapeutic implications for Canavan disease. **Ann Neurol** 48:27–38, 2000.

48. Kaplitt MG, Leone P, Samulski RJ, et al.: Long-term gene expression and phenotypic correction using adeno-associated virus vectors in the mammalian brain. **Nat Genet** 8:148–154, 1994.

49. During MJ, Samulski RJ, Elsworth JD, et al: In vivo expression of therapeutic human genes for dopamine production in the caudates of MPTP-treated monkeys using an AAV vector. **Gene Ther** 5:820–827, 1998.

50. Bankiewicz KS, Eberling JL, Kohutnicka M, et al: Convection-enhanced delivery of AAV vector in parkinsonian monkeys; in vivo detection of gene expression and restoration of dopaminergic function using pro-drug approach. **Exp Neurol** 164:2–14, 2000.

11

Cellular Therapies for Neurodegenerative Diseases

DOUGLAS KONDZIOLKA, M.D., M.Sc., F.R.C.S.C,
ELIZABETH TYLER-KABARA, M.D., Ph.D.,
AND CRISTIAN ACHIM, M.D., Ph.D.

THE BASIS OF NEUROTRANSPLANTATION

Modern restorative neurosurgery began over 25 years ago when neurosurgeons and neurobiologists envisioned the possibility of replacing human neurons in neurodegenerative diseases like Parkinson's disease and Huntington's disease. Early clinical trials were based first on a direct approach targeting the replacement of missing specific neurotransmitters rather than regenerating the damaged neuronal circuitry. More recently, with the advent of therapeutic strategies developed from experimental work with stem and progenitor cells, there is hope that the final goal of reconstructing neuronal pathways may be achieved. We can summarize the goals of this field as replacement, release, and regeneration. Dead neurons have to be replaced, the grafts have to be able to release neurotransmitters and circuits have to be rebuilt. Of course, all these goals can be fulfilled only if our understanding of molecular mechanisms of disease will keep up the pace with the development of new bioengineering strategies. Since the pioneering work of Björklund et al., almost three decades ago (1–3) much progress was made (4–6).

The field of neural transplantation for the treatment of neurologic diseases first showed therapeutic potential in 1979 when Björklund (3) and Perlow (26) showed that transplantation of dopamine-containing neurons in rat striatum improved functional deficits induced by damage to the nigrostriatal pathway. Since that time advances in neural transplantation has moved from the animal model to the human model with varying degrees of success. Animal models encompass a wide variety of disease states from degenerative diseases to trauma and stroke models. Tissue used for transplantation ranges from fetal tissue to tumor lines to stem cells. In some models, implants provide a source of neurotrophic factors. Successes in animal models have led to transplant trials in the human population. Patient trials include transplantation for Parkinson's disease, Huntington's disease, spinal cord injury, and stroke. As research in animal models progresses, transplant trials may be initiated for the treatment of multiple sclerosis, traumatic brain injury, cerebral palsy, amyotrophic lateral sclerosis (ALS), Alzheimer's disease, hereditary ataxias, and other disorders.

NEURAL TRANSPLANTATION: CLINICAL TRIALS AND EXPERIMENTAL MODELS

Background

The concept of using dissociated central nervous system (CNS) tissues for transplantation was promoted by Schmidt et al. (7) who argued that this protocol may be used for intraparenchymal implantation. The same group of investigators has later shown, including detailed methodology, that mesencephalic, dopaminergic rich cell suspensions can be injected in various regions of lesioned rat brains and promote regeneration (8–12). Since these early attempts, a whole field has grown largely on the idea of using human fetal tissues to replace human degenerating neurons. Parkinson's disease (PD) has become the frontier in neurotransplantation.

The hypotheses tested and lessons learned from transplantation studies in PD have been extended to other problems like Huntington's disease (HD) and spinal cord regeneration. The therapeutic principles are largely similar and the obstacles to be conquered to secure graft survival and functional recovery, identical. For this reason, our chapter will emphasize PD studies as the benchmark for any new experimental approaches in CNS cell transplantation although promising advances have been reported in stroke. Among the challenges to any transplantation protocol are: source and preparation of donor tissue, surgical protocol, post-transplantation hypoxia, local toxic factors like free radicals and excitatory amino acids, deprivation of neurotrophic factors (NTF), necrosis and neuronal apoptosis (5). Any factors alleviating these limitations will have a significant impact on the cell transplantation protocol in any neurodegenerative disease.

CLINICAL TRIALS IN PARKINSON'S DISEASE: THE PROTOTYPE FOR CELL TRANSPLANTATION

Parkinson's disease is characterized primarily by the degeneration of dopaminergic neurons projecting from the substantia nigra to the corpus striatum. Logically, the first therapeutic approach in diseases associated with parkinsonian symptoms, for a long time equated primarily with rigidity, were based on replacing the natural neurotransmitter with precursors like levodopa. This has proved to be a highly effective treatment and is still the first choice in PD. Nevertheless, some of its limitations derived from extended use and coupled with the significant progress in developmental neurobiology have led to clinical trials using human fetal tissues as potential replacements for the degenerating adult dopaminergic neurons. For more than two decades, experimental and clinical data have accumulated to suggest that this can be a beneficial strategy for PD patients (especially those with poor response to traditional medication) and that dopamine replacement can be achieved through cell transplantation.

An important issue to be considered in brain cell transplantation is the availability and suitability of tissues from abortions. Besides the obvious ethical concerns, the basic science and clinical studies are still in progress and many questions have yet to be answered. For example, in an extensive study of five tissue banks funded by NIH, out of approximately 1500 embryonic donors, only 7 were considered suitable for transplantation in PD patients (13). Of course, this is based on the older concept that only first-trimester mesencephalic tissues from multiple donors are to be used for transplantation in one patient. Fortunately, more recent studies have shown that the use of multiple donors (14) or first-trimester tissues (15, 16) are not absolute requirements to generate long-term surviving human brain grafts. Furthermore, of great promise is the current work with stem cells, neuronal precursors, and cell lines that may soon replace the use of primary human brain cells as the main donors. Finally, as will be discussed below, the use of neurotrophic treatments along with viral vector technology is another exciting area in this field and may become an important approach to promote brain regeneration in PD.

Fetal mesencephalic transplants

The majority of current clinical trials are based on using human fetal mesencephalic tissues from first-trimester abortuses. In general, multiple donors are used and the tissues are cryopreserved before implantation. The use of tissue fragments is still popular. The clinical outcome of some of the studies discussed below depends more on the surgical technique and underlying host condition rather than quality of the donor tissue. The autopsy studies are few and the in vivo assessment of the grafts still limited by the accuracy of positron emission tomography (PET). Nevertheless, clinical symptoms do appear to improve in some patients, often for extended periods of time, and the overall results are encouraging. The investigators agree on the need of standardized tissue processing and implantation protocols as well as the need for more sensitive imaging techniques. Current discussion also centers on the number and topography of the implantation sites and the ongoing debate about the use of immunosuppressants.

The difficulty of using clinical improvement (measured on various standardized scales) or PET imaging in establishing the *direct* benefit from graft survival was overcome by Kordower et al. (17) who in a detailed autopsy report showed that in a PD patient who died of unrelated causes at 18 months post-surgery (bilateral grafts), the fetal mesencephalic tissue was surviving, relatively well integrated, and containing a significant number of dopaminergic neurons. Surprisingly, there was no host dopaminergic neuronal sprouting. This appeared to be in contrast to findings from adrenal medullary grafts which did not survive well but were accompanied by host dopaminergic sprouting (18). Nevertheless, the same group of investigators reported more recently that the use of abundant donor tissue (from seven donors) has resulted in significant clinical and PET improvement in one patient even in the absence of host dopaminergic sprouting in the graft (19). At autopsy, the majority of the host putamen receiving the graft was positive for tyrosine hydroxylase (TH) and this may explain the post-surgery benefits.

From various clinical trials using fetal mesencephalic tissues, one of the most interesting observations is that the grafts appear to survive for long periods of time even if the underlying disease affecting the host dopaminergic neurons does not change its course (20). These results are encouraging, to say the least. When we can overcome problems in generating reliable, high quality, thoroughly assessed grafting material (21), cell transplantation could become a standard adjuvant in pharmacotherapies for PD or other novel interventions like deep-brain stimulation (22). PET imaging is of utmost importance in assessing these therapeutic interventions. Traditionally, dopamine production was measured by imaging of fluorodopa but newer radiotracers like CFT (a dopamine transporter ligand), SCH (D1 receptor), and raclopride (D2 receptor), may give a more accurate picture of the disease progress (23, 24) and also the survival and function of the grafted cells (25).

Adrenal and Carotid Body Transplants in Parkinson's Disease

After early observations that adrenal chromaffin cells transplanted in rats can survive in the host brain (26), clinical trials were initiated in humans. The early results, encouraging to some extent (27, 28) were questioned later, especially due to poor graft survival (29). One of the proposed explanations was the contamination of adrenal grafts with non-chromaffin cells. When this was corrected, improved survival and graft function were noted (30). Purified chromaffin cells can be grown and differentiated in vitro preimplantation (31) or manipulated to express growth factors that may further benefit the graft in vivo (32). An intriguing but promising alternative is the use of carotid body cell aggregates that have been shown to be of significant benefit in parkinsonian rats (33) and more recently in pilot studies in monkeys (34).

Xenografts in Parkinson's Disease

Human xenografts have been used in animal models to study principles of neurotransplantation or mechanisms of brain degeneration (15, 35). More often, xenotransplantation has been tested with the goal to explore alternative sources of mesencephalic fetal tissues for grafting in the degenerating brain (36). Recent studies using porcine fetal cells in rats showed that the grafts survived and integrated successfully in the host (37–39). Currently, there are several ongoing clinical trials to assess the feasibility of porcine xenografts in PD and HD patients and the preliminary data suggest that this may be a safe procedure. The efficacy has still to be determined (40).

HUNTINGTON'S DISEASE

The rationale for intrastriatal grafting in HD patients is in many ways similar to PD (41) but the methodological challenges could be greater due to the more complex neurophysiologic substrate. Nevertheless, extensive efforts are under way to establish a series of large scale clinical trials and the preliminary data are currently under evaluation. More promising are the studies analyzing the benefits of cell grafts in primate models of HD (42). Like in PD, much hope is invested in developing neuronal cells that can be manipulated in vitro to promote their in vivo functional integration in the degenerating striatum of HD patients (43).

Based on successful animal models striatal transplantation for the treatment of Huntington's disease, human trials have been initiated. The first human transplant for Huntington's disease was performed in 1990 in Mexico using an open surgical procedure (44). Follow-up of this patient and a second treated by the same group showed slowed progression of their disease. Clinical studies have also been initiated in the United States. Twelve month follow-up showed increased striatal tissue volume by MRI and improved measures of mobility and cognition. Hopefully, as human trials for the treatment of Huntington's disease progress, large, organized, controlled studies will emerge that will effectively evaluate this treatment modality.

Other Disease Models

Animal models of other neurodegenerative diseases have been developed and transplantation studies are being initiated. Huntington's disease has been modeled by injections of excitotoxic agents into the rodent striatum. Several groups have investigated transplants of fetal striatal tissue in this model with good results. Studies conducted in the non-human primate model also showed improvement of motor function. In these studies transplanted neurons formed synaptic connections leading to restoration of function. Because Huntington's disease can be identified genetically, before the onset of symptoms or evidence of striatal degeneration, investigators have explored the potential of nerve growth factor to prevent striatal degeneration. Studies in the excitotoxic model and the mitochondrial dysfunction model show that grafts of fibroblasts genetically modified to secrete nerve growth factor protect striatal cells from degeneration. A murine model with Purkinje cell degeneration has been used to study hereditary ataxias. After transplantation of fetal cerebellar cells in these mice, transplanted cells migrated to the molecular layer and formed synaptic connections.

In addition to models of degenerative diseases, animal models of trauma and ischemia have been developed. Animal transplant studies in both traumatic brain and traumatic spine injuries have been initiated. Transplantation has also been evaluated in animal models of cortical infarcts and lacunar infarcts.

STROKE

Transplantation of human neuronal cells is a new approach for ameliorating functional deficits caused by central nervous system (CNS) disease or injury. Several investigators have evaluated the effects of transplanted fetal tissue, rate striatum, or cellular implants into small animal stroke models (45). One of the best studied models of brain ischemia is the murine hippocampal stroke that results in well-defined lesions, especially in the CA1 region. The standardization of this model is invaluable to the reliable testing of various experimental protective and regenerative therapies. Among them, cell transplantation of fetal hippocampal neurons has shown that they can survive and integrate in the ischemic brain (46). Methodological issues are still to be resolved since subsequent studies questioned the capacity of rat fetal neocortical tissues, implanted in an infarcted area, to integrate in the surrounding host tissue (47). However, it has been shown that the chronic ischemic region can support graft tissue.

Since the widespread clinical use of primary human tissue is likely to be extremely limited due to the ethical and logistical difficulties inherent in obtaining large quantities of fetal neurons, much effort has been devoted to developing alternate sources of human neurons for use in transplantation. One alternate source is the Ntera 2/cl.D1 (NT2) human embryonic carcinoma-derived cell line. These cells proliferate in culture and differentiate into pure, postmitotic human neuronal cells (LBS-Neurons) upon treatment with retinoic acid (RetA) (48, 49). Thus, NT2 precursor cells appear to function as CNS progenitor cells with the capacity to develop diverse mature neuronal phenotypes. When transplanted, these neuronal cells survive, extend processes, express neurotransmitters, form functional synapses, and integrate with the host (50, 51). The final product is >95% pure populations of human neuronal cells that appear virtually indistinguishable from terminally differentiated, post-mitotic neurons (52). The cells are capable of differentiation to express different neuronal markers characteristic of mature neurons, including all three neurofilament proteins (NFL, NFM, and NFH); microtubule associated protein 2 (MAP2), the somal/dendritic protein; and tau, the axonal protein. Their neuronal phenotype makes them a promising candidate for replacement in CNS disorders, as a virtually unlimited supply of pure, postmitotic, terminally differentiated human neuronal cells.

In support of different mechanisms for efficacy, animal transplantation studies of LBS-Neurons revealed graft survival, mature neuronal phenotype, and integration into host brain in vivo (52). LBS-neurons grafted into different regions of the CNS of nude mice showed viable cells in 90% of recipients, with some grafts surviving for up to 14 months. Transplanted neurons formed synapse-like structures and elaborated dendrites and axons. Thus, transplanted LBS-Neurons demonstrated survival for at least 14 months post-implantation, a fully mature neuronal phenotype in vivo, and integration with the host CNS.

The LBS-Neurons expressed multiple neurotransmitter synthetic enzymes upon maturation, including choline acetyltransferase (ChAT), glutamic acid decarboxylase (GAD), and tyrosine hydroxylase (TH). They also displayed diverse neurotransmitter phenotypes, including acetylcholine, glutamate, and GABA. They transcribed all nine known non-NMDA glutamate receptor genes, expressed functional NMDA and non-NMDA glutamate receptor channels, showed glutamate-induced neurotoxicity, and generated low-amplitude slow action potentials similar to primary CNS neurons. Synaptogenesis of LBS-Neurons was demonstrated in vitro using co-cultures of LBS-Neurons and primary astrocytes (which enhanced the formation of functional synapses), a milestone of neuronal differentiation. When plated on astrocytes, LBS-Neurons formed both glutamatergic excitatory (70%) and GABAergic (30%) functional synapses that displayed electrophysiological synaptic currents consistent with functional neurotransmission (e.g., currents representing the release of individual quanta of neurotransmitter).

In patients disabled by stroke, the concept of restoring function by transplanting human neuronal cells into the brain is innovative (53, 54). Research in a rat model of transient focal cerebral ischemia demonstrated that transplantation of fetal tissue restored both cognitive and motor functions. Sanberg, Borlongan, and colleagues were the first to show that transplants of LBS-Neurons could also reverse the deficits caused by stroke (45, 56). The preclinical studies of LBS-Neurons were carried out in a model of transient focal, rather than global, ischemia in order to maximize the chances of functional recovery. Animals received ischemic insults to the striatum and were tested for behavioral deficits 1 month later. Animals that showed significant behavioral deficits received neuronal transplantation, and then were periodically reevaluated during the 6 month posttransplantation period. Animals that received transplants of LBS-Neurons (and cyclosporine treatment) showed amelioration of ischemia-induced behavioral deficits throughout the 6-month observation period. They demonstrated complete recovery in the passive avoidance test, as well as normalization of motor function in the elevated body swing test. In comparison, control groups receiving transplants of rat fetal cerebellar cells, medium alone, or cyclosporine failed to show significant behavioral improvement. A second study that evaluated response in comparison to the number of cells transplanted confirmed the efficacy of transplanted LBS-Neurons in reversing the behavioral deficits resulting from transient ischemia in an MCA occlusion rat model. The percentage of surviving cells was approximately 15% at the highest dose of 160×10^3 LBS-Neurons. This is comparable to the 5 to 10% survival rates reported for human fetal tissue. It appears from this and other studies that a small percentage of surviving cells may be sufficient to enhance behavioral recovery.

The initial objectives of the first clinical study performed at the University of Pittsburgh was to demonstrate the safety and feasibility of the neuronal-cell implantation procedure (54). These goals were met, in that no adverse events related to the implantation have occurred in at least 27 months of follow-up in 12 patients. The adverse events that did occur in these patients were thought to be unrelated to the implantation of the neuronal cells, and can be considered typical of a population with known cardiovascular disease and advanced age. This study was also intended to provide some information on the efficacy of neuronal-cell implantation in improving stroke-related neurologic deficits. Like any phase 1 study, problems with limited blinding, information on patient selection, adequate cell number, location of the brain implantation sites, use of immunosuppression, lack of a control group, and knowledge of the optimal evaluation of the response, was lacking. The small number of patients enrolled in the first study precluded any attempt at reaching a conclusion regarding efficacy, but some trends were discerned. In both treatment groups, mean NIHSS (National Institutes of Health Stroke Scale) total scores decreased and mean ESS (European Stroke Scale) total scores increased; both changes indicated improvement. For the ESS, the increases tended to be larger in the group of four patients receiving 6 million cells, both in the total scores and in the composite motor subscale scores. Both the Barthel Index and the SF-36 scores decreased in the group receiving 2 million cells and increased in the group receiving 6 million cells. All outcomes measurements were consistent in identifying a trend toward improved scores in the group of patients who received 6 million neuronal cells. The PET scan results also provided a suggestion of efficacy, in that increased activity at the area of the stroke was seen in 6 patients. An optimistic interpretation of these data would be that they indicate the return of viable neuronal cells to the areas of infarction. Other possibilities include an increased metabolic activity due to an inflammatory process rather than normal cellular function, although no changes suggestive of inflammation were noted on MRI.

The neuronal cells could improve neurologic function through a number of different mechanisms. These include provision of neurotrophic support (acting as local pumps to support cell function), provision of neurotransmitters, reestablishment of local interneuronal connections, cell differentiation and integration, and improvement of regional oxygen tension. Transplanted cells also may act to limit the reactive glial response and to limit retrograde degeneration, although this may be less feasible in a chronic injury. We believe that axonal reconnections through the grafted cells (serving as a "bridge") over large distances is less likely, although this phenomenon has been observed in spinal cord injury models. Phase 2 dose-response trials in patients are currently planned to evaluate further the role of neurotransplantation for patients with chronic motor deficits caused by basal ganglia region infarction.

TRANSPLANTATION STRATEGIES TO MAXIMIZE CELL SURVIVAL

Significant progress has been made in the transplantation protocol itself but we have much to learn about the intrinsic potential of various donor brain tissue preparations and the in vivo cues of the to determine the fate of the neuroglial graft. In general, it is still believed that first-trimester human fetal mesencephalic tissue is the best source for harvesting and grafting of dopaminergic neurons. This "window" can be somewhat extended (comparable numbers of surviving TH positive grafted neurons) if cell suspensions are used instead of solid grafts (55).

This finding was confirmed by different groups in various animal models and most data suggest that if survival of TH positive cells is used as the main criterion of assessing the grafting efficacy, the younger embryonic tissues are superior to older fetal donors. Nevertheless, as discussed before, there are several reports that challenge this concept.

The influence of host age on graft survival merits discussion for identifying potential in vivo cues that are responsible for the integration of the implanted cells. One of the first observations made was that in the neocortical transplants in older rats both types of grafts, with high (early embryonic) or low (late embryonic) growth potential, survived and integrated to similar extend vs. clear in vivo differences when younger host animals were used (57). Further studies have confirmed that migration of donor cells (58) and integration of the grafts decreases in older hosts (59). On the other hand, studies analyzing host dopaminergic sprouting in the graft, in general very limited, is not significantly different in young vs. adult rats (60). Furthermore, these results were confirmed by functional studies showing that even if the cytoarchitecture of the grafts in hosts of various ages may be different, the benefits are comparable (61). It is interesting to speculate on the clinical implications of these observations since several authors agree that the host responses are most critical to the functional benefits of fetal grafting.

Cell Processing

The first limiting factor in the success of cell grafting is the availability of suitable cells. Banking cryopreserved tissues (62) is still employed and is considered to be feasible by several authors (63). In the future, techniques for in vitro processing of fresh tissues in order to obtain long-term survival should become standard (64). The University of Pittsburgh stroke transplantation trial was the first to use a cryopreserved cell line in patients. Another approach is to maintain fetal cells as aggregates in long term suspension cultures that may even allow their expansion (65). However, this approach may not be feasible for processed neuronal cell lines.

There are benefits to in vitro processing of brain cells before implantation. First, processing may select for a viable, better characterized neuronal donor population. Second, it can help identify the donor glial-neuronal interactions that are critical in vivo, potentially protecting the graft from detrimental host reactions (66). Third, in can offer a setting for trophic (67) and genetic manipulations that will enhance in vivo survival and integration. Finally, neuronal apoptosis in fetal grafts is well described and appears to be significant during the first 10 to 15 days postimplantation (68). The mechanisms of neuronal death are predominantly mediated by caspases (69) and inhibitors of this process may have important benefits in improving the viability of the grafts (70).

Implantation Techniques

The majority of the TH positive neurons (around 90%) within fetal grafts appear to die within the first week after implantation (71). Perhaps changes in implantation protocols may have an important impact on the survival of the graft. One approach is to include a biologic adjuvant at the time of implantation, often as a co-graft of peripheral nerve which may offer continuous trophic support, promoting the survival and differentiation of the donor dopaminergic cells (72, 73). Over the past decade, this approach was tested several times and the results, while mixed, are in general positive. Another bioengineering protocol, proposed by Brecknell et al. (74) is based on providing a "bridge" for the implanted dopaminergic neurons to grow into the striatum by using cells transformed to secrete growth factors. At present, stereotactic techniques are used to deposit cells at distances such that the "sphere of influence" of each graft might determine the distance between individual graft locations.

The most direct strategies to increase transplant integration in the host dopaminergic pathways is the use of co-grafts of mesencephalic and striatal donor cells (75), or simultaneous mesencephalic grafts in the nigra and striatum of the host (76). Both these interesting approaches are currently explored in clinical trials in PD patients. Finally, the idea of using the nigra (vs. striatum) as a site of dopaminergic fetal cell grafting has gained again momentum and recent studies propose it as a feasible alternative in PD (77, 78).

Host Immune Response

Another potentially serious limiting factor in cell survival, despite optimal in vitro tissue processing and efficient implantation protocol, is the host rejection of the graft. While the brain is still considered to be an organ with a limited immune response (historically called "immunoprivileged"), rejections of grafted tissues can occur through the classic cell mediated immune response. The immune reactions to neural grafts have been studied extensively (79) but the necessity of immune suppression is still debated. A recent review by Widner emphasizes the complexity of the immune response in the brain and also questions the impact of immunosupressive therapies on allo or even xenograft survival. Furthermore, it should be noted that another host reaction, the degeneration of the graft mediated by brain macrophages, that does not involve the presence of lymphocytes, can also be considered a form of rejection. The role played by reactive microglia in graft survival is currently the object of dispute. Finally, following an interesting observation in rats implanted with fetal dopamine cells, Hudson et al. (80) suggested that host immunocompetence to the allogeneic graft is necessary but not sufficient to cause rejection.

Early studies in rats showed that immunosupression with cyclosporin A (CsA) was critical for graft survival and function of dopaminergic human xenografts (81). The benefit of CsA was confirmed in other animal xenograft models (82) but the graft degeneration in nontreated animals was not evident (83). Furthermore, the lack of a detectable systemic immune response in primates with embryonic brain grafts (84) raised the possibility that aggressive immune suppression (85) may not be necessary and local immune modulation or evasion strategies can be developed (86). Assuming that the immune response is exclusively detrimental, which is not clear yet (87), methods proposed to modulate it include the co-grafting of Sertoli cells that seem to have both a trophic effect and a surprising immunosuppressive activity on the host response (88, 89). Another proposed approach is to use specific anti-T-cell antibodies capable of inducing immune tolerance (90) or, as suggested in an interesting report, a short course of treatment with an anti IL-2 receptor antibody (CD25) which may be as effective as long-term CsA (91).

Trophic Support of the Graft

An important factor deciding the fate of the future graft is the trophic support offered by the intrinsic milieu, the host environment, or administered in vivo postgrafting. Neurotrophic factors (NTF) have been the focus of intense studies discussing them as therapeutic agents in neurodegenerative diseases (92, 93). In the field of neurotransplantation, the studies proposing NTF as in vitro and in vivo adjuvants to the graft have been significantly more successful. Overwhelming evidence from developmental neuroscience experiments demonstrated that growth factors are crucial in the differentiation of neural progenitor cells (94), or in general, less differentiated cells that are abundant in the fetal grafts. Among these factors, epidermal and fibroblast growth factors (FGF) were most important in promoting the mitogenic capacity of neuroglial progenitors. While work by Gage and colleagues established FGF as a principal mitogenic factor in the developing neuronal population (95), other growth factors may participate in the expansion and differentiation of the neuronal precursor cell population as demonstrated by in vitro and in vivo experiments with insulin-like growth factor (96) and hepatocyte growth factor. Interestingly, the latter seems to function as a primer for other trophic signals.

Hepatocyte growth factor is only one of the newer trophins for the CNS. Today, the family of growth and trophic factors proposed to affect the survival and development of neuroprogenitor cells is probably the largest in this ever-expanding field. Factors like cytokines, once considered to be exclusively neurotoxic (e.g., TNF) are now studied for neurotrophic properties. Among them, leukemia inhibitory factor (LIF) and ciliary neurotrophic factor (CNTF), in addition to more traditional growth factors like platelet-derived growth factor (PDGF), are considered to be potent promoters of neuroprogenitor cell proliferation and eventually differentiation (97). In vivo, CNTF produced by reactive astrocytes (98) can prevent the degeneration of dopaminergic neurons in adult rats (99). Astrocytes and endothelial cells surrounding or infiltrating the transplant are susceptible to the effects of PDGF, which may control the survival of graft through neovascularization (100).

In addition to the proliferative support offered to neuroprecursor cells, NTF are key players in their differentiation to the mature phenotype. This function may be critical for the graft integration in the host environment. It was shown that, at least when cell lines were used (e.g., PC12), in vitro pretreatment with NGF is crucial for the in vivo phenotype of the graft: differentiated (NTF treated cells) vs. nondifferentiated, tumor-like (nontreated cells) (101). The in vivo effects of NGF become even more obvious when fetal grafts are continuously treated through in situ injection (102) or regeneration is promoted through gene delivery using transformed cells (103).

Brain-Derived Neurotrophic Factor

Brain derived neurotrophic factor (BDNF), another member of the neurotrophin family (that includes NGF, NT-3 and NT-4/5), has been shown to have great potency in modulating the growth and survival of dopaminergic cells and their precursors. It is now widely accepted that the pluripotent BDNF and its high affinity receptor trkB are widely distributed both in the developing and mature nervous system. Our increasing understanding of neurotrophin binding to their receptors, signal transduction following trk and p75 dimerization and activation has lead to a series of exciting developments in designing experimental models to test novel trophic treatments. In addition to dopaminergic cells, BDNF was found to be potent on cholinergic and glutamatergic motor and sensory neurons, both in the central and peripheral nervous system.

In spinal cord injuries, neurotrophin treatments are proposed to present significant clinical benefits. For example, BDNF infused at the site of spinal cord injury in rats showed a positive but transient effect on local reflexes (104). The most dramatic impact of BDNF occurred in fully transected spinal cords. When these chronic infusions were stopped, the behavioral effects disappeared. BDNF was also shown to stimulate sprouting of cholinergic fibers at the injury site, but did not effect serotonergic fibers or total axon density. In an effort to promote directional regeneration, cells transformed to secrete BDNF were grafted in trails in the transected spinal cord and the results showed a significant positive effect on axons from trkB expressing neurons (105). In another study by Menei et al. it was shown that in spinal cord transplants, addition of BDNF increased axonal outgrowth of axotomized neurons (106).

Interestingly, some reports suggested that BDNF enhanced the function rather than survival of the grafts enriched with dopamine cells (107, 108). In vitro, BDNF can protect dopaminergic neurons from hydroxy dopamine toxicity (109). In vivo, similar protective functions were observed in rats with BDNF producing grafts, after being challenged with the active metabolite of the dopaminergic toxic MPTP (110). The regenerative capacity of BDNF on dopaminergic projections was shown to be both direct and indirect, mediated through improved fetal grafts (111). Still, only a subpopulation of nigral dopaminergic cells may be susceptible to these effects, depending on their capacity to express the high affinity receptor trkB (112). Furthermore, there are some concerns about the effects of long-term in situ delivery of BDNF in vivo, at least in the rat striatum (113). Currently, it still appears that the most consistently positive use of BDNF in cell transplantation is to promote dopaminergic differentiation preimplantation. When rate and human nigral fetal cell aggregates were treated with BDNF, the number of TH positive neurons increased significantly (114). These effects were further enhanced when GDNF was used in combination with BDNF.

Glial-Derived Neurotrophic Factor

In general, GDNF has similar or even enhanced trophic functions on dopaminergic neurons and their precursors. In vivo, GDNF was also shown to be relatively potent in animal models of dopaminergic protection or regeneration but human clinical trials have not been so encouraging (115). Nonetheless, its potential use in PD has made GDNF the prime candidate for NTF treatments in association with fetal mesencephalic transplants of dopaminergic neurons.

GDNF, a related member of the TGF-b family was first identified and characterized in 1993 by Lin et al. (116). From the beginning it was evident that GDNF has a potent but specific/selective activity on dopaminergic neurons, inducing their differentiation in the absence of overt neuroglial proliferation. Shortly after, in vivo studies demonstrated that GDNF injected into the substantia nigra produced a significant decrease in the motor deficits associated with 6-OHDA lesioning in rats (117). When GDNF was injected in developing or mature mesencephalic grafts, in oculo, its primary effect was to promote dopaminergic neuritic growth, rather than survival of TH positive cells (118). Interestingly, administration of GDNF in a murine MPTP parkinsonian model had both protective and regenerative effects (119). The in vivo protective effects were also demonstrated in a rat nigral axotomy model suggesting again that GDNF has a high specificity for dopaminergic neurons (120).

Further in vitro studies showed that a mixture of slow release GDNF, fibrin glue, and fetal mesencephalic neuroglial cells resulted in a significant increase in the number of TH positive cells and neuritic density (121). Another in vitro study indicated that GDNF may protect from continuous cell death after removal of toxins and even stimulate dopaminergic fiber regrowth (122). When another neurotoxin, quinolinic acid, was used, GDNF showed selective protection of dopaminergic neurons against excitotoxicity (123).

In vivo studies using fetal mesencephalic grafts showed that injections of GDNF in the vicinity of the rat brain implant resulted in significantly increased survival and growth of TH positive cells accompanied by marked functional improvement (124). The improved survival and differentiation of dopaminergic fetal grafts treated with GDNF pre- or postimplantation has been independently confirmed in numerous studies focused on the therapeutic benefits in parkinsonian models (125–128). A more recently identified member of this family of growth factors, neurturin, was found to be similarly potent in preventing dopaminergic cell death but lacked the support for TH positive neuritic growth associated with GDNF treatments (129). Finally, in clinical studies, two patients with PD who received fetal dopaminergic implants pretreated in vitro with GDNF showed increased graft survival (130). The benefits of GDNF treatments in PD patients appear to be restricted to association with fetal grafts. When GDNF was injected in the cerebroventricular system of a PD patient that did not receive a graft, the results appeared detrimental (115). Further research is continuing on this approach.

Other Protective and Trophic Factors

In addition to the beneficial effects of neurotrophic factor treatments, the ganglioside GM1 has been shown to enhance effects even at minimal concentrations of BDNF (131). The lazaroids are another intriguing class of compounds that demonstrated a strong trophic effect on promoting the survival of embryonic mesencephalic tissues and their development in vivo (132, 133). Interestingly, the lazaroids promoting in vivo survival of dopaminergic neurons (134) but did not increase target striatal innervation (135).

Mechanisms of grafted cell death include excitotoxicity and apoptosis. Among the excitotoxic inhibitors, the calcium channel/NMDA receptor antagonist MK-801 is one of the most studied. In vivo, this compound was not able to enhance dopaminergic neuronal survival in the graft, suggesting that cell death in the grafts may not be due to excitotoxicity (136). The other mechanism of cell death in transplants, apoptosis, is currently under intense scrutiny since caspase inhibitors seem to reduce neuronal death in the grafts. Furthermore, the combination of pretreatment with a caspase inhibitor and a lazaroid may have a significantly higher positive effect on transplanted dopaminergic neurons (137).

Finally, recent debates in neural cell grafting gravitate around the potentially beneficial effects of new generation immunosupressive drugs that have been shown to be less toxic to the brain (138). A representative member of this family is the FK 506 drug. This compound, together with CsA and rapamycin (recently approved for clinical trials), bind to receptors called immunophilins (139). Many of the immunophilin ligands have be shown to posses neurotrophic activities (140). This field is under intense scrutiny, especially since immunophilins have been proven to be abundant in the brain (141). Among the newer members of the immunophilin ligand family, the nonimmunosuppressive drug GPI-1046 shows much promise in promoting regenerative neuritic growth from surviving neurons in various CNS lesions (142). Furthermore, the immunophilin ligand V-10,367 has been shown to specifically increase the growth of dopaminergic neurons (mostly neurite branching) and protect against MPTP lesioning (143), in a manner superior to FK-506.

Non-Neuronal Primary Human Cells

Based on the observations discussed above, regarding the importance of the trophic host response in promoting regeneration post-transplantation, often independent of graft survival or function, some investigators have proposed alternate sources of donor cells that will primarily serve as promoters of host regeneration. Among the non-neuronal brain cells, astrocytes are prime candidates. A study of neuroglial cell grafting in a murine model of lesion-induced memory deficits showed that astrocytic grafts induced a significantly higher improvement compared to the cholinergic neuronal grafts (144). Another interesting method is based on transplanting activated macrophages to promote CNS regeneration. This approach was discussed also above, in the section about the host response. One of the rationales is that grafted macrophages may compensate for the failure of host macrophages to provide trophic support or potentially overcome their inhibitory activity. Finally, one of the most intriguing sources of donor cells is the bone marrow stroma. Azizi and colleagues (145) have shown that human marrow stromal cells grafted in the rat brain can survive, spread, and differentiate into a neuroglial phenotype in the absence of a host immune response or any signs of rejection. An important comment is that the donor cell mixture may include a significant population of nonhematopoietic tissue precursors. If any of these methods proves to be consistent among various laboratories and disease models, they could become a powerful strategy for promoting a "natural" regeneration or an important platform for delivering gene therapy.

STEM CELLS AND NEURONAL PRECURSORS

The recent advances in our ability to manipulate embryonic stem cells has opened a whole new spectrum of potential therapies in tissue regeneration in general, and brain in particular (146). It has also reignited the interest in brain stem cells and neuroprecursors that show many analogies with the considerably better characterized hematopoietic system (147). The definition of brain stem cells vs. neural precursors is increasingly more precise and tends to delineate better the distinction between toti-potent, multipotent, and lineage committed. Comprehensive reviews about the potential of using stem cells in regeneration were published recently (148, 149). The reports that stem cells are present not only in the developing brain but can be identified also in adults have further contributed to the excitement about new possibilities to promote CNS regeneration.

Many of the early studies have often reported successful harvesting of progenitor cells from various regions of the brain (the subventricular zone being the most popular but not singular) that can be expanded in vitro and then differentiate in vivo into functional neurons. The challenge is still to better identify the neural progenitor cells and understand the mechanisms of growth and differentiation from embryonic stem cells. An important characteristic of neuroepithelial stem cells, described more than a decade ago and still widely used, is expression of the intermediate filament protein, nestin (150). More recently, new markers of neuronal progenitor cells, conserved in their evolution and useful for early lineage selection, include Musashi-1 (151) and an epitope recognized by the 2F7 monoclonal antibody (152). The mechanisms of progenitor cell maturation appear to be similar in various brain regions (153) and seem to depend primarily on a cascade of signals mediated by specific combinations of growth factors (154) and molecules (like noggin) that can modulate their activity (155).

Understanding the dynamics of gene expression and specific protein production in the development of the neural lineage from stem cells is critical for designing new isolation and purification methods to be used in vitro for preimplantation neuronal enrichment of future grafts. In addition to the traditional marker nesting, Li and colleagues reported that the transcription factors Sox1 and Sox2 could identify with higher specificity progenitor cells restricted to the neural lineage (156). Furthermore, expression of neuron-specific promoter (like Hu and TuJ1/beta-III tubulin), offers another opportunity to intervene through gene engineering in the development of neural progenitor cells and select for this cell phenotype (157).

Regardless of their origin, fetal or adult, neural precursor cells show much promise in brain repair. They can survive and differentiate in the host lesioned brain (158, 159) although it seems that their predominant differentiation in vivo, posttransplantation, is along the astrocytic lineage (160). Not surprisingly, the migration and differentiation of the grafted precursor cells is significantly influenced by local cues (161). Nonetheless, the potential for in vivo survival of grafted neural precursor cells can be fully exploited when they are used as platforms for gene delivery or engineered to modulate the neurotrophic factor environment in the host brain (162).

Neuronal Cell Lines

The use of "primitive" neuroglial cell lines that preserve their mitotic potential in vitro but can differentiate in vivo (163) was proposed for a long time as being a feasible alternative to primary cell cultures. While the PC12 line is well established as the work horse of a plethora of in vitro experiments studying neurotoxic or neurotrophic mechanisms in the CNS, its capacity to differentiate and integrate in vivo in the host brain is limited, at best. Since the usefulness of this cell line in humans may be seriously hampered by its uncontrolled capacity to proliferate in a nondifferentiated state, significant efforts were made to identify new human neuronal cell lines that will overcome this obstacle. One of the candidates, that under certain conditions can differentiate into a "mature neuronal phenotype," is the human cortical neuronal cell line HCN-1 which has many of the characteristics of immature neuroepithelial cells but, interestingly, does not respond to traditional growth factors for CNS cells, like bFGF (164). Another example is the human neuroblastoma cell line SH-SY5Y that can synthesize dopamine in vitro and differentiate in vivo. Still, a puzzling observation, seen, as discussed above, with primary cell grafts too, is that in Parkinsonian animal models the functional benefit postgrafting may not be due to dopamine release by the implanted cells (165). Recently, the use of immortalized primary cell cultures has become a popular approach. Experiments with SV40 tumor antigen immortalized dopaminergic cells showed that they can be used for in vitro analysis (e.g., the SN4741 line) of the effects of BDNF on mesencephalic cultures. In vivo, similar immortalized dopaminergic cells (the 1RB3AN27 clone) survived for more than 1 year in grafts and were associated with clinical improvement but, again, did not show significant differentiation and integration in the host brain (166).

Currently, one of the most studied neuronal cells are the NT2 line derived from a human teratocarcinoma that can differentiate in vitro, following treatment with retinoic acid (50), into cells with a mature neuronal phenotype, known as "hNT" or, the older designation "NT2N" cells. In vivo, grafted hNT cells acquired a mature phenotype (including growth of neuritic processes and synaptic contacts) and could survive for more than a year in the mouse CNS (51). Interestingly, later studies showed that in vitro treatments of NT2 cells are not critical to their in vivo differentiation (167). One of the most convincing applications of using these cells in transplantation comes from experiments using a rat CNS ischemic model where hNT cells induced a more robust recovery than fetal rat striatal grafts (45). In the rate 6-OHDA parkinsonian model, hNT cells grafted into the striatum and substantia nigra were shown to survive in the host parenchyma and generate TH immunoreactivity when pretreated with LiCl (168). When made for human use, these cells are called LBS-Neurons.

Polymer Encapsulation

As discussed above, one of the major challenges to graft survival in the CNS is modulation of the host immune response. Most neuroglial cells (including in vitro adapted lines like PC12 (169, 170) could, at least theoretically, benefit from protection against the host immune response and rejection by using an encapsulating physical barrier. While many grafted cells can survive, the connectivity between the host and implanted neurons is limited and a significant number of donor cells die. In an early study by Jaeger et al., dopaminergic cell lines survived within a semipermeable membrane (171). Shortly after, Winn et al. proposed that polymer-encapsulated cells may provide a means of neurotransmitter and growth factor delivery in vivo (172). This approach was proposed early on as an alternative treatment in PD and its feasibility was demonstrated in animal models (173). In MPTP monkeys that showed clinical improvement after grafting, encapsulated cell implants were shown to be able to uptake and metabolize dopamine (174).

Another promising application of this approach is the delivery of trophic factors in the regenerating brain. The main problem with using genetically engineered cells for in vivo delivery of growth factors in their uncontrolled growth in the host brain. This can be readily solved when the donor cells, modified to secrete trophic factors, are encapsulated in a semipermeable membrane (175). Intrastriatal implants of polymer encapsulated cells producing NGF induced a significant increase in the cholinergic neuronal immunoreactivity at the site of implantation (176). The long-term production of NTF by encapsulated grafts is physiologically relevant and associated with a positive host response in the absence of any detectable side effects. In parkinsonian animal models, encapsulated grafts engineered to produce GDNF added a significant functional benefit to the dopaminergic co-grafts (177).

SUMMARY

We are confident that neurodegenerative diseases will be managed by an array of pharmacologic and cellular therapies. These may involve oral or intravenous preparations, surgical cell deliveries, or infusion through cerebral delivery systems. Achievements in neuroscience over the past three decades have redefined some of the rules for basic and clinical research in neurotransplantation. Restorative neurosurgical procedures will develop from different directions, and it is likely that a combination of approaches will be necessary to maximize patient outcomes.

REFERENCES

1. Björklund A, Stenevi U: Growth of central catecholamine neurones into smooth muscle grafts in the rat mesencephalon. **Brain Res** 31(1):1–20, 1971.
2. Björklund A, et al: Re-establishment of functional connections by regenerating central adrenergic and cholinergic axons. **Nature** 253:446–448, 1975.
3. Björklund A, Stenevi U: Reformation of the severed septohippocampal cholinergic pathway in the adult rat by transplanted septal neurons. **Cell Tissue Res** 185(3):289–302, 1977.
4. Tabbal S, Fahn S, Frucht S: Fetal tissue transplantation [correction of transplantation] in Parkinson's disease. **Curr Opini Neurology** 11(4):341–349, 1998.
5. Brundin P, et al: Improving the survival of grafted dopaminergic neurons: a review over current approaches [In Process Citation]. **Cell Transplant** 9(2):179–195, 2000.
6. Freeman TB, Widner H: Cell transplantation for neurological disorders: Toward reconstruction of the human central nervous system. **Contemp Neuroscience** Totowa, NJ: Humana Press. 1998, pp xviii, 350.
7. Schmidt RH, Bjorklund A, Stenevi U: Intracerebral grafting of dissociated CNS tissue suspensions: a new approach for neuronal transplantation to deep brain sites. **Brain Res** 218(1–2):347–356, 1981.
8. Gage FH, et al: Intracerebral grafting of neuronal cell suspensions. VIII. Survival

and growth of implants of nigral and septal cell suspensions in intact brains of aged rats. **Acta Physiol Scand Suppl** 522:67–75, 1983.

9. Björklund A, et al: Intracerebral grafting of neuronal cell suspensions. II. Survival and growth of nigral cell suspensions implanted in different brain sites. **Acta Physiol Scand Suppl** 522:9–18, 1983.

10. Björklund A, et al: Intracerebral grafting of neuronal cell suspensions. VII. Recovery of choline acctyltransferase activity and acetylcholine synthesis in the denervated hippocampus reinnervated by septal suspension implants. **Acta Physiol Scand Suppl** 522:59–66, 1983.

11. Björklund A, et al: Intracerebral grafting of neuronal cell suspensions. VI. Survival and growth of intrahippocampal implants of septal cell suspensions. **Acta Physiol Scand Suppl** 522:49–58, 1983.

12. Björklund A, et al: Intracerebral grafting of neuronal cell suspensions. I. Introduction and general methods of preparation. **Acta Physiol Scand Suppl** 522:1–7, 1983.

13. Branch DW, et al: Suitability of fetal tissues from spontaneous abortions and from ectopic pregnancies for transplantation. Human Fetal Tissue Working Group [see comments]. **JAMA** 273(1):66–68, 1995.

14. Sladek JRJC, Elsworth J, Roth D, Taylor H, Jane R, and Redmond DE Jr: Intrastriatal grafts from multiple donors do not result in a proportional increase in survival of dopamine neurons in nonhuman primates. **Cell Transplantation** 7(2):87–96, 1998.

15. Achim CL, et al: In vivo model of HIV infection of the human brain. **Dev Neurosci** 15(6):423–432, 1993.

16. Sanders VJ, et al: A murine model of HIV encephalitis: xenotransplantation of HIV-infected human neuroglia into SCID mouse brain. **Neuropathol Appl Neurobiol** 24(6):461–467, 1998.

17. Kordower JH, et al: Neuropathological evidence of graft survival and striatal reinnervation after the transplantation of fetal mesencephalic tissue in a patient with Parkinson's disease [see comments]. **N Engl J Med** 332(17):1118–1124, 1995.

18. Kordower JH, et al: Dopaminergic transplants in patients with Parkinson's disease: neuroanatomical correlates of clinical recovery. **Exp Neurol** 144(1):41–46, 1997.

19. Kordower JH, et al: Fetal nigral grafts survive and mediate clinical benefit in a patient with Parkinson's disease. **Mov Dis** 13(3):383–393, 1998.

20. Lindvall O: Update on fetal transplantation: the Swedish experience. **Mov Disord** 13(Suppl 1):83–87, 1998.

21. Mamelak AN, et al: Fatal cyst formation after fetal mesencephalic allograft transplant for Parkinson's disease [see comments]. **J Neurosurg** 89(4):592–598, 1998.

22. Kupsch A, and Earl C: Neurosurgical interventions in the treatment of idiopathic Parkinson disease: neurostimulation and neural implantation. **J Mol Med** 77(1):178–184, 1999.

23. Ouchi Y, et al: Presynaptic and postsynaptic dopaminergic binding densities in the nigrostriatal and mesocortical systems in early Parkinson's disease: a double-tracer positron emission tomography study. **Ann Neurol** 46(5):723–731, 1999.

24. Brownell AL, Jenkins BG, Isacson O: Dopamine imaging markers and predictive mathematical models for progressive degeneration in Parkinson's disease [In Process Citation]. **Biomed Pharmacother** 53(3):131–140, 1999.

25. Piccini P, et al: Dopamine release from nigral transplants visualized in vivo in a Parkinson's patient [see comments]. **Nat Neurosci** 2(12):1137–1140, 1999.

26. Perlow MJ, Kumakura K, Guidotti A: Prolonged survival of bovine adrenal chromaf-

fin cells in rat cerebral ventricles. **Proc Natl Acad Sci USA** 77(9):5278–5281, 1980.

27. Petruk KC, et al: Treatment of refractory Parkinson's disease with adrenal medullary autografts utilizing two-stage surgery. **Prog Brain Res** 82:671–676, 1990.

28. Luquin MR, et al: [Adrenal transplantation and Parkinson's disease]. **Rev Med Univ Navarra** 38(4):174–180, 1994.

29. Ahlskog JE: Cerebral transplantation for Parkinson's disease: current progress and future prospects. **Mayo Clin Proc** 68(6):578–591, 1993.

30. Schueler SB, et al: Robust survival of isolated bovine adrenal chromaffin cells following intrastriatal transplantation: a novel hypothesis of adrenal graft viability. **J Neurosci** 13(10):4496–4510, 1993.

31. Drucker-Colin R, et al: Transplant of cultured neuron-like differentiated chromaffin cells in a Parkinson's disease patient. A preliminary report. **Arch Med Res** 30(1):33–39, 1999.

32. Chalmers GR, et al: Adrenal chromaffin cells transdifferentiate in response to basic fibroblast growth factor and show directed outgrowth to a nerve growth factor source in vivo. **Exp Neurol** 133(1):32–42, 1995.

33. Espejo EF, et al: Cellular and functional recovery of Parkinsonian rats after intrastriatal transplantation of carotid body cell aggregates. **Neuron** 20(2):197–206, 1998.

34. Luquin MR, et al: Recovery of chronic parkinsonian monkeys by autotransplants of carotid body cell aggregates into putamen. **Neuron** 22(4):743–750, 1999.

35. Wictorin K, et al: Long distance directed axonal growth from human dopaminergic mesencephalic neuroblasts implanted along the nigrostriatal pathway in 6-hydroxydopamine lesioned adult rats. **J Comp Neurol** 323(4):475–494, 1992.

36. Isacson O, et al: Transplanted xenogenic neural cells in neurodegenerative disease models exhibit remarkable axonal target specificity and distinct growth patterns of glial and axonal fibres. **Nat Med** 1(11):1189–1194, 1995.

37. Jacoby DB, et al: Long-term survival of fetal porcine lateral ganglionic eminence cells in the hippocampus of rats. **J Neurosci Res** 56(6):581–594, 1999.

38. Deacon T, et al: Pig fetal septal neurons implanted into the hippocampus of aged or cholinergic deafferented rats grow axons and form cross-species synapses in appropriate target regions. **Cell Transplant** 8(1):111–129, 1999.

39. Barker RA, et al: Fetal porcine dopaminergic cell survival in vitro and its relationship to embryonic age. **Cell Transplant** 8(6):593–599, 1999.

40. Fink JS, et al: Porcine xenografts in Parkinson's disease and Huntington's disease patients: preliminary results [In Process Citation]. **Cell Transplant** 9(2):273–278, 2000.

41. Peschanski MP, Cesaro P, Hantraye P: Rationale for intrastriatal grafting of striatal neuroblasts in patients with Huntington's disease. **Neuroscience** 68(2):273–285, 1995.

42. Kendall AL, et al: Functional integration of striatal allografts in a primate model of Huntington's disease [see comments]. **Nat Med** 4(6):727–729, 1998.

43. Hurlbert MS, et al: Neural transplantation of hNT neurons for Huntington's disease. **Cell Transplant** 8(1):143–151, 1999.

44. Madrazo I, Franco-Bourland RE, Castrejon H, et al: Fetal striatal homotransplantations for Huntington's disease: First two cases reports. **Neurol Res** 17, 312–315, 1995.

45. Borlongan CV, et al: Cerebral ischemia and CNS transplantation: differential effects of grafted fetal rat striatal cells and human neurons derived from a clonal cell line. **Neuroreport**, 9(16):3703–3709, 1998.

46. Aoki H, et al: Neural grafting to ischemic CA1 lesions in the rat hippocampus: an autoradiographic study. **Neuroscience** 56(2):345–354, 1993.

47. Grabowski M, Johansson BB, Brundin P: Neocortical grafts placed in the infarcted brain of adult rats: few or no efferent fibers grow from transplant to host. **Exp Neurol** 134(2):273–276, 1995.

48. Trojanowski JW, Mantione JR, Lee LJ, Seid DP, You T, Lee VMY: Neurons derived from a teratocarcinoma cell line establish molecular and structural polarity following transplantation into the rodent brain. **Exp Neurol** 122:283–294, 1993.

49. Pleasure SJ, Lee VMY: Ntera-2 cells: A human cell line which displays characteristics expected of a human committed neuronal progenitor cell. **J Neurosci Res** 35:585–602, 1993.

50. Andrews PW: Retinoic acid induces neuronal differentiation of a cloned human embryonal carcinoma cell line in vitro. **Dev Biol** 103(2):285–293, 1984.

51. Kleppner SR, et al: Transplanted human neurons derived from a teratocarcinoma cell-line (ntera-2) mature, integrate, and survive for over 1 year in the nude-mouse brain. **J Comp Neurology** 357(4):618–632, 1995.

52. Trojanowski JQ, Kleppner SR, Hartley RS, Miyazono M, Fraser NW, Kesari S, Lee VMY: Transfectable and transplantable postmitotic human neurons: a potential platform for gene therapy of nervous system diseases. **Exp Neurol** 144:92–97, 1997.

53. Thompson T, Lunsford LD, Kondziolka D: Restorative neurosurgery: Opportunities for restoration of function in acquired, degenerative, and idiopathic neurological diseases. **Neurosurgery** 45:741–752, 1999.

54. Kondziolka D, Wechsler L, Goldstein S, Meltzar C, Thulborn K, Gebel J, Jannetta P, DeCesare S, Elder E, McGrogan M, Reitman M, Bynum L: Transplantation of cultured human neuronal cells for patients with stroke. **Neurology** 55:565–569, 2000.

55. Freeman TB, et al: The influence of donor age on the survival of solid and suspension intraparenchymal human embryonic nigral grafts. **Cell Transplantation,** 4(1):141–154, 1995.

56. Borlongan CV, Koutouzis TK, Jorden JR, et al: Neural transplantation as an experimental treatment for cerebral ischemia. **Neurosci Biobehavior Rev** 21:79–90, 1997.

57. Hallas, BH, Das GD, Das KG: Transplantation of brain tissue in the brain of rat. II. Growth characteristics of neocortical transplants in hosts of different ages. **Am J Anat,** 158(2):147–159, 1980.

58. Andersson C, Tytell M, Brunso-Bechtold J: Transplantation of cultured type 1 astrocyte cell suspensions into young, adult and aged rate cortex: Cell migration and survival. **Int J Dev Neurosci,** 11(5):555–568, 1993.

59. Olsson M, et al: Extensive migration and target innervation by striatal precursors after grafting into the neonatal striatum. **Neuroscience** 79(1):57–78, 1997.

60. Chkirate M, Vallee A, Doucet G: Host striatal projections into fetal ventral mesencephalic tissue grafted to the striatum of immature or adult rat. **Exp Brain Res** 94(2):357–62, 1993.

61. Abrous DN, Torres EM, Dunnett SB: Dopaminergic grafts implanted into the neonatal or adult striatum: comparative effects on rotation and paw reaching deficits induced by subsequent unilateral nigrostriatal lesions in adulthood. **Neuroscience** 54(3):657–668, 1993.

62. Redmond DE Jr, et al: Cryopreservation, culture, and transplantation of human fetal mesencephalic tissue into monkeys. **Science** 242(4879):768–771, 1988.

63. Collier TJ, Gallagher MJ, Sladek CD: Cryopreservation and storage of embryonic

rate mesencephalic dopamine neurons for one year: Comparison to fresh tissue in culture and neural grafts. **Brain Res** 623(2):249–256, 1993.

64. Meyer M, et al: Comparison of mesencephalic free-floating tissue culture grafts and cell suspension grafts in the 6-hydroxydopamine-lesioned rat. **Exp Brain Res** 119(3):345–355, 1998.

65. Svendsen CN, Smith AG: New prospects for human stem-cell therapy in the nervous system. **Trends Neurosci** 22(8):357–364, 1999.

66. Bronstein DM, et al: Glia-dependent neurotoxicity and neuroprotection in mesencephalic cultures. **Brain Res** 704(1):112–116, 1995.

67. White MG, et al: Neuron-enriched second trimester human cultures: growth factor response and in vivo graft survival. **Cell Transplant** 8(1):59–73, 1999.

68. Mahalik TJ, et al: Programmed cell death in developing grafts of fetal substantia nigra. **Exp Neurol** 129(1):27–36, 1994.

69. D'Sa-Eipper C, Roth KA: Caspase regulation of neuronal progenitor cell apoptosis. **Dev Neurosci** 22(1–2)116–124, 2000.

70. Schierle GS, et al: Caspase inhibition reduce apoptosis and increases survival of nigral transplants. **Nat Med** 5(1):97–100, 1999.

71. Emgard M, et al: Patterns of cell deaths and dopaminergic neuron survival in intrastriatal nigral grafts. **Exp Neurol** 160(1):279–288, 1999.

72. Kordower JH, et al: NGF-like trophic support from peripheral nerve for grafted rhesus adrenal chromaffin cells. **J Neurosurg** 73(3):418–428, 1990.

73. Collier TJ, Springer JE: Co-grafts of embryonic dopamine neurons and adult sciatic nerve into the denervated striatum enhance behavioral and morphological recovery in rats. **Exp Neurol,** 114(3):343–350, 1991.

74. Brecknell JE, et al: Functional and anatomical reconstruction of the 6-hydroxydopamine lesioned nigrostriatal system of the adult rat. **Neuroscience** 71(4)913–925, 1996.

75. Costantini LC, Lin L, and Isacson O: Medial fetal ventral mesencephalon: a preferred source for dopamine neuron grafts. **Neuroreport,** 8(9–10)2253–2257, 1997.

76. Mendez I, Sadi D, Hong M: Reconstruction of the nigrostriadal pathway by simultaneous intrastriatal and intranigral dopaminergic transplants. **J Neurosci** 16(22):7216–7227, 1996.

77. Starr PA, et al: Intranigral transplantation of fetal substantia nigra allograft in the hemiparkinsonian rhesus monkey. **Cell Transplant** 8(1):37–45, 1999.

78. Bentlage C, et al: Reformation of the nigrostriatal pathway by fetal dopaminergic micrografts into the substantia nigra is critically dependent on the age of the host. **Exp Neurol** 159(1):177–190, 1999.

79. Bakay RA, et al: Immunological responses to injury and grafting in the central nervous system of nonhuman primates. **Cell Transplant** 7(2):109–120, 1998.

80. Hudson JL, et al: Allogeneic grafts of fetal dopamine neurons: behavioral indices of immunological interactions. **Neurosci Lett** 171(1–2)32–36, 1994.

81. Brundin P, et al: Human fetal dopamine neurons grafted in a rat model of Parkinson's disease: immunological aspects, spontaneous and drug-induced behaviour, and dopamine release. **Exp Brain Res** 70(1):192–208, 1988.

82. Finsen B, Poulsen PH, Zimmer J: Xenografting of fetal mouse hippocampal tissue to the brain of adult rats: Effects of cyclosporin A treatment. **Exp Brain Res** 70(1):117–133, 1988.

83. Howard OM, et al: Small molecule inhibitor of HIV-1 cell fusion blocks chemokine receptor-mediated function. **J Leukoc Biol** 64(1)6–13, 1998.

84. Ansari AA, et al: Lack of a detectable systemic humoral/cellular allogeneic response in human and nonhuman primate recipients of embryonic mesencephalic allo-

grafts for the therapy of Parkinson's disease. **Transplant Proc** 27(1)1401–1405, 1995.

85. Pedersen EB, Zimmer J, Finsen B: Triple immunosuppression protects murine intracerebral, hippocampal xenografts in adult rat hosts: Effects on cellular infiltration, major histocompatibility complex antigen induction and blood-brain barrier leakage. **Neuroscience** 78(3):685–701, 1997.

86. Borlongan CV, et al: CNS immunological modulation of neural graft rejection and survival. **Neurol Res** 18(4):297–304, 1996.

87. Kordower JH, et al: Fetal grafting for Parkinson's disease: Expression of immune markers in two patients with functional fetal nigral implants. **Cell Transplant** 6(3)213–219, 1997.

88. Saporta S, et al: Microcarrier enhanced survival of human and rat fetal ventral mesencephalon cells implanted in the rat striatum. **Cell Transplant** 6(6):579–584, 1997.

89. Sanberg PR, et al: Testis-derived Sertoli cells survive and provide localized immunoprotection for xenografts in rat brain [see comments]. **Nat Biotechnol** 14(13)1692–1695, 1996.

90. Okura Y, et al: Treatment of rat hemiparkinson model with xenogeneic neural transplantation: Tolerance induction by anti-T-cell antibodies. **J Neurosci Res** 48(5):385–396, 1997.

91. Honey CR, Shen H: Immunosuppression for neural xenografts: a comparison of cyclosporin and anti-CD25 monoclonal antibody. **J Neurosurg** 91(1):109–113, 1999.

92. Elkabes S, Diciccobloom EM, Black IB: Brain Microglia Macrophages Express Neurotrophins That Selectively Regulate Microglial Proliferation and Function. **Journal of Neuroscience** 16(8):2508–2521, 1996.

93. Hefti F: Neurotrophic factor therapy for nervous system degenerative diseases. **Journal of Neurobiology** 25(11):1418–1435, 1994.

94. Olson L: Toward Trophic Treatment In Parkinsonism—A Primate Step. **Nat Med** 2(4):400–401, 1996.

95. Gage FH, et al: Survival and differentiation of adult neuronal progenitor cells transplanted to the adult brain. **Proc Natl Acad Sci U S A** 92(25):11879–1183, 1995.

96. Arsenijevic Y, Weiss S: Insulin-like growth factor-I is a differentiation factor for postmitotic CNS stem cell-derived neuronal precursors: Distinct actions from those of brain-derived neurotrophic factor. **J Neurosci** 18(6):2118–2128, 1998.

97. Maina F, Klein R: Hepatocyte growth factor, a versatile signal for developing neurons. **Nat Neurosci** 2(3):213–217, 1999.

98. Galli R, et al: Regulation of neuronal differentiation in human CNS stem cell progeny by leukemia inhibitory factor. **Dev Neurosci** 22(1–2):86–95, 2000.

99. Asada H, et al: Time course of ciliary neurotrophic factor mRNA expression is coincident with the presence of protoplasmic astrocytes in traumatized rat striatum. **Journal of Neuroscience Res** 40(1):22–30, 1995.

100. Hagg T, Varon S: Ciliary neurotrophic factor prevents degeneration of adult rat substantia nigra dopaminergic neurons in vivo. **Proc Natl Acad Sci USA** 90(13):6315–6319, 1993.

101. Ballagi AE, et al: Platelet-derived growth factor receptor expression after neural grafting in a rat model of Parkinson's disease. **Cell Transplant** 3(6):453–460, 1994.

102. Chen XL, Roisen FJ, Gupta M: The effect of prior in vitro exposure of donor cells to trophic factors in neurotransplantation. **Exp Neurol** 138(1):64–72, 1996.

103. Mouton PR, Olson L: Nerve growth factor increases the size of intracortical cholinergic transplants. **Acta Neurol Scand** 87(5):376–381, 1993.

104. Wells DG, et al: Neurotrophins regulate agrin-induced postsynaptic differentiation. **Proc Natl Acad Sci USA** 96(3):1112–1117, 1999.

105. Jakeman LB, et al: Brain-derived neurotrophic factor stimulates hindlimb stepping and sprouting of cholinergic fibers after spinal cord injury. **Exp Neurol** 154(1):170–184, 1998.
106. Menei P, et al: Schwann cells genetically modified to secrete human BDNF promote enhanced axonal regrowth across transected adult rat spinal cord. **Eur J Neurosci** 10(2):607–621, 1998.
107. Mogi M, et al: Brain-derived growth factor and nerve growth factor concentrations are decreased in the substantia nigra in Parkinson's disease. **Neurosci Lett,** 270(1):45–48, 1999.
108. Sauer H, et al: Brain-derived neurotrophic factor enhances function rather than survival of intrastriatal dopamine cell-rich grafts. **Brain Res** 626(1–2):37–44, 1993.
109. Zhou J, Bradford HF, Stern GM: Influence of BDNF on the expression of the dopaminergic phenotype of tissue used for brain transplants. **Dev Brain Res** 100(1):43–51, 1997.
110. Skaper SD, et al: Brain-derived neurotrophic factor selectively rescues mesencephalic dopaminergic neurons from 2,4,5-trihydroxyphenylalanine-induced injury. **Journal of Neuroscience Res** 34(4):478–487, 1993.
111. Frim DM, et al: Implanted fibroblasts genetically engineered to produce brain-derived neurotrophic factor prevent 1-methyl-4-phenylpyridinium toxicity to dopaminergic neurons in the rat. **Proc Nat Acad Sci USA** 91(11):5104–5108, 1994.
112. Yurek DM, et al: BDNF enhances the functional reinnervation of the striatum by grafted fetal dopamine neurons. **Exp Neurol** 137(1):105–118, 1996.
113. Mufson EJ, et al: Distribution and retrograde transport of trophic factors in the central nervous system: Functional implications for the treatment of neurodegenerative diseases. **Prog Neurobiol** 57(4):451–484, 1999.
114. Rubio F, et al: BDNF gene transfer to the mammalian brain using CNS-derived neural precursors. **Gene Ther** 6(11):1851–1866, 1999.
115. Kordower JH, et al: Clincopathological findings following intraventricular glial-derived neurotrophic factor treatment in a patient with Parkinson's disease [In Process Citation]. **Ann Neurol** 46(3):419–424, 1999.
116. Lin LF, et al: GDNF: A glial cell-line derived neurotrophic factor for midbrain dopaminergic neurons [see comments]. **Science** 260(5111):1130–1132, 1993.
117. Hoffer BJ, et al: Glial cell-line derived neurotrophic factor reverses toxin-induced injury to midbarin dopaminergic neurons in vivo. **Neurosci Lett** 182(1):107–111, 1994.
118. Johansson M, et al: Effects of glial cell line derived neurotrophic factor on developing and mature ventral mesencephalic grafts in oculo. **Exp Neurol** 134(1):25–34, 1995.
119. Tomac A, et al: Protection and repair of the nigrostriatal dopaminergic system by GDNF in vivo [see comment]. **Nature** 373(6512)335–339, 1995.
120. Beck KD, et al: Mesencephalic dopaminergic neurons protected by GDNF from axotomy-induced degeneration in the adult brain [see comments]. **Nature** 373(6512):339–41, 1995.
121. Cheng H, et al: The effect of glial cell line-derived neurotrophic factor in fibrin glue on developing dopamine neurons. **Exp Brain Res** 104(2):199–206, 1995.
122. Hou JG, Lin LF, Mytilineou C: Glial cell-line derived neurotrophic factor exerts neurotrophic effects on dopaminergic neurons in vitro and promotes their survival and regrowth after damage by 1-methyl-4-phenylpyridinium. **J Neurochemi** 66(1)74–82, 1996.

123. Perez-Navarro E, et al: Intrastriatal grafting of a GDNF-producing cell line protects striatonigral neurons from quinolinic acid excitotoxicity in vivo. **Eur J Neurosci** 11(1):241–249, 1999.

124. Rosenblad C, Martinez-Serrano A, Bjorklund A: Glial cell line-derived neurotrophic factor increases survival, growth and function of intrastriatal fetal nigral dopaminergic grafts. **Neuroscience** 75(4):979–985, 1996.

125. Wang Y, et al: GDNF triggers fiber outgrowth of fetal ventral mesencephalic grafts from nigra to striatum in 6-OHDA-lesioned rates. **Cell Tissue Res** 286(2):225–233, 1996.

126. Granholm AC, et al: Glial cell line-derived neurotrophic factor improves survival of ventral mesencephalic grafts to the 6-hydroxydopamine lesioned striatum. **Exp Brain Res** 116(1):29–38, 1997.

127. Zawada WM, et al: Growth factors improve immediate survival of embryonic dopamine neurons after transplantation into rats. **Brain Res** 786(1–2):96–103, 1998.

128. Mehta V, et al: Enhancement of graft survival and sensorimotor behavioral recovery in rats undergoing transplantation with dopaminergic cells exposed to glial cell line-derived neurotrophic factor [see comments]. **J Neurosurg** 88:1088–1095, 1998.

129. Nakao N, et al: Promotion of survival and regeneration of nigral dopamine neurons in a rat model of Parkinson's disease afer implantation of embryonal carcinoma-derived neurons genetically engineered to produce glial cell line-derived neurotrophic factor. **J Neurosurg** 92(4):659–670, 2000.

130. Akerud P, et al: Differential effects of glial cell line-derived neurotrophic factor and neurturin on developing and adult substantia nigra dopaminergic neurons. **J Neurochem** 73(1):70–78, 1999.

131. Fadda E, et al: Ganglioside GM1 cooperates with brain-derived neurotrophic factor to protect dopaminergic neurons from 6-hydroxydopamine-induced degeneration. **Neurosci Lett** 159(1–2):147–150, 1993.

132. Grasbon-Frodl EM, Nakao N, Brundin P,: The lazaroid U-83836E improves the survival of rat embryonic mesencephalic tissue stored at 4 degrees C and subsequently used for cultures or intracerebral transplantation. **Brain Res Bull** 39(6):341–347, 1996.

133. Othberg A, et al: Tirilazad mesylate improves survival of rat and human embryonic mesencephalic neurons in vitro [published erratum appears in Exp Neurol 1998 Nov; 154(1):260]. **Exp Neurol** 147(2):498–502, 1997.

134. Björklund L, Spenger C, Stromberg I: Tirilazad mesylate increases dopaminergic neuronal survival in the in Oculo grafting model. **Exp Neurol** 148(1)324–333, 1997.

135. Björklund L, Vidal N, Stromberg I: Lazaroid-enhanced survival of grafted dopamine neurons does not increase target innervation. **Neuroreport** 9(12):2815–2819, 1998.

136. Schierle GS, Karlsson J, Brundin P: MK-801 does not enhance dopaminergic cell survival in embryonic nigral grafts. **Neuroreport** 9(7):1313–1316, 1998.

137. Hansson O, et al: Additive Effects of Caspase Inhibitor and Lazaroid on the Survival of Transplanted Rat and Human Embryonid Dopamine Neurons. **Exp Neurol** 164(1):102–111, 2000.

138. Lopez OL, Martinez AJ, Torre-Cisneros J: Neuropathologic findings in liver transplantation: A comparative study of cyclosporing and FK 506. **Transplant Proc** 23(6):3181–3182, 1991.

139. Schreiber SL: Chemistry and biology of the immunophilins and their immunosuppressive ligands. **Science** 251(4991):283–287, 1991.

140. Hamilton GS, Steiner JP: Immunophilins: beyond immunosuppression. **J Med Chem** 41(26):5119–5143, 1998.
141. Snyder SH, Lai MM, Burnett PE: Immunophilins in the nervous system. **Neuron** 21(2):283–294, 1998.
142. Steiner JP, et al: Neurotrophic immunophilin ligands stimulate structural and functional recovery in neurodegenerative animal models. **Proc Natl Acad Sci USA,** 94(5):2019–2024, 1997.
143. Costantini LC, et al: A novel immunophilin ligand: Distinct branching effects on dopaminergic neurons in culture and neurotrophic actions after oral administration in an animal model of Parkinson's disease. **Neurobiol Dis** 5(2):97–106, 1998.
144. Bradbury EJ, et al: Astrocyte transplants alleviate lesion induced memory deficits independently of cholinergic recovery. **Neuroscience** 65(4):955–972, 1995.
145. Azizi SA, et al: Engraftment and migration of human bone marrow stromal cells implanted in the brains of albino rats—similarities to astrocyte grafts. **Proc Natl Acad Sci USA** 95(7):3908–3913, 1998.
146. Gearhart J: New potential for human embryonic stem cells [comment]. **Science** 282(5391):1061–1062, 1998.
147. Scheffler B, et al: Marrow-mindedness: a perspective on neuropoiesis. **Trends Neurosci** 22(8):348–357, 1999.
148. Fuchs E, Segre JA: Stem cells: A new lease on life. **Cell** 100(1):143–155, 2000.
149. Weissman IL: Stem cells: units of development, units of regeneration, and units in evolution. **Cell** 100(1):157–68, 2000.
150. Lendahl U, Zimmerman LB, McKay RD: CNS stem cells express a new class of intermediate filament protein. **Cell** 60(4):585–595, 1990.
151. Kaneko Y, et al: Musashi1: an evolutionally conserved marker for CNS progenitor cells including neural stem cells. **Dev Neurosci** 22(1–2):139–153, 2000.
152. Schubert W, et al: Characterization and distribution of a new cell surface marker of neuronal precursors. **Dev Neurosci** 22(1–2):154–166, 2000.
153. Burrow RC, Lillien L, Levitt P: Mechanisms of progenitor maturation are conserved in the striatum and cortex. **Dev Neurosci** 22(1–2):7–15, 2000.
154. McKay R: Stem cells in the central nervous system. **Science** 276(5309):66–71, 1997.
155. Li W, LoTurco, JJ: Noggin is a negative regulator of neuronal differentiation in developing neocortex. **Dev Neurosci** 22(1–2):68–73, 2000.
156. Li M, et al: Generation of purified neural precursors from embryonic stem cells by lineage selection. **Curr Biol** 8(17):971–974, 1998.
157. Wang S, et al: Promoter-based isolation and fluorescence-activated sorting of mitotic neuronal progenitor cells from the adult mammalian ependymal/subependymal zone. **Deve Neurosci** 22(1–2):167–176, 2000.
158. Svendsen CN, et al: Long-term survival of human central nervous system progenitor cells transplanted into a rat model of Parkinson's disease. **Exp Neurol** 148(1):135–146, 1997.
159. Snyder EY, et al: Multipotent neural precursors can differentiate toward replacement of neurons undergoing targeted apoptotic degeneration in adult mouse neocortex. **Proc Natl Acad Sci USA** 94(21):11663–11668, 1997.
160. Lundberg C, et al: Survival, integration, and differentiation of neural stem cell lines after transplantation to the adult rat striatum. **Exp Neurol** 145(2 Pt 1):342–360, 1997.
161. Fricker RA, et al: Site-specific migration and neuronal differentiation of human neural progenitor cells after transplantation in the adult rat brain. **J Neurosci** 19(14):5990–6005, 1999.

162. Andsberg G, et al: Amelioration of ischaemia-induced neuronal death in the rat striatum by NGF-secreting neural stem cells. **Eur J Neurosci** 10(6):2026–2036, 1998.

163. De Vitry F: Growth and differentiation of a primitive nervous cell line after in vivo transplantation into syngeneic mice. **Nature** 267(5607):48–50, 1977.

164. Poltorak M, et al: Human cortical neuronal cell line (HCN-1): further in vitro characterization and suitability for brain transplantation. **Cell Transplant** 1(1):3–15, 1992.

165. Morton AJ, et al: The morphology of human neuroblastoma cell grafts in the kainic acid-lesioned basal ganglia of the rat. **J Neurocytol** 24(8):568–584, 1995.

166. Clarkson ED, et al: Improvement of neurological deficits in 6-hydroxydopamine-lesioned rats after transplantation with allogeneic simian virus 40 large tumor antigen gene-induced immortalized dopamine cells. **Proc Natl Acad Sci USA** 95(3):1265–1270, 1998.

167. Trojanowski JQ, et al: Transfectable and transplantable postmitotic human neurons: a potential "platform" for gene therapy of nervous system diseases. [Review] [36 refs]. **Exp Neurol** 144(1):92–97, 1997.

168. Baker KA et al: Intrastriatal and intranigral grafting of hNT neurons in the 6-OHDA rat model of Parkinson's disease. **Exp Neurol** 162(2):350–360, 2000.

169. Ono T, et al: Evaluation of intracerebral grafting of dopamine-secreting PC12 cells into allogeneic and xenogeneic brain. **Cell Transplant** 6(5):511–513, 1997.

170. Aebischer P, et al: Long-term cross-species brain transplantation of a polymer-encapsulated dopamine-secreting cell line. **Exp Neurol** 111(3):269–275, 1991.

171. Jaeger CB, et al: Polymer encapsulated dopaminergic cell lines as "alternative neural grafts." **Prog Brain Res** 82:41–46, 1990.

172. Winn SR, et al: Behavioral recovery following intrastriatal implantation of microencapsulated PC12 cells. **Exp Neurol** 113(3):322–329, 1991.

173. Emerich DF, Winn SR, Lindner MD: Continued presence of intrastriatal but not intraventricular polymer-encapsulated PC12 cells is required for alleviation of behavioral deficits in Parkinsonian rodents. **Cell Transplant** 5(5):589–596, 1996.

174. Subramanian T, et al: Polymer-encapsulated PC-12 cells demonstrate high-affinity uptake of dopamine in vitro and 18F-Dopa uptake and metabolism after intracerebral implantation in nonhuman primates. **Cell Transplant** 6(5):469–477, 1997.

175. Hoffman D, et al: Transplantation of a polymer-encapsulated cell line genetically engineered to release NGF. **Exp Neurol** 122(1):100–106, 1993.

176. Kordower JH, et al: Intrastriatal implants of polymer encapsulated cells genetically modified to secrete human nerve growth factor: trophic effects upon cholinergic and noncholinergic striatal neurons. **Neuroscience** 72(1):63–77, 1996.

177. Sautter J, et al: Implants of polymer-encapsulated genetically modified cells releasing glial cell-line neurotrophic factor improve survival, growth, and function of fetal dopaminergic grafts. **Exp Neurol** 149(1):230–6, 1998.

12

Technology from the Military

Pre-Hospital and Battlefield Care

JAMES M. ECKLUND, M.D., F.A.C.S., LTC, M.C., U.S.A.,
ROSS R. MOQUIN, M.D., C.DR., U.S.N.,
AND GEOFFREY LING, M.D., PH.D., LTX, M.C., U.S.A.

HISTORICAL PERSPECTIVE

A number of medical and neurosurgical advances have historically emerged from the military experience. The military neurosurgeon is exposed to a vast number of injured patients during wartime. This situation creates an opportunity for rapid professional growth of the surgeon and progressive refinements in medical and surgical techniques. As early as 400 BC Hippocrates commented that war is the only real school for the surgeon. One of the first successful applications of Lister's principles of antisepsis was during the Russo-Turkish War of 1877 by Ernst von Bergmann (1, 2). In the American Civil War the ambulance system introduced by Domenique-Jean Larrey during the Napoleonic Wars, was expanded by Jonathon Letterman (4). Later this concept was applied to the Korean and Vietnamese conflicts where air-mobile evacuation was extensively utilized, and today it is incorporated into most civilian trauma systems. In World War I, COL Harvey Cushing demonstrated how impeccable surgical technique could vastly improve operative mortality as he reduced it from 54% to 28% in 3 months (3, 5).

During World War II antibiotics, transfusions, and improved techniques were used on a large scale by neurosurgeons to further improve this mortality to 14.5% (6). The Seddon nomenclature and Sunderland classification of peripheral nerve injury grew out of the vast experience from the casualties during World World War II (7–9). Within the first 6 months of the Korean Conflict, LTC Arnold Mierowsky recognized the importance of having neurosurgical support far-forward as the MASH concept was born (10, 11). In Vietnam, a comprehensive data collection effort by military neurosurgeons enabled re-evaluation of the appropriate extent of surgical debridement in penetrating head injury (12, 13); and through later experience in the Israeli-Lebanese conflict (14, 15),

Iran-Iraq conflict (16), and others (17), this area of our practice has been refined. A similar data collection system has been established for use in future conflicts by a joint effort of the Defense and Veterans Brain Injury Program and AANS/CNS Joint Committee of Military Neurosurgeons.

UNIQUE MISSION

Several hundred of our Congress members have served proudly in the military during the World Wars, Korea, Vietnam, Desert Storm, other smaller conflicts, and peacetime. What all past, present, and future military neurosurgeons share is the honor of caring for the brave men and women who defend our nation's shores. The military neurosurgeon has the unique responsibility to provide care for the soldiers, sailors, airman, and marines during combat and in remote environments. Intrinsic to this mission is the responsibility to champion research efforts addressing neurosurgical care before the patient reaches a fixed hospital facility.

To effectively address this mission it must be recognized that warfare is changing. As CNN broadcast Desert Storm, the public was astounded at the advanced weaponry modern warfare brings. Bayonets and lower velocity slugs have been replaced by nuclear, biological, and chemical weapons and computerized ordinance delivery systems. With changes in warfare the practice of military neurosurgery must respond to meet new demands. Injuries have and will continue to become more complex.

The battlefield and enemy are often less defined as we deal with more urban conflicts and terrorism threats. Evacuation of casualties in urban warfare often takes much longer than traditional horizontal front line conflicts, because helicopters have difficulty landing between tall city structures and are easily shot down by snipers in nearby buildings (18). Threats of terrorism are more prevalent, and the potential of mass casualty scenarios close to home is a reality. Medical support in these situations requires close collaboration between local civilian and military hospitals.

Deployments are steadily becoming more austere. While civilian trauma systems are designed to deliver care within a regional network, the military must be prepared to deliver care throughout the entire world, often in very remote locations and under extreme conditions.

DEVELOPING TECHNOLOGIES

A major emphasis for technology development in the military is to improve care delivery to an injured soldier or sailor, who may be in the middle of a firefight, aboard a submarine, on a mission in Antarctica, or any number of remote locations. While we all like to think that technological advances will save more lives and improve our care, we have to remember that when the rubber meets the road we have a young medic crawling up to a wounded soldier to do an initial evaluation. The Glascow Coma Scale is a wonderful tool to use in a hospital environment, but it is unrealistic to expect a young 18-year-old medic to administer this exam while under fire.

The Marine Corps is investigating the development of a more basic clinical evaluation tool that can be reliably administered in the heat of battle and easily place the neurologically injured marine into three categories—evacuate, return to battle, or expectant. This examination consists of a six-point scale. One point is awarded for each of the following: disorientation, any weakness, seizure, pupil abnormality, scalp laceration, obvious skull fracture. A retrospective review of 146 patients has been completed using this tool and a very high correlation with outcome has shown. A prospective study is currently in progress to further validate and possibly modify the exam. It is also important to note that scalp lacerations alone did not have any prognostic implications on the retrospective review. It is still premature to translate these data into the categories above that will be pragmatically useful to the marines (J Blanchard, unpublished data).

After his initial evaluation, the medic must then independently manage the patient until such a time that he can be evacuated to the next echelon of care at either a battalion aid station, which has a physician, and ultimately, if the tactical situation permits, to a field hospital or hospital ship with a neurosurgeon. Depending on the tactical situation, evacuation can be quite delayed, requiring the combat medic to provide continued care with the limited equipment contained in his aid bag. In Desert Storm, a war in which the Allied Forces had complete air dominance, medical evacuation time averaged 4.5 hours (19). Understanding this dilemma, military research laboratories, like their civilian counterparts, continue to do active research in brain protection and inflammatory cascades looking for the ultimate neurococktail medics could administer to the neurologically injured patient in the field. The military is also actively investigating artificial blood substrates like substituted hemoglobin and the use of fibrin bandages. These advances can aid the treatment and prevention of shock at the first evaluation in the field. A noninvasive hydration instrument currently undergoing trials in the neurotrauma lab at the Uniformed Services University of the Health Sciences shows promise for determining the degree of shock. This instrument when applied to the gum measures tissue turgor, and early results suggest it provides an accurate estimation of shock and the need for hydration (G Ling, unpublished data).

When the patient reaches the first line of more sophisticated medical support his electronic dog tag or Personnel Identification Card (PIC) will be placed into a modified disc and then inserted into a laptop computer. The PIC contains the patients entire medical history, including medications, lab tests, X-rays, and EKG (20, 21). In order to image the brain currently the patient must be evacuated to a field hospital that has a portable CT capability. At the Neurotrauma lab at USUHS a handheld Radiofrequency Triage System (RAFTS), which uses high frequency radio wave to detect intracranial hematomas, pneumothorax, and compartment syndromes, is being developed. The RAFTS operates between 1–6 gigahertz and uses .01 watt of power. In comparison, a cell phone operates at 1–3 gigahertz and requires 1 watt. Animal trials have been completed, and this instrument can reliably detect as little as 2 cc of intracranial blood (22). Currently, human use approval is pending to continue investigation of this instrument which holds promise as a handheld trauma management tool.

When the patient needs to be evacuated to the next echelon of care either within the field environment or back to a fixed hospital stateside, the portable ICU termed Life Support for Trauma and Transport or "LSTAT" is used. This self-contained unit mounts inside a Blackhawk helicopter or C130 with a cover that protects the patient when flying through NBC contaminated areas. It has a ventilator with every mode, suction, IV pumps the size of cigarette cases that each pump up to 6 liters per hour, monitors capable of reading vitals, end-tidal CO_2, ICP, and CPP. This data can be transmitted via telemedicine links to a physician who can then direct the flight crew on patient management issues (M Caulkins, personal communication, 23). When the patient finally arrives at either a field hospital with neurosurgeons or a hospital ship, the capability and equipment is quite good. A full selection of surgical instruments including power drills and operating microscopes is standard in all the DEPMEDS and hospital ship operating rooms.

When the tactical situation doesn't allow timely evacuation or when the need for evacuation isn't clear, telemedicine can be utilized to consult and sometimes avoid the need for evacuation. Telemedicine helps keep the soldier and sailor on the job while reducing the forward deployment of medical personnel and equipment. The distance learning capability is also utilized to transmit CME conferences and facilitate education of physicians assigned to more remote sites.

On an attack submarine, store and forward technology is utilized with a digital camera, video camcorder, optical camera, electronic stethoscope, and digital vital signs. These submarines have independent duty corpmen who are exceptionally trained, but no physician is on board. They will gather and store the data on a patient and then rise to a depth where they can deliver what's called a "data burp." They can then drop back to tactical depths while the data is reviewed and a response is generated. They will then rise again to receive a data burp containing guidance from a specialist (R Bakalar, personal communication). During the summer of 2000, relay buoys were deployed at appropriate depths in select locations to allow submarines to remain at more tactical depths while exchanging information.

On the USS George Washington aircraft carrier, which has approximately 5000 hands and 10 physicians, the store and forward technique is used for nonemergent consultations. Real-time consultation is also available for complex and emergent cases. A 3 meter satellite antenna is used for real time consultation. One of the challenges when using real time transmission is maneuvering the ship and positioning the planes in such a way that the signal is not blocked. Heavy seas can also compromise transmission and reception. An example of the utilization of telemedicine is seen in data taken from a 6 month deployment of the USS George Washington in 1997–1998. There were 60 consults for 10 specialties including neurosurgery. Over 400 radiology studies were transmitted for interpretation. The medical evacuation rate was down to 7 per month from a historical average of 12 per month. As a result of the telemedicine capability, sicker patients were managed on-board and the in-patient census was up 30% (M Krentz, personal communication).

Telepresence surgery combines real-time telemedicine with robotics technology. Visual and audio stimuli are transmitted to the surgeon via real-time telemedicine signals. The biggest obstacle in telepresence surgery is refining the haptics. Haptics is the ability to feel the tissue interaction with your instruments as if you were actually holding them. That feel has improved dramatically, but still requires a substantial amount of refinement and will likely limit our deployment of this technology for several years. A laboratory at USUHS has developed an early prototype instrument where two robotic arms hold instruments that are controlled by a surgeon sitting in an adjacent room. The surgeon places his hands inside two gloves, looks into a pair of goggles that display the image from the camera, and directs his assistants who are with the patient through a microphone. Vessels and lacerations have been experimentally sutured and appendectomies have been performed with this apparatus (24).

If this technology continues to progress and the haptics is significantly improved, a future battlefield could include the following scenario. A casualty is evacuated to a far forward medical unit which has what is termed a Warfighter Information Network for Telemedicine, real-time consultation is performed, the patient is then placed in an armored medical vehicle where a technician assists a surgeon in performing a telepresence life-saving operation.

CONCLUSION

The military has traditionally been and will continue to be a leader in technological innovation; specifically as it applies to the military mission. As mentioned in the earlier battlefield scenario with the medic, the usefulness of technological advance is limited by the capability to augment the practical efforts of our most valuable resource, our people. Today there are 38 neurosurgeons on active duty in the US Armed Forces, stationed at 15 different hospitals worldwide. There are approximately 60 neurosurgeons in the reserves. Retention in both active duty and reserve ranks remains a significant problem primarily because of reimbursement and administrative support issues. While the vast number of neurosurgeons express reluctance to join the Armed Forces, the majority frequently express that "If our troops are ever in trouble and need help, you call me, and I'm there." Neurosurgeons are by definition industrious, service-oriented, patriotic individuals. With this in mind, the health of our nation and neurosurgical care of our military remains secure.

REFERENCES

1. Hannigan W, Ragen W, Ludgera M: Neurological surgery in the nineteenth century: The principles and techniques of Ernst von Bergmann. **Neurosurgery** 30(5):750–757, 1992.
2. Power D, Spencer W, Gask G: *Plarr's Lives of the Fellows of the Royal College of Surgeons of England.* Vol. 1. London: John Wright & Sons Ltd., 1930, pp 715–716.
3. Hanigan WC: Neurological surgery during the Great War: The influence of Colonel Cushing. **Neurosurgery** 23(3):283–294, 1988.
4. Zellem RT: Wounded by bayonet, ball, and bacteria: Medicine and neurosurgery in the American Civil War. **Neurosurgery** 17(5):850–860, 1985.
5. Cushing H: Notes on penetrating wounds of the brain. **Br Med J** 1:221–226, 1918.
6. Matson D: The management of acute craniocerebral injuries due to missiles, in Spurling G, Woodhall B (eds):*Surgery in World War II: Neurosurgery.* Washington, DC, Office of the Surgeon General, Department of the Army, 1958, pp 123–182.
7. Naff N, Ecklund J: The history of peripheral nerve surgery techniques. **Neurosurg Clin N Am** 12.1:197-210, 2001.
8. Seddon, H., *Three Types of Nerve Injury.* Brain, 1943. 66: p. 237.
9. Sunderland S: A classification of peripheral nerve injuries producing loss of function. **Brain** 74:491, 1951.
10. Meirowsky A, Barnett J: Mobile neurosurgical team. **Ann Surg** 138:178–185, 1953.
11. Meirowsky A: Penetrating cerebral trauma. Observations in Korean War. **JAMA** 154:666–669, 1954.

12. Rish BL, et al.: Analysis of brain abscess after penetrating craniocerebral injuries in Vietnam. **Neurosurgery** 9(5):535–541, 1981.

13. Myers P, B J, Salazar A, et al.: Retained bone fragments after penetrating brain wounds: Long-term follow-up in Vietnam veterans. **J Neurosurg** 70:319A(abstract), 1989.

14. Brandvold B, et al.: Penetrating craniocerebral injuries in the Israeli involvement in the Lebanese conflict, 1982–1985. Analysis of a less aggressive surgical approach. **J Neurosurg** 72(1):15–21,1990.

15. Taha JM, Saba MI,Brown JA: Missile injuries to the brain treated by simple wound closure: results of a protocol during the Lebanese conflict. **Neurosurgery** 29(3):380–383, 1991; discussion p 384.

16. Aarabi B, et al.: Central nervous system infections after military missile head wounds. **Neurosurgery** 42(3):500–507, 1998; discussion pp 507–509.

17. Chaudhri K, Choudhury A, Al Moutaery K, Cybulski G: Penetrating craniocerebral shrapnel injuries during Operation Desert Storm: Early results of a conservative surgical treatment. **Acta Neurochir** 126:120–123, 1994.

18. Leitch R: The medical implications of urban conflict. **U.S.Medicine** 22–27, 2000.

19. Leedham C, Blood C, Newland C: A desriptive anaysis of wounds among US Marines treated at second-echelon facilities in the Kuwaiti Theater of Operations. **Military Medicine** 158(8):508–512, 1993.

20. Chappelle J: Medical dog tag gets test at Ft Hood, in *The Mercury*. 2000, p 6.

21. Slabodkin G: Absolute patient focus Q & A (interview with Army Surgeon General, LTG Ron Blank). **Military Medical Technology** 1999, pp 20–22.

22. Ling G, Riechers R, Pasala K, et al.: diagnosis of subdural and intraparenchymal intracranial hemorrhage using a microwave based detector. **SPIE** 4037:212–217, 2000.

23. McNaughton C, 212th MASH takes "smart litter" to Kosovo, in *The Mercury*. 2000, p 2.

24. Kaufmann C, Rhee P, Burris D: Telepresence surgery system enhances medical student surgery training, in Westwood J, et al. (eds): *Medicine Meets Virtual Reality*, IOS Press 1999, pp 174–178.

13

Proof Before Practice

The Practice of Neurosurgery Must Change to Thrive.

STEPHEN J. HAINES, M.D.

DEFINING THE PROBLEM

The fundamentals driving the national organization of health care in the United States at the start of the 21st century are three simple facts:

1. The demand for health care services continues to rise.
2. The cost of providing health care services continues to rise.
3. The resources available to pay for health care services are limited.

Under these circumstances, in a free market, the price of health care services would rise dramatically resulting in rationing according to ability to pay. As the medical profession and American society do not consider it appropriate to strictly ration health care on this basis, and many consider at least basic health care to be a right rather than a privilege, health care services in the United States operate in a regulated marketplace that constrains availability, utilization, and price differently depending on location, employment, health status, age, and numerous other factors. In such an environment, the inevitable result of the operation of the three fundamentals listed above is increasing regulation to hold down the cost of and demand for health care services.

Rising Demand

The aging of the U.S. population coupled with an increasing life expectancy will increase the need for health care services over the next several decades regardless of other factors. Increased expectation that health care intervention can improve and prolong life will contribute to an even greater per capita demand than we presently see. Further breakthroughs in biomedical research are likely to open therapeutic avenues to previously untreatable diseases and to prolong life even further, creating additional demand.

Increasing Cost

Biomedical research and the interventions it produces are increasingly dependent on very sophisticated technology that is very expensive to develop and deploy. While widespread adoption of some techniques will bring costs down, the medical market for therapeutic (as opposed to preventive) interventions is not a true "mass market" and, coupled with high development, safety, and liability costs, the forces will tend to keep costs of new interventions high. Health care delivery also remains highly dependent on human labor, the cost of which continually rises.

Limited Resources

The demand for health care cost containment clearly demonstrates that American society feels that it is close to the limit on the percentage of its income (the Gross Domestic Product) that it is willing to spend on health care. As stark evidence of this, note that federal spending for health care services is being severely constrained at the moment when the United States is wealthier than it has ever been and is projecting very large federal budget surpluses. Medicare is the largest controllable portion of federal governmental expenditures, and therefore the biggest target for reductions. American business has identified rising health care costs, paid as benefits to its employees, as a major drain on profitability and a target for cost control. Those who pay for the bulk of health care in America have declared that they have reached the limit on their willingness to spend.

The Inevitable Result

In this environment, the payers look for rational ways to determine which health care services to purchase. Unfortunately, they find a chaotic mass of providers with conflicting ideas about the efficacy and effectiveness of various interventions and remarkably little sound data upon which to base decisions about quality and cost-effectiveness. It isn't hard to understand why they resort to arbitrary criteria based on their cost (something they **can** measure) to bring those costs under control.

In a situation in which an increasing amount of costly care **must** be provided with limited resources, pressure to drive down unit cost (reimbursement) and utilization is inevitable. Where apparently equally qualified practitioners show wide variations in the utilization of health care interventions, the payers will understandably choose the lowest rate of utilization as their benchmark until it is proven that a higher rate of utilization is superior. As Wennberg has said: "Unless the medical profession accepts the responsibility for the question of which rate [of surgical utilization] is right and addresses these issues within the current cost containment context, others will see to it that the 'least is always best' theory dominates by default" (1).

WHAT IS PROOF?

If payers will demand proof of effectiveness before paying for procedures in practice, what constitutes proof? Stated simply, proof is *bias-free evidence replicated by independent investigators, that the recommended intervention predictably produces better outcome than other treatment options.*

Bias-Free Evidence

No evidence will be completely free of bias. However, the techniques of controlling bias are well known and well developed. Basic bias control techniques include measures to assure that observations are made objectively, free of distortions caused by the expectations of the observer, treating physician, or patient. The use of blinded observers, validated measurement scales, and instruments and avoiding conflicts of interest are all examples of objectivity techniques.

Bias can be introduced into a study when data are collected before the study is designed. In this circumstance, the best objective measurement tools may not have been used, it may not be possible to measure certain aspects of care because data were not accumulated and other factors may be associated with the intervention being studied in a way that their effect cannot be separated from that of the intervention. Prospective data collection avoids these complicating factors.

Changes in medical practice that occur over time are a very well-known source of bias when patients of one epoch are compared to those in another. The best method of controlling for this type of bias is to compare patients treated contemporaneously. The use of concurrent control populations is a fundamental bias control technique.

No matter how much we know about a certain condition, there are bound to be unsuspected factors that influence outcome. It would be wonderful, almost magical, if there were a way to keep these factors from distorting the results of a study, but how could you control the effects of something you don't even know about? There is a way, and it's called **randomization.** The great power of randomized allocation of patients to intervention groups in clinical studies is that it equalizes the chance that unknown factors may influence the outcome in the intervention groups. No other technique exists that has this powerful effect in eliminating bias from studies. This is the reason that randomization is the gold standard of clinical trial design: it confers a degree of freedom from bias not otherwise attainable.

Replication

A single observation is always at risk of being valid only in the unique circumstances in which it was made. Clinical evidence is valuable only if it is generalizable: applicable to other patients in similar circumstances. Evidence supporting an intervention cannot be considered generalizable unless the observations have been replicated by independent investigators. This may occur through the conduct of more than one clinical study by separate investigation groups in different locations or by conducting the investigation at multiple sites (a multicenter trial). Even one replication markedly reduces the possibility that an observation is in error. If each study is conducted so that probability of an erroneous conclusion is 0.05, and both reach the same conclusion, the probability that both studies have made the same error is 0.0025, a twenty-fold reduction in risk of error.

Other Intervention Options

Proof that an intervention should be used implies that it is better than something. All too often enthusiastic physicians and patients forget that the natural progression of many disorders is one of improvement. Proving an intervention effective means, at a minimum, proving that it is better than the natural history of the disorder. This of course implies that the natural history of the disorder must be known if an intervention is to be proposed. For many conditions that we treat (the "black disc" for example) the natural history is poorly defined.

For most conditions some form of nonsurgical treatment exists to which any new intervention should be compared. If there is good evidence that such treatment is effective, it is appropriate to use patients treated in that way as the contemporaneous controls for the investigation of the effectiveness of the intervention under study. The same applies to alternative surgical interventions.

The Dimensions of Outcome

Finally, proof requires careful consideration of the dimensions of outcome. To prove that an intervention deserves the allocation of limited resources, the outcome obtained must be relevant to the needs of those who will purchase the service. Outcome science has defined four basic dimensions of outcome that need to be assessed to prove the effectiveness of an intervention: medical (technical) efficacy, effect on health functional status, patient satisfaction, and cost-effectiveness.

Most clinical studies in the past have focused on medical or technical efficacy. For example, studies of spinal fusion techniques that use radiographic demonstration of fusion as the endpoint. The literature is replete with studies showing that, under specified circumstances, certain physiologic effects can be produced, but when the observation was put into clinical practice it did not have an ultimately beneficial effect for the patient.

Assessments of improvement in functional status have received a good deal of attention over the past 20 years. Some have been shown to be applicable to a wide range of diseases and some more appropriate to specific disease entities. They share the quality of assessing whether a successful technical result is translated into a change in the patient's ability to function, a step toward meeting the patient's goals rather than just focusing on the physician's goals.

Assessment of patient satisfaction is inherently subjective and many factors beyond the treating physician's control can affect patient satisfaction. Nonetheless, an unsatisfied patient may feel that a technically and functionally successful intervention was not worthwhile. Patient satisfaction is a measure of the concordance of patient and physician goals, an important aspect of providing health services. Therefore, the measurement of patient satisfaction is important to those who purchase health services.

Assessing cost-effectiveness also has many subjective components. Ultimately, it is this assessment that determines if patients and payers will purchase our services. The scope of cost assessed (direct provider reimbursement versus direct costs plus lost wages and productivity, for example) can drastically affect the analysis as can the choice of outcome measures used to assess effectiveness. Valuation of time and function lost to illness is very subjective and highly controversial. There is much art in cost-effectiveness analysis, but bringing these analyses into the open informs the discussion in important ways.

> **The Patient and Payer Question for the 21st Century: "If you can't show me that what you propose to do predictably succeeds and makes me function and feel better at a reasonable cost, why should I pay you for it?"**

DOESN'T TIME TELL THE ANSWER?

Confronted with demands for proof of efficacy and effectiveness, many neurosurgeons are befuddled. Don't we already have this information? This is what we are taught to do. It seems to work for our patients. If it doesn't work we wouldn't keep doing it, would we?

Unfortunately, the history of medicine is littered with interventions promoted as effective that continued to be used long after they were shown to be ineffective or replaced by more effective methods (2). It is true that ineffective interventions will gradually disappear when a more attractive alternative comes along. However, the newer intervention is not necessarily any more effective, it may just be cheaper, easier, or apparently safer.

It is possible to compare the evaluation paradigm of putting an intervention into practice, having practitioners refine it in their own way, and waiting for multiple evaluations to lead to a consensus (a paradigm we will call "Time Will Tell") against the scientific paradigm of Phase I (determine safety and technique or dosage), Phase II (estimate safety and efficacy), and Phase III (randomized clinical) trials by reviewing in retrospect several neurosurgical interventions that were evaluated in both ways (3). In *Table 13.1,* the questions of antifibrinolytic therapy for aneurysmal subarachnoid hemorrhage, chemonucleolysis, antibiotic prophylaxis for clean elective neurosurgical operations, extracranial-intracranial bypass, and carotid endarterectomy are examined. In each case large numbers of patients were evaluated in the "Time Will Tell" paradigm without reaching a clear conclusion. When randomized clinical trials were performed, unambiguous conclusions about effectiveness resulted. Perhaps as important, in the scientific paradigm, far fewer patients (50% to 1% of the number evaluated in the "Time Will Tell" paradigm) were exposed to the less effective therapy.

CAN INNOVATION SURVIVE?

In an environment that requires proof before practice, can innovation survive? Our traditional method of introducing innovative surgical procedures is to do them and expect to be paid as if they were procedures of proven effectiveness. This raises complex issues of financing, ethics, and regulation. The bold surgeon, the willing patient, and the open operating room has produced some of the most dramatic advances in surgery. It has also produced some disastrous outcomes, ethical lapses, and the useless expenditure of millions of dollars.

Table 13.1
*Comparison of Evaluation by Uncontrolled ("Time Will Tell")
and Randomized Controlled Trials*

Content Area	"Time Will Tell"		RCT		Ratio uncontrolled
	# studies	N	# studies	N	RCT
Antifibrinolytic therapy	21	3,398	8	479	7.1
Chemonucleolysis	>20	>20,000	3	234	>85.5
Antibiotic prophylaxis	15	13,787	5	2,713	6.3
EC-IC bypass	23	2,662	1	1,377	1.9
Carotid endarterectomy	51	17,484	3	1,626	10.8

Done in this way, surgical innovation is not subject to scientific or ethical oversight. In the absence of funding for evaluation of the procedure from a third party, there is no requirement for review of the treatment proposal by anyone other than the surgeon and the patient. The surgeon's desire to develop an effective intervention and the patient's desire to be relieved of their disorder introduce insurmountable obstacles of bias except in the treatment of rapidly fatal diseases with highly effective treatments.

To be sure, review of indications by third party payers places some restraint on the most radical departures from conventional therapy, but this is economic rather than ethical, medical, or scientific oversight. It is inconsistent among payers.

This lack of oversight has shifted much surgical innovation out of academic centers, where NIH oversight rules are often applied to innovation regardless of funding source. It has also had the insidious effect of eliminating any apparent need for organized capital investment in the development and evaluation of surgical intervention.

Should there be a serious effort to impose ethical and scientific review on innovative surgical procedures, or even a demand for proof of effectiveness to support reimbursement, the present system would not sustain any significant amount of innovation in surgical procedures. Unfortunately, this is likely to happen.

Pharmaceutical innovation is highly regulated. Despite the time and expense required, the pharmaceutical industry is one of the most profitable in the U.S. The safety record of drug introduction into the U.S. is enviable. This has been accomplished through the application of scientific principles to the process.

On the surgical side, regulation is limited to the introduction of new devices. Much of this is avoided through use of the 510(k) loophole (which exempts devices shown to be "substantially similar" to devices already in use). In the absence of a new device or drug to be surgically implanted, there are no large corporations to support clinical surgical research or to be subject to regulation in introducing new procedures. The only accessible control point is payment for performing the procedure.

Ethical Issues in Neurosurgical Innovation

The introduction of innovative surgical procedures in the present environment of fiscal constraint poses ethical issues to the forward-thinking neurosurgeon. When resources are limited, how do we justify payment for procedures of unproven value? When procedures of unproven value are done outside of formal trials, how do we assure informed consent or the scientific usefulness of any data that might be generated?

The present system poses a number of barriers to ethical behavior if progress is to be made. At present, practitioners do get paid for innovative procedures not identified as part of a clinical trial so long as they seem to resemble an existing procedure. As soon as the procedure is part of an identifiable clinical trial, it may no longer be eligible for reimbursement, even if it is reimbursed in standard practice. The disincentive to participate in a trial under these circumstances is obvious. The Medicare Program has recently taken a big step in ruling that procedures done in certain trials of accepted quality will be paid for under certain circumstances. However, a much larger initiative in this direction is required if we are to remove the disincentive to high quality clinical research.

It is also clear that collecting the data required to evaluate new procedures adds cost to surgical practice. This must be taken into account if we are to expect large scale trials to precede the introduction of surgical innovations into standard practice.

The Fate of Surgical Innovation in the U.S.

In the present setting of limited resources, economic and procedural disincentives to clinical research of high quality reimbursement for the performance of innovative procedures will become more and more difficult to obtain, no alternative mechanism for financing the development of surgical innovation will develop, and surgical innovation will increasingly be done outside of the U.S. health care system.

POSSIBLE SOLUTIONS

We could continue to practice as we have in the past: treat by economics rather than evidence, waiting for the inevitable imposition of external controls. We could support the early imposition of an external control system like the FDA for new surgical procedures. This would likely involve strict rules of evidence-based payment and would be run by payers— private, governmental, or both. Neither plan seems likely to promote the rapid evaluation of surgical innovation with translation to standard neurosurgical practice.

I propose an alternative solution that requires both neurosurgeons and payers to recognize their responsibilities for the rapid, scientific and ethical evaluation and introduction into practice of innovative neurosurgical procedures.

Such a partnership would have four critical components.

1. Both neurosurgeons and payers would accept the principle that payment for procedures in neurosurgical practice would be based on accepted rules of evidence.

2. Procedures of unproven value would be paid for only if carried out within an approved clinical efficacy or effectiveness trial.
3. Such trials would be funded by their beneficiaries, payer organizations, and patients, through health insurance premiums.
4. Crucially, any neurosurgical practitioner meeting eligibility criteria and willing to submit the necessary data would be able to participate in these trials.

In such a partnership, we could balance the needs of the three major stakeholders in the process: patients, payers, and providers. Patients would have assurance that procedures that are routinely reimbursed have been shown to be effective. Payers would be able to minimize the administrative investment in reviewing such procedures, and providers would experience minimal interference with the process of care for such interventions of proven effectiveness. For unproven procedures, patients would have wider access with better oversight than the present system allows, because any willing practitioner could participate in a well-run study of the procedure. Payers would gain in two ways: the utilization of unproven procedures would be limited by the requirements of the study, and they would have assurance that they would know the value of the intervention within a reasonable period of time. Neurosurgeons' practice environment would improve because there would be less administrative work required to perform procedures of proven value, there would be less risk of severe restrictions on the practice of innovative neurosurgery, and the system for evaluating new procedures would be open to all who are willing to provide data.

CONCLUSION

We are entering the most exciting time clinical neuroscience has ever seen. Treatments are improving rapidly, untreatable disease is becoming treatable. In the next several decades, a host of novel neurosurgical interventions will be developed. We have a great opportunity to rapidly and accurately assess the efficacy and effectiveness of these new treatments, assuring that the valuable ones are rapidly incorporated into practice and the ones that don't work are rapidly discarded. We must change our present methods of evaluation if we are to accomplish these goals in an environment of severe cost containment, but by keeping the principles of science, the goal of improved health for our patients, and the spirit of cooperation in the forefront we can accomplish this difficult task.

REFERENCES

1. Wennberg J: Which rate is right? [editorial] **N Engl J Med** 314:310–311, 1986.
2. Paauw DS: Did we learn evidence-based medicine in medical school? Some common medical mythology, in Geyman JP, Deyo RA, Ramsey SD (eds): *Evidence-based Clinical Practice: Concepts and Approaches.* Boston, Butterworth Heinemann, 2000, pp 13–19.
3. Haines SJ: How do you know? **Clin Neurosurg** 44(1):1–15, 1997.

III

General Scientific
Session III
Spinal Surgery Outcomes:
The Basis of Practice

14

The Need for Outcome Studies

What Are We Doing in Neurosurgery?

PAUL C. MCCORMICK, M.D., M.P.H.

The surgical management of patients with benign spinal conditions such as herniated intervertebral disc and spinal stenosis has been an integral part of neurosurgery since its inception. The empiric efficacy of these procedures in relieving pain and restoring function seems undeniable. Neurosurgeons are also aware, however, that not all patients benefit equally from these procedures, some patients benefit not at all, and in some patients, the benefit is short lived. These tempering realizations do not call into question the efficacy of these surgical procedures but, instead, challenge neurosurgeons to better define, characterize, and select those patients most likely to benefit from an appropriately determined and successfully achieved surgical objective.

Yet government agencies, which set policy and allocate scarce societal resources, third-party payers, who shoulder the costs of these treatments, and patients, who choose from a variety of treatment options and providers, have different perspectives. They see the high cost of spinal disorder treatment, significant failure rates for many spinal procedures, and wide treatment variation among surgeons reflecting uncertainty as to indications and benefits of many spinal surgical procedures (3). Indeed, public agencies have scrutinized our science and peer reviewed literature regarding these treatments and have concluded that, while there is not proof of absence of the efficacy of these procedures, there is, nevertheless, an absence of proof that these commonly performed spinal procedures provide greater, or even equivalent, benefit to patients than alternative treatments or no treatment at all.

The recently completed evidence-based report on the treatment of degenerative lumbar stenosis by the Agency of Health Care Research and Quality, for example, concludes that, "Definitive evidence-based statements about the treatment of spinal stenosis await the results of well designed trials" (1).

In commenting on the recently funded $13.5 million dollar SPORT study Steven Katz, Director of the National Institute of Arthritis and Musculoskeletal and Skin Diseases (NIAMS) stated: "Based on this (SPORT) trial, we shall, for the first time, have scientific evidence regarding the relative effectiveness of surgical versus nonsurgical treatment of these commonly diagnosed spinal conditions (i.e., herniated lumbar disc, lumbar stenosis, and degenerative spondylolisthesis. (4)"

The need for high quality outcome studies from neurosurgery to validly address these concerns has, therefore, never been more real or compelling for our specialty and the patients we treat. Similarly, the need for high quality outcome studies to evaluate new treatments and technologies will be critical if neurosurgery is to maintain leadership and advance the field of spinal surgery in service to our patients. Finally, for the spine surgeon practicing in an increasingly competitive and cost-conscious environment, outcome assessment can be a valuable tool to manage the effectiveness and efficiency of their care. Adequately integrated into their practice, these tools can improve the quality of their care, efficiency and effectiveness of its delivery, and serve as an important source of competitive advantage.

WHAT ARE WE DOING IN NEUROSURGERY?

The Joint Spine Section, under the guidance of the AANS/CNS Outcomes Committee and with the full support of the parent organizations, has empowered its own outcomes committee to comprehensively address the needs and opportunities of outcomes measurement for organized neurosurgery and its practitioners. The mission of the outcomes committee was simple: To develop the tools, infrastructure, and methodology to establish efficacy of current spinal surgery treatments, critically assess new treatments and technologies, and allow the individual practitioner to quantify and continuously improve the value of their care.

To accomplish this mission the committee set four objectives. First, to design validated instruments for outcomes measurement that would serve as the standards for spinal outcomes research and assessment. These instruments would share a common core data set with additional condition specific modifications. Secondly, to develop a coordinated mechanism for centralized data collection, scoring, analysis, and auditing which could be easily accessed and utilized by all practicing neurosurgeons. Third, to provide meaningful feedback of data, both with respect to content and timeliness, to practicing physicians for continuous quality improvement. Finally, the committee would assist individuals, institutions, and consortia in hypothesis development and study design as well as provide methodological support for outcomes research.

To further develop and achieve these objectives, the committee initiated a pilot study on lumbar disc herniation in the latter half of 1999.

The primary purpose of this study was to gain organizational experience with data collection and management utilizing an online Internet-based format. We contracted with Outcome Sciences from Boston to perform the data management functions. In addition, we hoped to gain meaningful feedback from surgeons and patients to refine our instrument and streamline our processes. Finally, while we did anticipate generating valid scientific data for peer reviewed publication as a prognosis with treatment study, it was not intended to be an efficacy study.

Lumbar disc herniation was chosen for study because of the frequency of the condition and the homogeneity with respect to diagnostic criteria, surgical indications and technique, and expected outcomes. Forty neurosurgeons from private practice and academics were invited to prospectively enroll 10 consecutive patients undergoing surgery for lumbar disc herniaton. A baseline patient and surgeon assessment would be followed by patient follow-up at 6 weeks, 3 months, and 1 year postoperatively.

The surgeon accesses the Outcome Sciences Website directly or through a link through the Neurosurgery://On-Call Website *(Fig. 14.1)*. Only the surgeon has access to review or enter data on their patients through their unique user name and password

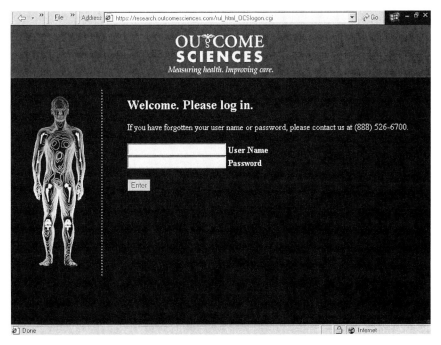

FIG. 14.1 Computer screen appearance of password-protected entry page to lumbar disc pilot study on the Outcome Sciences Website.

The surgeon selects the appropriate form for data entry or review with a simple 'point and click' on the computer screen. The outcome instruments can be completed online or downloaded, completed by hand and uploaded *(Fig. 14.2)*. The patient baseline instrument is 5 pages in length and takes about 10 minutes for the patient to complete and less than 5 minutes to upload. The baseline instrument includes the SF-36, the Oswestry disability scale, a neurogenic symptom scale, comorbidity assessment, and various demographic and socioeconomic items known to be associated with spinal surgery outcomes.

The instrument is practical and has been validated (2). It captures multiple dimensions of outcomes important to patients with spinal disorders. It discriminates among patients with varying disease severity and allows comparison of disease burden to both population norms as well as other nonspinal chronic diseases. Additional data sets include a 1-page surgeon operative and 6-week postoperative form and patient forms at 6 weeks, 3 months, and 1 year postoperatively which includes the SF-12, and items related to satisfaction, expectation, costs of care, and return to work.

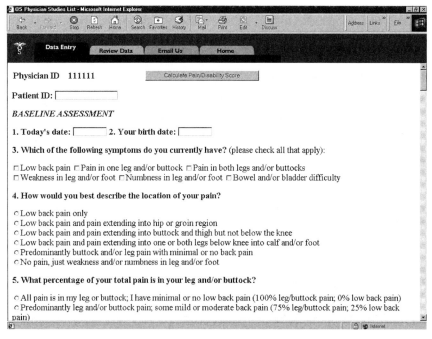

FIG. 14.2 Computer screen appearance of patient baseline instrument. The instrument can be completed and scored online or downloaded for 'paper/pencil' completion.

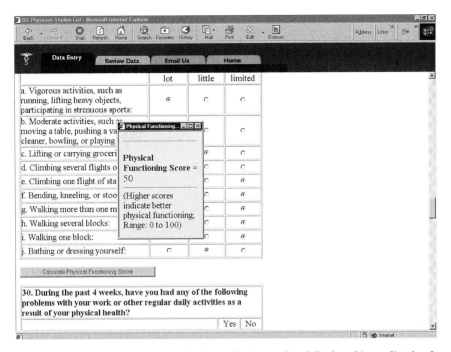

FIG. 14.3 The SF-36 physical functioning scale is scored and displayed immediately after form completion.

The instrument is automatically scored online to provide the patient's score for the disability scale, the neurogenic symptom scale, and the physical functioning, the role functioning, and bodily pain scales of the SF-36 *(Fig. 14.3)*. The surgeon also has instantaneous access to comparative data between their data and the aggregate data from all study patients with respect to demographics and outcomes *(Fig. 14.4)*.

PRELIMINARY RESULTS

Three hundred and twelve patients from 22 physicians have been enrolled to date. There is a greater than 80% retention rate at 6-week follow-up. The preliminary results are more or less what we would anticipate. The vast majority of disc herniations were at L4–5 or L5-S1 *(Fig. 14.5)*. Most patients had symptoms greater than 12 weeks prior to surgery with less than 10% undergoing surgery less than 4 weeks following the onset of symptoms *(Fig. 14.6)*. Over one third of patients were unable to work because of their symptoms while about one third of patients continued to work full time.

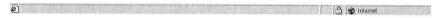

PATIENT-BASED MEASURES: BASELINE AND POSTOPERATIVE MEAN SCORES

Physician ID: 99051610				
	This Physician		All Physicians	
	Baseline	3 Month	Baseline	3 Month
Lumbar Specific: (Note: Higher scores indicate worse health)				
Neurogenic Symptoms	15.15	7.15	15.01	8.14
Pain/Disability	34.09	14.73	33.83	17.25
General Health (SF-36 Scales): (Note: Higher scores indicate better health)				
Physical Functioning	29.54	79.45	28.33	69.89
Role Functioning-physical	11.36	75	9.15	57.75
Bodily Pain	29.17	79	29.98	70.88

FIG. 14.4 Comparative data of individual physician's patients average scores to the combined aggregate scores of all other physician's patients in the study.

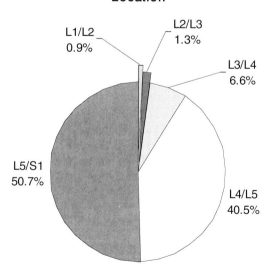

FIG. 14.5 Pie chart shows distribution of the level of lumbar disc herniation in 312 patients.

Duration of Symptoms

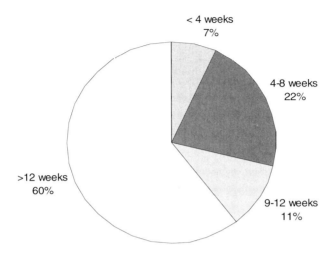

FIG. 14.6 Pie chart demonstrates distribution of preoperative symptom duration.

A significant improvement in the neurogenic symptoms and pain/disability scores was measured at 3 months *(Fig. 14.7)*. Most, but not all, of this improvement was realized by 6 weeks and the outcomes were more or less maintained at 1 year *(Fig. 14.8)*.

The pattern was similar for the SF-36 scales with significant improvements in physical functioning, role functioning, and bodily pain at 3 months *(Figs. 14.9 and 14.10)*.

For the most part there was general agreement between surgeon and patient assessment of outcome *(Fig. 14–11)*.

Patient satisfaction with the processes and points of care was generally good but did identify opportunities for improvement, particularly at the hospital level *(Fig. 14.12)*.

Ninety percent of patients reported that they would have definitely or probably have chosen the same treatment *(Fig. 14.13)*.

In summary, this pilot study has demonstrated the feasibility and widespread applicability of Internet-based outcomes assessment. Indeed, this lumbar disc study is now available to all neurosurgeons for participation. Surgeon 'buy-in' remains an obstacle and was the primary reason why the American Academy of Orthopedic Surgery walked away from their 3 million dollar "Modems" outcomes initiative. The Joint Spine Section will continue to refine these assessment instru-

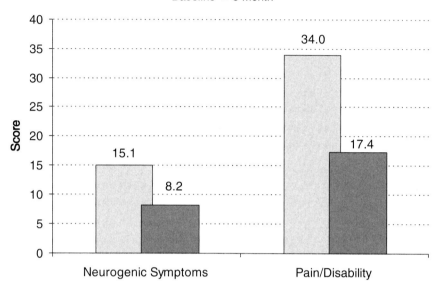

FIG. 14.7 Bar graph of baseline preoperative and 3-month postoperative neurogenic symptom and pain/disability scale scores of all patients. A significant improvement was noted in both outcome dimensions at 3 months postoperative.

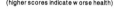

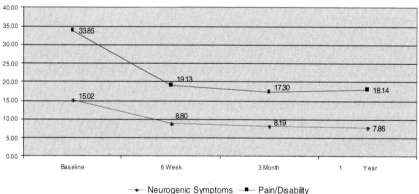

FIG. 14.8 Graph of the time course of average neurogenic symptom and pain/disability scores. Most improvement was noted by 6 weeks postoperative and maintained at 1-year follow-up

SF-36 Scales

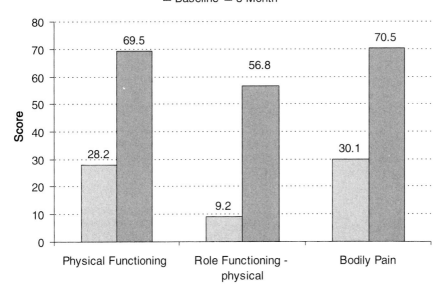

FIG. 14.9 Bar graph shows improvement in SF-36 scales at 3 months postoperative.

General Health SF-36 Scales

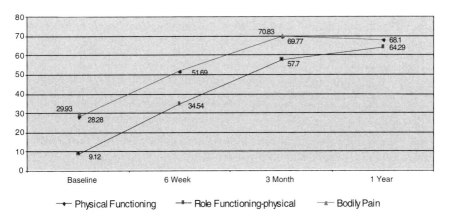

FIG. 14.10 Graph of time course of average SF-36 scale scores.

Patient Outcome at 6 Weeks

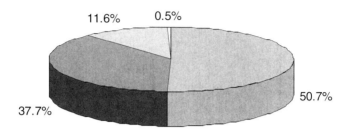

☐ Excellent ☐ Good ☐ Fair ☐ Poor

FIG. 14.11 Pie chart of the distribution of the surgeons' nonquantitative assessment of patient outcome following surgery.

PATIENT SATISFACTION

	Very Satisfied	Somewhat Satisfied	Neutral	Slightly Dissatisfied	Very Dissatisfied
Doctor's office or clinic	83%	12%	2%	2%	2%
Office staff	87%	9%	1%	1%	1%
Doctor	88%	7%	1%	1%	1%
Hospital facility	71%	19%	5%	3%	2%
Hospital staff	76%	12%	4%	7%	1%

FIG. 14.12 Patient satisfaction survey results at 3-months postoperative follow-up

ments and data collection processes to be more relevant and valuable for incorporation into the surgeon's practice. We will continue to develop modifications to the core instrument for other spinal conditions such as cervical radiculopathy, mechanical back pain, myelopathy, and spinal cord injury. Finally, we are planning to institute efficacy and effectiveness studies for lumbar stenosis, lumbar fusion, cervical disc herniation, and cervical spondylotic myelopathy.

If you could go back in time and make the decision again, would you choose the same treatment for your condition? N=171

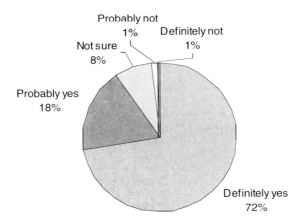

FIG. 14.13 Pie chart of distribution of patients' perception of treatment expectations.

ACKNOWLEDGMENT

The lumbar disc herniation pilot study was supported in part by a financial grant from The William E. Bradley Scientific and Medical Foundations, Seattle Washington. This support is gratefully acknowledged.

REFERENCES

1. Agency of Health Care Research and Quality: Treatment of degenerative lumbar stenosis: An evidenced-based summary and analysis of the literature. 2000 Draft Copy.
2. Deyo RA, Battie M, Beurskens AJHM, et al.: Outcome measures for low back pain research. A proposal for standardized use. **Spine** 23:2003–2013, 1998.
3. McCormick PC: Selection criteria for degenerative lumbar instability. **Clin Neurosurg** 44:29–40, 1997.
4. National Institute of Arthritis and Musculoskeletal and Skin Diseases: Press release regarding funding of Spine Patient Outcome Research Trial (SPORT), James Weinstein, Principal Investigator, 1999.

CHAPTER

15

Do Current Outcomes Data Support the Technique of Lumbar Interbody Fusion?

BRIAN R. SUBACH, M.D., REGIS W. HAID, M.D.,
GERALD E. RODTS, JR., M.D., AND MARK R. MCLAUGHLIN, M.D.

*"It's not what you don't know that hurts you. . . .
It's what you know that just ain't so."*

-Leroy Satchel Paige

ABSTRACT

Over the past 20 years, significant technical advances in spinal surgery have made the concept of interbody fusion a reality. The procedure, whether approached anteriorly or posteriorly, appears to improve patient satisfaction and radiographic fusion rates in selected cases. The lack of a randomized, prospective study and difficulty in comparing outcomes between studies has made it difficult to draw such a conclusion from the literature.

INTRODUCTION

The role of fusion procedures in spine surgery has characteristically been the treatment of painful joints and the correction of skeletal deformity. Fusion, or arthrodesis, may be simply defined as the surgical obliteration of an unstable spinal motion segment. Instability, as defined by White and Panjabi, is the loss of the ability of the spine under physiologic load to maintain the relationship between vertebrae in such a way that there is neither initial damage nor subsequent irritation to the spinal cord or nerve root and, in addition, there is no development of incapacitating deformity or pain related to the structural changes (53). In 1911, Hibbs and Albee first reported the use of spinal fusion in the treatment of instability related to Pott's disease (1). By surgically accelerating the natural course of ankylosis occurring as a part of the disease, they reasoned that healing and pain relief might occur more rapidly. Fusion was shortly thereafter applied to the correction of scoliotic deformities. Early noninstrumented fusion techniques were soon replaced by fusion methods employing internal fixation with hardware.

The use of implantable devices has subsequently increased dramatically as surgeons attempt to provide greater degrees of deformity correction, enhanced early stabilization, and higher rates of bony consolidation. The relatively broad indications for spinal fusion coupled with the improved accessibility of instrumentation have led to both significant technical advances in surgical technique as well as allegations of unnecessary procedures by critics. Given the recent undue emphasis placed upon health care costs, it is not surprising that the numerous treatment strategies have been compared on the basis of both cost and patient outcome. As such, efficacy and outcome studies have attained a heightened degree of importance in patient selection and management.

Unfortunately, there are significant problems in attempting to organize clinical studies designed to evaluate patients after surgical intervention. The most difficult problems are cost, randomization, and choice of outcome measure. The enormous financial burden of a prospective study must be carried by either federal sources or often by private corporations with a vested interest in the results of the study being funded. Given the obvious impracticality and ethical questions of subjecting patients to control or placebo surgical procedures, truly randomized treatment groups are unfeasible. Instead, most surgeons choose to review their data and report their results retrospectively, which unfortunately weakens the power of the study. Finally, the choice of outcome measure, whether some form of pain reduction scale or functional score, remains highly subjective and difficult to generalize to a larger population.

In deciding the relative value of the various reported therapies or interventions in the literature, one must be able to clearly understand the nature of each study and the methods of data collection utilized. Evidence obtained from clinical studies may be classified as three distinct categories based upon the method of data collection (Classes I–III). Class I evidence, which is obtained from prospective, randomized, and controlled trials, represents the most valuable type of data. Class II evidence, representing clinical studies with prospective data collection and retrospective analyses based on clearly reliable data, is derived from most cohort studies, observational, and case-control studies. Class III evidence comes from studies solely based on retrospectively acquired data. As such, clinical series, reviews, and case reports represent the weakest supportive evidence.

The goal of this work is three-fold. The first goal is to briefly describe the anterior and posterior lumbar interbody fusion procedures, indications, and contraindications, as well as the advantages over older, more accepted fusion techniques. The second goal is to define the current tools used to quantify outcomes after lumbar fusion surgery as well as their limitations. Finally, the third goal is to review the current literature to decide if the outcomes data clearly support the use of interbody fusion techniques.

ANTERIOR LUMBAR INTERBODY FUSION (ALIF)

Although initial reports of spinal fusion dealt solely with posterior approaches, in the 1930s, anterior surgery became an accepted method of treatment. In 1932, Capener, Burns, and Mercer first described the anterior approach to lumbar fusion for spondylolisthesis (8, 27). Since that time, ALIF has been widely used in the treatment of degenerative disease of the lower lumbar spine, intractable discogenic back pain, and deformity correction. It is particularly applicable to conditions affecting the anterior and middle columns of the spine, in cases of previously attempted posterolateral fusion procedures, and in cases of marked kyphosis. The procedure may be performed through either a laparoscopic or open approach via a transperitoneal or retroperitoneal approach (35). Extensive discectomy and careful endplate preparation are followed by implantation of threaded titanium cages, corticocancellous dowels, or blocks of various composition (57). Strength of the construct is obtained through interspace distraction and subsequent tension placed upon the annulus (10). The need for supplemental posterior instrumentation with posterolateral arthrodesis for single level ALIF has been debated. There is evidence, however, in multilevel ALIF that supplemental posterolateral fusion enhances the overall fusion rate of the construct(19, 25, 56).

The most common indications for ALIF include segmental disc deterioration at L4-L5 or L5-S1 with corresponding mechanical back pain. Concomitant foraminal stenosis with radicular complaints may or may not be present in such patients. Other indications include degenerative lumbar instability, stable grade I spondylolisthesis, iatrogenic lumbar instability after posterior decompression, and pseudarthrosis after attempted posterior arthrodesis. Relative contraindications include evidence of posterior pathology such as hypertrophic facet arthropathy, lateral recess stenosis, or herniated disc fragments. Prior abdominal surgery, radiation therapy, age greater than 60 years, and the presence of systemic atherosclerotic disease cause difficulty with exposure of the target interspace and may preclude an anterior approach.

Possible complications of the procedure include damage to the iliac vessels, injury to the presacral plexus leading to retrograde ejaculation in men, retroperitoneal hemorrhage, ureteral injury, and intestinal perforation. Despite the associated risks, the allure of ALIF lies in the decreased postoperative pain, direct fixation of the diseased motion segment, and relative ease of exposure in experienced hands.

POSTERIOR LUMBAR INTERBODY FUSION (PLIF)

The concept of lumbar interbody fusion from an entirely posterior approach was first introduced by Cloward in 1945 and later popularized by Lin in 1977 (33). Although other surgeons had reported results of the PLIF procedure in the 1940s, Cloward reported the outcomes of his first 100 patients in 1947 at the Cushing Meeting. Laminectomy and medial or complete facetectomy are followed by extensive disc removal and placement of bone graft with or without "spacers" (42, 55). The posterior approach to interbody fusion shares technology with the anterior approach in terms of implant selection. Although the risk of injury to retroperitoneal structures is present, it is lower than that reported for anterior approaches. The risk of root and cauda equina neuropraxia at the upper lumbar levels, however, remains significant and necessitates aggressive facetectomy to minimize the need for retraction of the neural structures. Injury to the supporting musculature in the lumbar region combined with rigid fixation may account for the significant incidence of postoperative back pain. Similarly, the use of the posterior approach allows for both treatment of posterior pathology and fusion through a single incision. The use of supplemental posterolateral fusion with pedicle screw fixation allows for more extensive facetectomy and subsequently, less nerve root retraction (17, 40). This approach allows for disc space distraction, anterior arthrodesis, decompression of the neural elements, cancellous graft harvest, and posterolateral arthrodesis through a single incision. Unfortunately, there is evidence to suggest that the incidence of postoperative stenosis adjacent to the posterior fusion mass is higher (30%) when compared to that observed with the anterior approach (2.5%) (32).

Common indications for PLIF surgery include refractory mechanical low back pain secondary to intrinsic or iatrogenic disc degeneration, multiple recurrent disc herniation, mobile grade I or II spondylolisthesis, postlaminectomy segmental instability, reconstruction for failed back syndrome, and bilateral disc herniation. All involve loss of interspace height with varying degrees of foraminal stenosis, instability, and pain refractory to conservative management. Other complications include excessive blood loss due to epidural or end-plate sources, intraabdominal vascular injury, graft retropulsion, pseudarthrosis, epidural scar formation, arachnoiditis, infection, and dural tears.

OUTCOMES

The difficulty in assessing patient outcomes from spinal surgery lies not in quantifying fusion results or identifying complications, but in reliably correlating postoperative levels of functioning as related to the surgical procedure (24). Multiple attempts have been made to create scales and assessment devices, which allow objective comparisons to be made regarding the most subjective of variables—back pain (5). Deyo et al. classified the currently available outcome measures into seven categories: (1) functional questionnaires, (2) global satisfaction ratings, (3) timed activities and obstacle courses, (4) employment status, (5) disability days, (6) patient diaries, and (7) electronic monitors (14, 15). In evaluating the usefulness of such outcome scales, one must apply three principles: validity, reliability, and sensitivity. Validity of a test quite simply refers to the accuracy of the modality in describing the variable it is designed to measure. In other words, does the scale measure what it is supposed to? Reliability is the consistency of the test in arriving at the same rating each time it is used, or the reproducibility of the test despite the possibility of random error. Finally, the sensitivity of the testing modality is the ability of the scale to detect subtle differences in clinical status over a reasonable time period. For example, longer questionnaires are more reliable in terms of testing, but less appealing to patients. Scales designed to measure a wide range of disabilities may be very sensitive in identifying subtle differences between levels of moderate disability, while sacrificing validity at the ends of the spectrum.

There are a large number of scales, which have become widely accepted. Some of these focus specifically on the quality and severity of back pain such as the McGill Pain Questionnaire, the Oswestry Low Back Pain Disability Questionnaire, and the North American Spine Society Questionnaire (18, 26). Some scales focus on the quantification of physical disability and handicap, such as the Barthel Index, the Prolo Scale, and the Functional Status Index (41). Finally, others are considered generic quality-of-life measures and may be used to examine the impact of a variety of treatments upon a wide range of diseases, such as the Short Form -36 (SF-36) Health Survey and the Sickness Impact Profile (SIP) (16). With so many different available means of scoring outcomes available, two obvious problems arise. First, no scale has been shown to be superior by independent observers. Secondly, how does one compare two outcomes studies which utilize different means of quantification? The errors inherent in any study may be magnified or reduced simply by the choice of an alternate outcome scale. Attempts to rectify this problem have also met with variable success (19, 22). For example, Dionne et al. performed a prospective study to compare pain, functional limitations, and work status indices as measures of outcome in a group of back pain patients over a 2-year period (16). The study found that the three indices were related but clearly not interchangeable. Given such difficulties, there is a desperate need for a single, unifying classification system that is valid, reliable, and sensitive in describing a patient's functional status; is acceptable to surgeons, rehabilitation specialists, and therapists alike; and that may be easily administered to patients and readily quantified by researchers. Until that time, however, the difficulty in comparing outcomes remains.

REVIEW OF THE LITERATURE

There are numerous descriptions of the various surgical fusion techniques and patient outcomes in the literature. The fusion rates and extent of patient improvement vary considerably among published reports between 60 and 100% (2, 7, 12, 20, 21). The differences in the observed results may be attributed to variations in patient population, procedure choice, implant selection, and post-operative management. Even the method of evaluation has been found to affect the results of such studies. For example, Howe and Frymoyer identified a significant difference in outcome based solely upon the choice of evaluation technique used (22). The use of subjective criteria in post-operative questionnaires, such as patient satisfaction, tended to falsely elevate success rates when compared to more objective measures, such as doctor visits or employment status. Similarly, the reporting of fusion results may be influenced by the specific criteria used. Kumar found a 20% disparity in fusion rates for patients undergoing ALIF based solely on differences in radiographic interpretation (29).

In 1992, Turner published a review of the literature reporting the outcomes from lumbar fusion surgery (53). Between 1966 and 1991, 47 articles were identified which met minimal follow-up and outcome criteria. In none of the studies were patients randomized to different treatments, nor were any surgical techniques directly compared in the same population. There appeared to be no statistically significant difference in clinical outcome based on fusion technique. This included posterior, posterolateral, anterior interbody, and posterior interbody methods. In this review, the interbody techniques did demonstrate significantly higher fusion rates than the other two methods employed, however, populations in the responsible studies differed slightly.

In regard to ALIF, a review of the literature demonstrates nine articles with both adequate follow-up periods and quantifiable outcome measures (*Table 15.1*). Two studies performing ALIF with allograft alone (no supplemental posterior fixation) documented the lowest fusion rates (60%, 73%), although Kim et al. identified a 90% fusion rate with the same procedure (4, 25, 54). Studies using autograft alone, or allograft supplemented by autograft described fusion rates from 89 to 100% (11, 38). The addition of posterolateral fixation to allograft ALIF

Table 15.1
Current Outcomes Data Regarding Anterior Interbody Fusion

Study Name	Ant or Post	Implant Type	Year	Patients	Outcomes of Study	Study Class	Comment
Barrick	ALIF	allograft	2000	20	pain better 16/18 (89%) satisfied 16/18 (89%) return to work 5/15 (33%) fusion rate 18/18 at 6.4 mos	III	
Gertzbein	ALIF	allograft with PL fusion	1996	67	pain score 7.1 improved to 2.1 return to work (77%) fusion 65/67 (97%)	II	multicenter, prospective
Vamvanij	ALIF	allograft	1998	11	satisfied 4/11 (36%) return to work 3/11 (31%) fusion 6/10 (60%)	III	
		ALIF/BAK and PL fusion	1998	16	satisfied 10/16 (63%) return to work 6/16 (38%) fusion 14/16 (88%)	III	
Blumenthal	ALIF	ALIF/allograft	1988	34	return to work 25/34 (74%) fusion 24/34 (73%)	III	
Newman	ALIF	ALIF/auto	1992	36	return to work 31/36 (86%) fusion 32/34 (89%)	III	

Author	Technique	Material/Comparison	Year	N	Results	Level
Kuslich	ALIF PLIF	BAK cages BAK cages	1998 1998	591 356	return to work (91%) total ALIF fusion 2 yrs out (98%) PLIF fusion 2 yrs out (94%)	II
Whitecloud	ALIF	aalograft with PL fusion	1998	35	pain better 23/35 (66%) return to work 4/29 (14%) fusion (97%)	III
Cohen	ALIF	ALIF for pseudarth tricortical autologous crest femoral ring with autograft	2000	33 20	return to work (28%) fusion 32/33 (97%) return to work (36%) fusion 20/20 (100%)	II
Kim	ALIF	ALIF vs PL fusion/screws ALIF PL fusion/screws	1999	20 20	satisfied (85%) fusion (90%) satisfied (90%) fusion (95%)	III

procedures increased the fusion rate to 97% (20, 56). The use of threaded cages for the ALIF, in place of a structural allograft, may improve fusion rates slightly to 98% at 2 years (30). The addition of supplemental posterior fixation to the cage ALIF, however, was associated with a lower fusion rate of only 88% (54).

Functional outcome of the ALIF procedures varied similarly with satisfaction ratings from 36 to 89% (3, 25, 54, 56) and return-to-work status varying between 28% and 91% (3, 4, 11, 20, 30, 38, 54, 56, 57). With such variation in results, it is difficult to draw conclusions that are relevant to clinical practice.

In regard to PLIF, a review of the literature demonstrates 18 articles with both adequate follow-up periods and quantifiable outcome measures (Table 15.2). Nine of the studies performed single-level PLIF with allograft alone with documented fusion rates ranging from 81 to 95% (6, 12, 31, 34, 36, 41, 45–48). In the report by Mitsunaga, single level fusions were associated with higher fusion rates (81%) than two level PLIFs, which had a documented fusion rate of only 66% (36). Studies using autograft alone described fusion rates from 88 to 98% (23, 33, 49, 51, 52). Although such numbers appear to show increased fusion rates with autograft bone, Rish directly compared the efficacy of allograft to autograft in 250 patients undergoing PLIF surgery. The 1989 study found no statistically significant difference in fusion rates between the two groups (44). Takeda investigated the use of autograft by comparing unicortical and bicortical illiac crest grafts in 96 patients (51). The bicortical grafts demonstrated a higher fusion rate (98%) as compared to the 88% observed in unicortical grafts. The use of threaded cages for the PLIF, in place of a structural allograft, may improve fusion rates slightly to 90–96% (2, 43).

Functional outcome of the PLIF procedures varied similarly with satisfaction ratings from 60 to 95% (2, 6, 12, 17, 23, 31, 33, 34, 36, 41, 43–47, 50–52) and return-to-work status varying between 46% and 97% (1, 17, 31). With such variation in results, it is again difficult to draw conclusions that are relevant to clinical practice.

DISCUSSION

The optimal treatment of discogenic back pain remains controversial. This is primarily due to the lack of understanding of its anatomic origin, lack of acceptance of current provocative testing modalities, and lack of randomized, prospective trials quantifying improved patient outcomes with surgery. We are faced with retrospective reviews of both diagnostic procedures and surgical interventions performed in a widely diverse population, with no means of uniform cross comparison. In or-

TABLE 15.2
Current Outcomes Data Regarding Posterior Interbody Fusion

Study Name	Ant or Post	Implant Type	Year	Patients	Outcomes of Study	Study Class	Comment
Lee	PLIF	allograft	1995	62	pain better 47/54 (87%) satisfied 48/54 (89%) return to work 44/54 (97%) fusion 58/62 (94%)	II	
Agazzi	PLIF	carbon cages/PL fusion	1999	71	satisfied 47/71 (67%) return to work (46%) fusion 76/84 (90%)	III	
Freeman	PLIF	PLIF/allo with PL fusion	2000	60	satisfied (83%) return to work (50%) "fixation" (100%)	III	
Rompe	PLIF	PLIF vs PLIF/PL fusion PLIF/allograft	1995	30	pain better 86% no statistical difference in outcome between groups	III	
		PLIF/PL fusion		55			
Branch	PLIF	PLIF keystone graft	1987	172	improved 84%/prolo 75% fusion NR	III	
Collis	PLIF	PLIF/"allogeneic" allograft	1985	750	improved 95%/prolo 52% fusion 90%	III	
Hutter	PLIF	PLIF/autograft iliac	1983	492	improved 82%/prolo 88% fusion 94%	III	
Lin	PLIF	PLIF/autograft iliac	1983	465	improved 82%/prolo 82% fusion 88%	III	
Ma	PLIF	PLIF/allograft	1985	100	improved 91%/prolo 74% fusion 85%	III	
Mitsunaga	PLIF	PLIF/allograft	1989	27	improved 81%/prolo 70% fusion 81%	III	2 level pseudarth 66%

(continued)

TABLE 15.2 (*CONTINUED*)
Current Outcomes Data Regarding Posterior Interbody Fusion

Study Name	Ant or Post	Implant Type	Year	Patients	Outcomes of Study	Study Class	Comment
Prolo	PLIF	PLIF/allograft	1986	34	improved 85%/prolo 85% fusion 94%	III	
Rish	PLIF	PLIF/auto vs allograft	1989	250	improved 60%/prolo 60% fusion 86%	III	auto = allo fusion rate
Schechter	PLIF	PLIF/allograft	1991	25	improved 89%/prolo 91% fusion 95%	III	
Sepulveda	PLIF	PLIF/allograft	1985	17	improved 85%/prolo 70% fusion 92%	III	after failed chemonucl
Simmons	PLIF	PLIF/autograft	1985	113	improved 79%/prolo 54% fusion 91%	III	morselized spinous pr
Takeda	PLIF	PLIF/autograft (unicortical)	1985	44	improved ?%/prolo ?% fusion 88%	III	bicortical ant iliac best
		PLIF/autograft (bicortical)	1985	52	improved ?%/prolo ?% fusion 98%		
Tunturi	PLIF	PLIF/autograft	1979	79	improved 60%/prolo 24% fusion 91%	III	
Ray	PLIF	PLIF/Ray cage-autograft	1995	236	improved 86%/prolo 86% fusion 96%	II	prospective FDA study

der to determine if current outcomes data truly support the concept of interbody fusion, we must build from the most basic of facts and assumptions.

Each spinal segment has three joints, which may each undergo deterioration and thus become pain generators or sources in an afflicted patient. When the facet joint is affected, hypertrophy is the adaptive response of the body in an attempt to resist micromotion of the joint and the associated pain. Disc degeneration, annular tears, and interspace collapse occurring as a result of repetitive biomechanical stresses and the aging process, are registered as pain by annular nocioceptors. Discography may be used to reproduce and intensify existing (concordant) pain to assist in the localization of the responsible pain generator (9, 13). Obliteration of the causative motion segment by surgical fusion is effective in relieving back pain in many patients. There is Class I evidence (randomized, prospective) supporting the use of instrumentation to improve lumbar fusion rates (58). There is further evidence that a relatively small number of patients fail to improve after instrumented posterolateral fusion, presumably due to micromotion at the collapsed disc space. This same population has been successfully treated with interbody fusion, via anterior approach (3). The interspace, when relatively devoid of endplates represents a significant, well-vascularized surface area of exposed cancellous bone. When coupled with a structural allograft or synthetic support, the interspace height is restored, fusion rates enhanced, and micromotion eliminated (57). Based on the results of interbody fusion in failed posterolateral fusion cases, the use of ALIF and PLIF as a primary fusion technique is justified.

The surgical results of ALIF and PLIF procedures demonstrate slightly improved fusion rates and equivalent patient outcomes when compared to conventional posterolateral instrumented fusion techniques. Therefore, the currently available outcomes data, despite the previously discussed shortcomings, do support the use of interbody fusion in selected populations.

CONCLUSION

Do current outcomes data support the technique of lumbar interbody fusion? The authors find it difficult to unequivocally answer the question. There is tremendous difficulty in comparing and contrasting results in the current literature. There are, unfortunately, no strict or uniform criteria for patient evaluation, no defined standards of care, and no consistent nomenclature for diagnosis or surgical interventions. Perhaps most importantly, the quantification of outcomes is extremely variable and noncomparable.

In response to these issues, a combined neurosurgical/orthopedic initiative was undertaken to quantify and standardize the evaluation of lumbar interbody fusion. The S.I.R.G. (Surgical Interbody Research Group) is currently accumulating data regarding fusion assessment, restoration of lordosis, nomenclature of disease and reconstructive techniques, and classification of outcomes. Hopefully, this undertaking will lead to a better understanding of the surgical treatment of degenerative lumbar disease.

REFERENCES

1. Albee FH: Transplantation of a portion of the tibia into the spine for Pott's disease. **JAMA** 57:885–886, 1911.
2. Agazzi S, Reverdin A, May D: Posterior lumbar interbody fusion with cages: an independent review of 71 cases. **J Neurosurg** 91(2 suppl):186–192, 1999.
3. Barrick WT, Schofferman JA, Reynolds JB, Goldthwaite ND, McKeehan M, Keaney D, White AH: Anterior lumbar fusion improves discogenic pain at levels of prior posterolateral fusion. **Spine** 25(7):853–857, 2000.
4. Blumenthal SL, Baker J, Dossett A, Selby DK: The role of anterior lumbar fusion for internal disc disruption. **Spine** 13(5):566–569, 1988.
5. Boden SD: Outcome assessment after spinal fusion: why and how? **Orthop Clin North Am** 29(4):717–728, 1998.
6. Branch CL, Branch CL Jr: Posterior lumbar interbody fusion with the keystone graft: technique and results. **Surg Neurol** 27(5):449–454, 1987.
7. Brodke DS, Dick JC, Kunz DN, McCabe R, Zdeblick TA: Posterior lumbar interbody fusion: A biomechanical comparison, including a new threaded cage. **Spine** 22:26–31, 1997.
8. Capener N: Spondylolisthesis. **Br J Surg** 19:374–386, 1932.
9. Carragee EJ: Is lumbar discography a determinant of discogenic low back pain: Provocative discography reconsidered. **Cur Rev Pain** 4(4):301–308, 2000.
10. Chen D, Fay LA, Lok J, Yuan P, Edwards T, Yuan H: Increasing neuroforaminal volume by anterior interbody distraction in degenerative lumbar spine. **Spine** 20:74–79, 1995.
11. Cohen DB, Chotivichit A, Fugita T, et al.: Pseudarthrosis repair. Autogenous iliac crest versus femoral ring allograft. **Clin Orthop** 371:46–55, 2000.
12. Collis JS: Total disc replacement: A modified posterior lumbar interbody fusion. Report of 750 cases. **Clin Orthop** 193:64–67, 1985.
13. Derby R, Howard MW, Grant JM, Lettice JJ, Van Peteghem PK, Ryan DP: The ability of pressure controlled discography to predict surgical and nonsurgical outcomes. **Spine** 24(4):364–371, 1999.
14. Deyo RA, Andersson G, Bombardier C, et al.: Outcome measures for studying patients with low back pain. **Spine** 19(18 suppl):2032S–2036S, 1994.
15. Deyo RA, Battie M, Beurskens AJ, et al.: Outcome measures for low back pain research. A proposal for standardized use. **Spine** 15:24(4):418, 1999.
16. Dionne CE, Von Korff M, Koepsell TD, et al.: A comparison of pain, functional limitations, and work status indices as outcome measures in back pain research. **Spine** 24(22):239–245, 1999.
17. Freeman BJ, Licina P, Mehdian SH: Posterior lumbar interbody fusion combined with instrumented posterolateral fusion: 5 year results in 60 patients. **Eur Spine J** 9:42–46, 2000.

18. Gerszten PC: Outcomes research: A review. **Neurosurgery** 43(5):1146–1156, 1998.
19. Gertzbein SD, Betz R, Clements D, et al.: Semirigid instrumentation in the management of lumbar spinal conditions combined with circumferential fusion. A multicenter study. **Spine** 21:1918–1926, 1996.
20. Gertzbein SD, Hollopeter M, Hall SD: Analysis of circumferential lumbar fusion outcome in the treatment of degenerative disc disease of the lumbar spine. **J Spinal Disord** 11:472–478, 1998.
21. Greenough CG, Peterson MD, Hadlow S, Fraser RD: Instrumented posterolateral lumbar fusion: results compared with anterior lumbar interbody fusion. **Spine** 23:479–486, 1998.
22. Howe J, Frymoyer JW: The effects of questionnaire design on the determination of end results in lumbar spinal surgery. **Spine** 10:804–805, 1985.
23. Hutter CG: Posterior intervertebral body fusion. A 25-year study. **Clin Orthop** 179:86–96, 1983.
24. Johnson L: Outcomes analysis in spinal research. How clinical research differs from outcomes analysis. **Orthop Clin North Am** 25(2):205–213, 1994.
25. Kim SS, Denis F, Lonstein JE, Winter RB: Factors affection fusion rate in adult spondylolisthesis. **Spine** 15:979–984, 1990.
26. Kopec JA, Esdaile JM: Functional disability scales for back pain. **Spine** 20(17):1943–1949, 1995.
27. Kostuik JP, Smith TJ: Pitfalls of biomechanical testing. **Spine** 16:1233–1235, 1991.
28. Kozak JA, O'Brien JP: Simultaneous combined anterior and posterior fusion: An independent analysis of a treatment for the disabled low back pain patient. **Spine** 15:322–328, 1990.
29. Kumar A, Kozak JA, Doherty BJ, Dickson BJ: Interspace distraction and graft subsidence after anterior lumbar fusion with femoral strut allograft. **Spine** 18:2393–2400, 1993.
30. Kuslich SD, Ulstrom, Griffith SL, Ahern JW, Dowdle JD: The Bagby and Kuslich method of interbody fusion: history, techniques, and 2 year follow up results of a United States prospective, multicenter trial. **Spine** 23:1267–1279, 1997.
31. Lee CK, Vessa P, Lee JK: Chronic disabling low back pain syndrome caused by internal disc derangements. The results of disc excision and posterior lumbar interbody fusion. **Spine** 20:356–361, 1995.
32. Lehman TR, Spratt KF, Tozzi JE, et al.: Long term follow up of lower lumbar fusion patients. **Spine** 12:97–104, 1987.
33. Lin PM, Cautilli RA, Joyce MF: Posterior lumbar interbody fusion. **Clin Orthop** 180:154–168, 1983.
34. Ma GW: Posterior lumbar interbody fusion with specialized instruments. **Clin Orthop** 193:57–63, 1985.
35. McLaughlin MR, Zhang JY, Subach BR, Haid RW, Rodts GE: Laparoscopic anterior lumbar interbody fusion. **Neurosurg Focus** 7:article 8, 1999
36. Mitsunaga MM, Chong G, Maes KE: Microscopically assisted posterior lumbar interbody fusion. **Clin Orthop** 263: 121–127, 1991.
37. Nachemson A, Zdeblick TA, O'Brien JP: Lumbar disc disease with discogenic pain. What surgical treatment is most effective? **Spine** 21(15):1835–1838, 1996.
38. Newman MH, Grinstead GL: Anterior lumbar interbody fusion for internal disc disruption. **Spine** 17:831–833, 1992.
39. Penta M, Fraser RD: Anterior lumbar interbody fusion: A minimum 10 year follow up. **Spine** 22:2429–2434, 1997.
40. Penta M, Sandhu A, Fraser RD: A long-term assessment of adjacent disc degeneration following anterior lumbar interbody fusion. **Spine** 20:743–747, 1995.

41. Prolo DJ, Oklund SA, Butcher M: Toward uniformity in evaluating results of lumbar spine operations. A paradigm applied to posterior lumbar interbody fusions. **Spine** 11(6):601–606, 1985.
42. Rapoff AJ, Ghanayem AJ, Zdeblick TA: Biomechanical comparison of posterior lumbar interbody fusion cages. **Spine** 22:2375–2379, 1997.
43. Ray CD: Threaded titanium cages for lumbar interbody fusion. **Spine** 22(6): 667–679, 1997.
44. Rish BL: A critique of posterior lumbar interbody fusion: 12 years experience with 250 patients. **Surg Neurol** 31:281–289, 1989.
45. Rompe JD, Eysel P, Hopf C: Clinical efficacy of pedicle instrumentation and posterolateral fusion in the symptomatic degenerative lumbar spine. **Eur Spine J** 4(4):231–237, 1995.
46. Schechter NA, France MP, Lee CK: Painful internal disc derangements of the lumbar spine: Discographic diagnosis and treatment by posterior lumbar interbody fusion. **Orthopaedics** 14:447–451, 1991.
47. Sepulveda R, Kant AP: Chemonucleolysis failures treated by PLIF. **Clin Orthop** 193:68–74, 1985.
48. Simmons JW: Posterior lumbar interbody fusion with posterior elements as chip grafts. **Clin Orthop** 193:85–89, 1985.
49. Simmons JW: Treatment of failed PLIF with pulsing electromagnetic fields. **Clin Orthop** 193:127–132, 1985.
50. Simmons JW, Andersson GBJ, Russell GS, Hadjipavlou AG: A prospective study of 342 patients using transpedicular fixation instrumentation for lumbosacral spine arthrodesis. **J Spinal Disord** 11(5):367–374, 1998.
51. Takeda M: Experience in posterior lumbar interbody fusion: unicortical versus bicortical autologous grafts. **Clin Orthop** 193:120–126, 1985.
52. Tunturi T, Kataja M, Keski-Nisula L, et al.: Posterior fusion of the lumbosacral spine. Evaluation of the operative results and the factors influencing them. **Acta Orthop Scand** 50:415–425, 1979.
53. Turner JA, Ersek M, Herron L, Haselkorn J, Kent D, Ciol MA, Deyo R: Patient outcomes after lumbar spinal fusion. **JAMA** 268:907–911, 1992.
54. Vamvanij V, Fredrickson BE, Thorpe JM, Stadnick ME, Yuan HA: Surgical treatment of internal disc disruption: An outcome study of four fusion techniques. **J Spinal Disord** 11(5):375–382, 1998.
55. Weiner BK, Fraser RD: Spine update lumbar interbody cages. **Spine** 23:634–640, 1998.
56. Whitecloud TS, Castro FP, Brinker MR, Hartzog CW, Ricciardi JE, Hill C: Degenerative conditions of the lumbar spine treated with intervertebral titanium cages and posterior instrumentation for circumferential fusion. **J Spinal Disord** 11:479–486, 1998.
57. Voor MJ, Mehta S, Wang M, Zhang YM, Mahan J, Johnson JR: Biomechanical evaluation of posterior and anterior lumbar interbody fusion techniques. **J Spinal Disord** 11(4):328–334, 1998.
58. Zdeblick TA: A prospective, randomized study of lumbar fusion. **Spine** 18: 983–991, 1993.

16

Intradiscal Electrothermy: Indications, Techniques, and Clinical Results

WILLIAM C. WELCH, M.D., F.A.C.S.,
PETER C. GERSZTEN, M.D., M.P.H., AND PAULA MCGRATH, R.N.

INTRODUCTION

A number of intradiscal techniques to shrink or remove disc material causing lumbar pain and radiculopathy have been described over the years. These techniques include interbody fusion, postero-lateral fusion, microdiscectomy, arthroscopic discectomy (1), automated percutaneous lumbar discectomy (2), chymopapain, and other procedures. In general, a trend toward minimally invasive techniques for the treatment of lumbar disc disease has evolved. Recently, a new technique has been developed which involves the percutaneous insertion of a thermal resistance probe with controlled heating of the disc material (3). This technique is designed to reduce back pain associated with discogenic pathology, including disc degeneration, annular disruption, and perhaps disc rupture. The technique is known as intradiscal electrothermy (IDET). The purpose of this paper is to describe a single institution's patient selection, technique, and clinical results using IDET.

MATERIALS AND METHODS

Study criteria

Twenty-three patients were enrolled into a non-randomized, prospective, longitudinal, observational trial to assess the technique and clinical outcomes of patients undergoing IDET in the treatment of discogenic lower back pain.[a] Patients presenting with lower back pain with or without radiculopathy were evaluated in an outpatient setting. A detailed history was taken on all patients followed by physical examination. MRI scans were reviewed on all patients.

---

[a]University of Pittsburgh Institutional Review Board #0002107.

Study inclusion criteria were as follows:

- Patients experiencing primarily lower back pain with less than a 40% component of radicular pain;
- Discogenic back pain as evidenced by pain with tasks requiring axial loading of the spine and relief of pain with recumbency;
- Evidence of discogenic disease on MRI scan including disc dessication, high-intensity zones in the disc, disc rupture, loss of disc height, concordant discography;
- Failure of non-surgical therapies in the prior 6 months including physical therapy and non-steroidal anti-inflammatory medicines, and steroidal treatments.

Exclusion criteria included evidence of instability on MRI scan or plain radiographs (greater than 5 mm of luxation), active infection, or malignancy.

Quality of life and disability data collections were taken while the patients were in the office. The outcome instrument used was the AANS/CNS Joint Section Lumbar Disc Herniation Study Questionnaire which included the SF-36. The instruments were obtained 6 weeks, 3 months, 6 months, and 1 year after treatment.

Patients meeting all eligibility and exclusion criteria were considered to have discogenic lower back pain and were offered the option of undergoing interbody fusion or IDET. Patients who chose to undergo IDET were offered entry into the study.

IDET Technique

A standardized IDET technique was performed on all patients. The technique consisted of placing the patient on a Jackson table[b] in a prone position. Intravenous sedation was given and C-arm fluoroscopy was utilized to obtain antero-posterior and lateral images. The treatment level was localized and local anesthesia was applied to the skin 6 to 9 cms lateral to the midline. The 17 gauge needle and stylet was directed toward the center of the disc under fluoroscopic guidance and the annulus was punctured. The thermal-resistance catheter was inserted through the needle into the disc, coiling within the disc as it was deflected by the annular fibers *(Fig. 16.1)*. The tip of the catheter was directed to the posterior aspect of the disc in such a manner that the heating elements of the catheter remained located on the symptomatic side. The catheter temperature was increased along an electronically programmed protocol over 13 minutes to 90° C and allowed to remain at

---

[b]Orthopedic Systems Incorporated (OSI), Union City, California

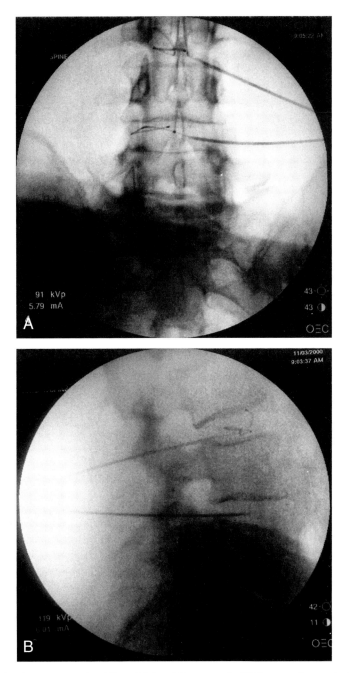

FIG. 16.1 Antero-posterior (A) and lateral fluoroscopic (B) images demonstrating the thermal catheter within the L_{3-4} and L_{4-5} disc spaces.

that temperature for 4 minutes. The catheter and needle was removed as a single unit.

Patients with multilevel disease underwent treatment at the other involved level(s) using the same protocol. New catheters and needles were used on each level. Patients with only back pain and no leg pain underwent treatment on the opposite disc side as well. The patients were discharged after 2 hours of observation. No standardized protocol was applied following the procedure and patients were instructed to resume their usual activities as tolerated.

Statistical Methods

The SF-36 summary scores were tabulated. Pre- and post-treatment mean scores were ascertained. A t test was used to determine whether the average difference between scores before and after treatment were statistically significant. Two-sided P values were reported.

RESULTS

A total of 23 (13 male) patients received IDET in the study period. The mean age of the study group was 39 years. Fifteen patients were on worker's compensation and eight patients had private insurance. Three patients had undergone prior microdiscectomy at the treated level.

Eight patients received pre-procedure MRI scanning as the sole diagnostic radiographic examination to evaluate the intervertebral disc. Nineteen patients underwent MRI scanning in combination with other studies including discography (14 patients). Thirteen patients were treated at a single level and 10 patients received treatment at multiple levels. Sixteen patients were treated on one side only and seven patients were treated on both sides of a single disc level. Six patients underwent treatment at L_{3}-$_4$, 15 patients at L_{4}-$_5$, and 12 patients were treated at the L_5-S_1 level.

Two patients experienced dural punctures during attempted needle placement. One patient had a prior microdiscectomy at the attempted IDET level. We were unable to slide the catheter into the L_5-S_1 disc space. The patient received an anterior lumbar interbody fusion (ALIF) 6 weeks later. Needle and catheter placement was successful in the other patient. No neurologic injury occurred in any patient.

Five patients went on to further surgery, including the patient with the failed catheter placement. All patients requiring further surgery were receiving worker's compensation. Surgical procedures included ALIF (three patients), and one patient received an intrathecal pump placement. Another patient was offered an ALIF but refused because of concerns about retrograde ejaculation. The patient ultimately underwent posterior lumbar interbody fusion.

Table 16.1
Three-month patient outcome (n=16).

• Levels Treated Compared to Outcomes:		
Number of Levels Treated	SF-36 Change (≥ 7 points)*	
Single Level (n=10)	5	(50%)
Multilevel (n=6)	0	(0%) P=.058

*Pre- and post-treatment comparisons at three months follow-up (n=16).

Three-month outcome data were available on 16 patients *(Table 16.1)*. Improvement in SF-36 score of seven or more points occurred in five of the ten patients treated at a single level and in no patients treated at multiple levels (P 0.058). No statistically significant difference was noted when symptom duration was compared to outcome *(Table 16.2)*. Pre- and post-treatment comparisons were most notable for improvement in the bodily pain score component of the SF-36 than in any other measure *(Table 16.3)*.

DISCUSSION

Thermal ablation of disc material has the potential to reduce pain by injuring free nerve endings, re-arranging collagen fibers, or in ways not completely understood. The IDET treatment method is designed to reduce pain due to discogenic pathology. This treatment is most correctly compared to surgical procedures designed for similar purposes.

Table 16.2
Three-month patient outcome with comparison of duration of symptoms (n=16).
Results: Outcomes

• Symptom Duration Compared to Outcomes:		
Duration of Symptoms	SF-36 Change (≥ 7 points)*	
Less than 12 mos. (n=10)	3	(30%)
Greater than 12 mos. (n=6)	2	(33%) P=.41

*Pre- and post-treatment comparisons at three months follow-up (n=16).

Table 16.3
Improvement in outcome scores (n=16). Results: Outcomes

• Data Pre- and Post-treatment Comparisons:			
Subsets	Baseline Mean Score	3 mos. Mean Score	% Change
(Higher score indicates improvement)			
SF-36 Physical functioning subscale	31	47	52%
SF-36 Bodily pain subscale	5	25	400%
SF-36 Role Functioning-physical	27	46	71%
(Lower score indicated improvement)			
Pain/Disability (Oswestry)	34	26	24%
Neurogenic Symptoms	15	13	13%

The surgical treatments include anterior, lateral, and posterior surgical approaches to the spine for interbody and posterior fusion. These techniques are highly invasive and require significant periods of rehabilitation. Also, the long-term outcome for patients undergoing fusion is fair (4).

The driving factor for percutaneous treatment of disc disorders is the minimally invasive nature of the techniques. Unfortunately, no percutaneous intradiscal technique has withstood the test of time and received general acceptance as an alternative to surgical techniques.

The purpose of this study was to examine the outcome of a group of patients with lower back pain due to discogenic pathologies such as disc degeneration, annular tears, and end-plate changes due to disc rupture treated with IDET. Previous studies have had similar patient inclusion criteria to those which we selected, such as disabling back pain for more than 6 months, normal neurologic examination and positive findings on provocative discography (5). We attempted to reduce the possibility of selection bias in this study by including only those patients willing to undergo surgical procedures such as ALIF or PLIF.

The greatest improvement in treatment scores was in the bodily pain scores. This component of the SF-36 is a valid scale for physical morbidity and suggests that patients treated with IDET do note reduced physical limitations following the treatment (6). Duration of symptoms was not a statistically significant finding. This was somewhat surprising as one would empirically expect that patients with shorter duration of symptoms fare better than those with long-standing problems.

The results of this study suggest that IDET may be most effective in treating patients with single level disc disease. This is not surprising as patients being treated for single level disc disease may be expected to fare better than those with multi-level disease. IDET may provide pain relief to patients with back pain due to discogenic disease. This procedure may provide an alternative to interbody fusion in a select group of patients and is deserving of long-term study (7).

CONCLUSIONS

IDET is a safe procedure. The technique is performed in an outpatient setting. IDET offers best results in patients with lower back pain of single-level discogenic origin.

REFERENCES

1. Derby R, Eek B, Chen Y, O'Neill C, Ryan D: Intradiscal electrothermal annuloplasty (IDET): A novel approach for treating chronic discogenic back pain. **Neuromodulation** 3:82–88, 2000.
2. Ware JE: SF-36 health survey update. **Spine** 25:3130–3139, 2001.

3. O'Neill C, Derby R, Kenderes L: Precision injection techniques for diagnosis and treatment of lumbar disc disease. **Semin Spine Surg** 11:104–118, 1999.

4. Turner JA, Ersek M, Herron L, Haselkorn J, Kent D, Ciol MA, Deyo R: Patient outcomes after lumbar spinal fusions. **JAMA** 268: 907–911, 1992.

5. Derby R, Eek B, Chen Y, O'Neill C, Ryan D: Intradiscal electrothermal annuloplasty (IDET): A novel approach for treating chronic discogenic back pain. **Neuromodulation** 3:82–88, 2000.

6. Ware JE: SF-36 health survey update. **Spine** 25:3130–3139, 2001.

7. O'Neill C, Derby R, Kenderes L: Precision injection techniques for diagnosis and treatment of lumbar disc disease. **Sem Spine Surg** 11:104–118, 1999.

CHAPTER

17

Acute Interventions in Spinal Cord Injury: What Do We Know, What Should We Do?

MICHAEL G. FEHLINGS MD, PH.D., F.R.C.S.(C),
AND LALI H.S. SEKHON M.B., B.S., PH.D., F.R.A.C.S.

INTRODUCTION

Spinal cord injury (SCI) occurs through various countries throughout the world with an annual incidence of 15 to 40 cases per million, with the causes of these injuries ranging from motor-vehicle accidents and community violence to recreational activities and workplace-related injuries. For a long time, the cornerstone of management of this devastating injury was skilled nursing care. Despite much work having been done, the only treatment to date known to ameliorate neurological dysfunction that occurs at or below the level of neurological injury has been intravenous methylprednisolone therapy. Despite intensive study, the precise roles of pharmacotherapy and surgery, and its timing, remain in dispute. This study examines the current state of play in terms of management of spinal cord injury, in particular the role of pharmacotherapy and surgical therapy and the controversies that surround each. A discussion of radiological studies in the evaluation of spinal cord injury, and an initial review of the processes associated with SCI are also addressed.

THE CONCEPTS OF PRIMARY AND SECONDARY MECHANISM

It is now generally accepted that acute SCI is a two-step process involving primary and secondary mechanisms. The primary mechanism involves the initial mechanical injury due to local deformation and energy transformation while the secondary mechanisms encompass a cascade of biochemical and cellular processes which are initiated by the primary process and which may cause ongoing cellular damage and even cell death (see *Table 17.1* and *Fig. 17.1*) (14). This concept of a secondary mechanism to acute SCI was first postulated by Allen in 1911 where he found that there was an improvement in neurological function after the removal of post-traumatic hematomyelia in dogs who underwent experimental acute SCI (5). Three years later, Allen specu-

Table 17.1

Primary and secondary mechanisms of acute spinal cord injury

Primary injury mechanism
  Acute compression
  Impact
  Missile
  Distraction
  Laceration
  Shear
Secondary injury mechanisms
  Systemic Effects
    Heart rate-brief increase, then prolonged bradycardia
    Blood pressure-brief hypertension, then prolonged hypotension
    Decreased
    Peripheral resistance
    Decreased cardiac output
    Increased catecholamines, then decreased
    Hypoxia
    Hyperthermia
    Injudicious movement of the unstable spine leading to worsening compression
  Local vascular changes
    Loss of autoregulation
    Systemic hypotension (neurogenic shock)
    Hemorrhage (especially gray matter)
    Loss of microcirculation
    Reduction in blood flow
      Vasospasm
      Thrombosis
  Electrolyte changes
    Increased intracellular calcium
    Increased intracellular sodium
    Increased sodium permeability
    Increased intracellular potassium
  Biochemical changes
    Neurotransmitter accumulation
      Catecholamines (*e.g.* norepinephrine, dopamine)
      Excitotoxic amino acids (*e.g.* glutamate)
    Arachidonic acid release
    Free-radical production
    Eicosanoid production
      Prostaglandins
    Lipid peroxidation
    Endogenous opioids
    Cytokines
  Edema
  Loss of energy metabolism
    Decreased adenosine triphosphate production
  Apoptosis
  Loss of neurotrophic factor support

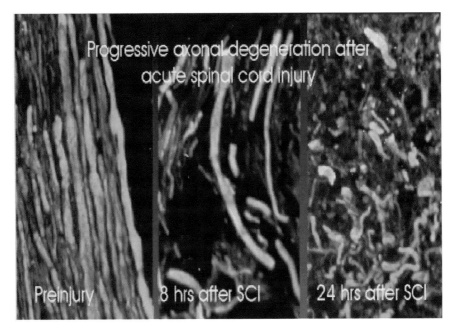

FIG. 17.1 Progressive axonal degeneration after SCI. Immunohistochemical flourescein labeling of spinal cord sections with anti-NF200 antibody. The normal spinal cord (*left*) shows progression 8 hours after injury (middle) with a substantial reduction in immunoreactivity and the presence of a few swollen axons. At 24 hours (*right*), the immunoreactivity is further reduced, with decreased axonal density and marked disorganization present.

lated that there was a putative "biochemical factor" that was present in the hemorrhagic necrosis material and which may be instigating ongoing damage (6). This concept of primary and secondary mechanisms and their duality in acute SCI has since been also embraced in the understanding of the pathophysiology of subarachnoid hemorrhage, cerebral and spinal ischemia, and head trauma.

Primary Mechanisms of Spinal Cord Injury

Primary SCI is most commonly a combination of the initial impact as well as subsequent persisting compression. This will typically occur with fracture dislocation, burst fractures, missile injuries, and acutely ruptured discs. Clinical scenarios where impact alone occurs without ongoing compression may include severe ligamentous injuries where the spinal column dislocates and then spontaneously reduces. Similarly, spinal cord laceration from sharp bone fragments or missile injuries can produce a mixture of spinal cord laceration, contusion and compression, or concussion (7).

Secondary Mechanisms of Spinal Cord Injury

The various theories of secondary mechanisms of SCI have undergone a process of maturation in the past 3 decades. In the 1970s, the free radical hypothesis, as advocated by Demopoulos et al. (8) was thought to be crucial to the injury process. Ten years later, focus shifted onto the role of calcium, opiate receptors, and lipid peroxidation. As we enter the new millennium, modern research is implicating apoptosis, intracellular protein synthesis inhibition, and glutaminergic mechanisms, among a myriad of pathophysiological pathways that mediate secondary injury mechanisms. There is considerable evidence that the primary mechanical injury initiates a cascade of secondary injury mechanisms that includes: (1) vascular changes including reduction in blood flow, loss of autoregulation, neurogenic shock, hemorrhage, loss of microcirculation, vasospasm, and thrombosis (see (9, 10) for reviews); (2) electrolyte shifts including increased intracellular calcium, increased extracellular potassium, and increased sodium permeability (11, 12); (3) neurotransmitter accumulation such as serotonin or catecholamines (13) and extracellular glutamate (14), the latter producing excitotoxicity (15); (4) arachidonic acid release, free radical production especially oxygen free radicals (16) eicosanoid production, especially prostaglandins and lipid peroxidation (17, 18); (5) endogenous opioids (19, 20); (6) edema formation (21); (7) inflammation; and (8) loss of energy metabolism especially decreased ATP production (22). These theories of secondary injury have been the subject of several recent reviews (2, 4, 23–25). The complexity and inter-relationship of these secondary mechanisms is now being embraced.

THE ROLE OF MRI AND CT IMAGING

Plain x-rays of the cervical spine in trauma have an important role. However, single cross-table lateral view has a sensitivity of less than 85% (26). Once this single x-ray is replaced by three standard views (lateral, anteroposterior, open-mouth odontoid view), the sensitivity for fractures increases to 90 to 100% (27). It is crucial that the relationship of C7 to T1 is identified, as, in some series, 18% of cervical fractures occur at C7 (28). Dynamic plain x-rays are also mandatory if ligamentous instability cannot be excluded on clinical grounds. CT scanning plays an important role in the assessment of spinal cord injury. In addition to allowing multiplanar views of fractures, CT scanning allows for complete assessment of the C1/C2 region. It can be used in critically unwell patients, and aids preoperative planning. CT scanning can also give some idea as to the status of the intervertebral disk at the site of injury. MRI scanning, the newest modality in the armamentarium available to assess spinal cord injury serves several important purposes. In neurologically intact patients, in whom dynamic flexion/extension views cannot be attained to exclude ligamentous injury, T2-weighted fast spin echo sequences incorporating frequency-selective fat saturation or with a short tau inversion recovery sequence have shown areas of ligamentous disruption (29). An evidence-based review of the radiological methods for assessing spinal canal compromise and cord compression in patients with cervical SCI is reported by Rao and Fehlings (30). In this review, 37 studies are reviewed, with the consensus that there are few quantitative, reliable radiologic outcome measures for assessing spinal canal compromise of cord compression in patients with acute cervical SCI. The authors put forth a quantitative outcome measure to assess spinal canal size/degree of cord compression. The also suggest that MRI is essential to the quantification of canal compromise.

HEMODYNAMIC RESUSCITATION

Early immobilization of the injured spine, rapid triage to specialty spinal surgical units, and the adequate resuscitation are all important measures in the management of SCI. Inferences made from scenarios seen in cerebral ischemia and after head trauma would suggest similar caveats regarding optimal hemodynamic resuscitation would apply to SCI, yet such viewpoints have not been readily embraced. Vale et al. (31) report a prospective study in 77 patients with cervicothoracic spinal cord injures, who were managed aggressively in terms of fluid volume and blood pressure parameters. A mean arterial pressure of 85 mmHg was maintained in this study for a minimum of 7 days. Review at 12 months suggests an improved outcome and these authors suggest that the secondary insults of spinal cord ischemia and aberrant autoregulation can be counteracted by aggressive hemodynamic resuscitation. The ideal target mean arterial blood pressure, as well as other hemodynamic parameters is still to be elucidated, and clearly this area is worthy of more detailed and systematic analysis.

PHARMACOLOGICAL THERAPY

Methylprednisolone

Recent studies of pharmacotherapy, such as the use of methylprednisolone, as recommended on the basis of the National Acute Spinal Cord Injury Studies (NASCIS-2 (32, 33) and NASCIS-3 (34, 35), have shown improved recovery in patients with SCI. Unfortunately, the improved neurological recovery observed to date has been modest with only slight improvement in the functional status.

Methylprednisolone has a number of neuroprotective effects, and the first National Acute Spinal Cord Injury Study (NASCIS-1) (36, 37) in 1984 compared the efficacy of 1000 mg/day with 100 mg/day of intravenous methylprednisolone semisuccinate (MPSS) administered for 10 days in patients with an acute SCI, within 48 hours of trauma. No placebo group was included. The results showed no difference between the two treatment arms, and because of this study, the use of steroids for acute SCI fell out of favor. NASCIS-2, (32, 33) in 1990, addressed the shortcomings of NASCIS-1. It was found that in patients treated within 8 hours of injury, MPSS therapy led to improved motor and sensory recovery at 6 weeks, 6 months, and 1 year, compared to naloxone or placebo. This group did, however, have a higher wound infection rate (7.1%) than the other groups. Despite criticisms, this landmark study established the role neuroprotective role of steroids in acute SCI.

NASCIS-3, in 1997, assessed the hypotheses that (1) ultra-early (within 3 hours) MPSS therapy was more effective than standard therapy; (2) prolonged infusion of MPSS for 48 hours improved functional recovery, and (3) that trilizad, a potent 21-aminosteroid with potent effects on lipid peroxidation and few corticosteroid effects, would be more effective than MPSS therapy (34, 35). Patients received either a 24-hour infusion of MPSS (5.4 mg/kg/hour), a 48-hour infusion of MPSS (5.4 mg/kg/hour), or tirilizad mesylate (2.5 mg/kg every 6 hours for 48 hours). The results showed that those patients who received drug treatment within 3 hours after SCI had similar neurological recovery in all treatment arms. In contrast, patients who received treatment within 3 to 8 hours, showed improved motor and functional independence. Tirilizad provided similar effects in terms of functional outcome to 24-hour infusion of MPSS. The 48-hour MPSS regimen was however associated with a higher rate of severe sepsis (2.6%) and pneumonia (5.8%), which, more recently, has been more recently suggested to occur with a greater frequency in those over 60 years of age (38). On the basis of NASCIS-2 and NASCIS-3 data, despite some contradictory studies (39), the current recommendation is for all adult patients with acute, nonpenetrating SCI to receive MPSS within 8 hours, and preferably within 3 hours, of trauma. Those receiving the initial bolus of MPSS between 3 and 8 hours, should receive a 48-hour infusion of MPSS rather than the standard 24-hour regimen. MPSS is not indicated in patients who present at greater than 8 hours after SCI.

GM-1

The gangliosides are a group of sialic acid-containing glycosphingolipids found in high concentration in the outer cell membranes of central nervous system (CNS) tissue. Monosialotetrahexosylganglio-side (GM-1) ganglioside, has been shown to have some neuroprotec-tive effect in animal models of SCI (40). GM-1 ganglioside works by an unknown mechanism of action, but it may exert a neurotrophic ef-fect. GM-1 ganglioside inhibits the neuroprotective effect of MPSS, probably via its effect on lipocortin and typically infusion of GM-1 ganglioside is delayed until MPSS infusion is completed. Early clinical studies are encouraging with suggestions that some improvement in functional outcome after SCI can be achieved (41). A large randomized trial evaluating GM-1 ganglioside has recently been completed by Geisler and colleagues. The results of this trail, which to date has not been published, suggest that GM-1 may promote earlier recovery of function.

SURGICAL THERAPY

Despite the widespread use of surgery in patients with acute SCI in North America, the role of this intervention in improving neurological re-covery remains controversial because of the lack of well-designed and ex-ecuted randomized controlled trials. There is strong experimental evi-dence from animal models that decompression of the spinal cord improves recovery after SCI (42–47). However, it is difficult to determine a time window for the effective application of decompression in the clinical set-ting from these animal models. To date, the clinical studies that have ex-amined the role of surgical decompression in SCI, are limited to Class II and III evidence except for one study of the timing of decompression.

The Role of Conservative Management

In order to evaluate the possible role of surgery in the management of SCI, it is important to examine the results of conservative, nonoper-ative treatment for comparative purposes. This approach has been ad-vocated by those who adhere to the tenets of Sir Ludwig Guttman, founder of the Stoke-Mandeville Hospital in England. Guttman used postural techniques combined with bedrest to achieve reduction and spontaneous fusion of the spine. Operative approaches were rarely used because of a higher incidence of neurological complications and impaired recovery with laminectomy (48–52) For example, Frankel et al reported on a cohort of 612 patients with "closed spinal injuries" who were treated by these techniques. Only four of these patients developed delayed instability and required operative fusion. However, a detailed description of the fractures and the criteria for determining spinal in-stability or failure of nonoperative management were not stated. Im-portantly, 29% of Frankel A patients (with complete motor and sensory

paralysis below the level of the injury) improved at least one grade during the course of their hospital stay.

The spontaneous improvement in neurological status with conservative therapy has been replicated in several subsequent studies (22, 50,
53–56). Accordingly, the comparative beneficial results of surgical
treatment need to weighed against the limited spontaneous recovery
which occurs after SCI. Indeed some authors have reported that neither spinal surgery nor anatomical realignment of the spinal column
improved neurological outcome in patients with acute SCI with the possible exception of bilateral locked facets (57, 58). To date, the studies of
nonoperative management are limited to non-controlled, retrospective
analyses of clinical databases and accordingly provide Class III evidence. Furthermore, it is now well recognized that laminectomy as the
sole surgical technique is contraindicated in most cases of acute SCI
because it usually fails to produce adequate decompression of the cord
and often causes spinal instability which itself can lead to neurological
deterioration.

The Role and Timing of Decompressive Surgery

While meticulous, conservative care remains the cornerstone of SCI
management, modern surgical techniques have evolved considerably
since the era of Guttman. Furthermore, there are major limitations to
using an exclusive policy of non-operative treatment of SCI. Up to 10%
of patients with incomplete cervical SCI who undergo an exclusively
conservative management protocol may neurologically deteriorate (59).
Consequently, the role of decompressive surgical management has been
explored more recently. Most studies, with a few notable exceptions are
retrospective, case series with historical controls (Class III evidence).
From these studies, there is no clear consensus as to the appropriate
timing of surgical intervention, nor is there compelling evidence that
decompression influences the neurological outcome after SCI (59–64).
The benefits of early reduction of dislocations of the spine by either
open or closed techniques are difficult to evaluate in the absence of randomization (60, 65–69).

Most studies examining the role of decompressive surgery, with a few
notable exceptions are retrospective, case series with historical controls
(Class III evidence). From these studies, there is no clear consensus as
to the appropriate timing of surgical intervention, nor is there compelling evidence that decompression influences the neurological outcome after SCI. For example, Aebi et al (60), Wiberg and Hauge (61),
Hadley et al (62), and Wolf et al (63) advocated early reduction (4–10
hrs) and operative fixation of spinal fractures associated with cord in-

jury. Suggestive evidence is presented in these studies that early decompression in selected patients may enhance neurological recovery. However, these studies are uncontrolled and the beneficial effects need to be considered in the context of spontaneous recovery which can occur in nonoperatively managed patients with SCI (59, 64).

The benefits of early reduction of dislocations of the spine by either open or closed techniques are difficult to evaluate in the absence of randomization (60, 65–69). Accounts of impressive neurological recovery in some cervical cases decompressed early by traction must be considered anecdotal (66). Moreover, several studies have not found any neurological benefit to reduction (57, 58, 69) with the possible exception of patients with bilateral facet dislocation (48). Burke and Berryman (70) described 76 patients with unilateral or bilateral dislocations of the cervical spine who were treated with closed reduction under general anesthesia, often with manipulation. Fifty percent of the patients were admitted to their center within 8 hours. These authors concluded that early reduction improved the neurological recovery of patients with incomplete SCI.

Aebi et al (60) examined the records retrospectively of 100 patients with cervical spine injuries and attempted to relate neurological recovery to the timing of the reduction by closed manual traction or open surgical reduction. A manual or surgical reduction was performed within the first 6 hours after the accident in only 25% of the cases, and within the first 24 hours in 57%. Overall, 31% of the 100 patients recovered, and 75% of the recoveries were in patients reduced manually or surgically within the first 6 hours. Cotler's group (67, 71) studied the safety and effectiveness of early reduction, and performed a prospective study of early reduction by traction in 24 patients. They found no neurological deterioration in any of the patients, most of whom were successfully reduced within 24 hours of injury, although the exact interval in hours between injury and reduction was not given. All of the patients were awake during reduction, although a muscle relaxant was used in some patients. Mirza et al (65) retrospectively reviewed 30 patients who sustained cervical spine injuries and underwent surgical decompression and stabilization either before, or after, 72 hours. They suggested that the early group had neurological improvement immediately postoperatively, without an increase in complication rate.

In contrast to the aforementioned studies of early decompression, Larson and coworkers (72) advocated operating a week or more after SCI to allow medical and neurological stabilization of the injured patient. This remains the practice in many institutions, particularly in light of early reports suggesting an increased rate of medical complications with early surgery (< 5 days after SCI) (73). Interestingly, a number of authors have documented recovery of neurological function after delayed decompression of the spinal cord (months to years) after the injury (72, 74–79). Although these studies are retrospective in design, the improvement in neurological function with delayed decompression in patients with cervical or thoracolumbar SCI who have plateaued in their recovery is noteworthy and suggests that compression of the cord is an important contributing cause of neurological dysfunction. Review of the literature yields six prospective, controlled studies of surgical decompression in acute SCI (31, 60, 63, 69, 72, 80–95). In a prospective, non-randomized case control study of 208 patients with acute spinal cord or cauda equina injury, Tator and colleagues compared the results of surgery (56% of patients) with non-operative management (44%) (92). Operative management was associated with a lower overall mortality rate (6.1%) than non-operative treatment (15.2%) despite a higher rate of thromboembolic complications in the surgical group. Overall, there was no difference between operated and non-operated patients in length of stay or neurological recovery.

In an analysis of the NASCIS-2 database (Class II evidence), Duh et al (86) reported that patients undergoing acute surgery (<25 hours after injury) had improved (though not statistically significant) outcomes (mean neurological change score of 17.8) when compared with a control cohort treated non-operatively (mean change score of 13.2). Interestingly, results of surgery were similar in the early (<25 hrs) and delayed (>200 hrs) groups. In contrast, in a series of prospective studies Vale et al (31), Vaccaro et al (93),and Waters et al (69) could not document a beneficial effect of surgical decompression. It is noteworthy, however, that all patients underwent delayed operative management in the study by Waters et al (69). Moreover, although the study by Vaccaro et al (93) was a prospective, randomized trial, 20 of the 62 patients were lost to follow-up and "early" surgery was defined as being within 72 hours after SCI. In view of the large number of patients lost to follow-up, we have considered the study by Vaccaro et al (93) to provide class II evidence. More recently, Chen et al (80) evaluated 37 patients with cervical spondylosis and incomplete cord injury to assess surgical versus non-surgical outcomes. They suggested that 13 of 16 patients treated surgically improved within 2 days of surgery, and overall, showed faster recovery of neurological function, better long-term neurological outcome, shorter hospital stays and few complications than the nonoperative group. Because of the lack of randomization, this study was classified as Class II evidence.

The Effect of Surgery on the Complication Rate and the Length of Stay after Spinal Cord Injury

There has been controversy about whether surgery, especially early surgery, increases the rate of complications in patients with SCI. Many SCI patients with high cervical complete injuries or significant associated injuries to the limbs or viscera are critically ill due to either hemodynamic or respiratory difficulties. Early investigators such as Guttman (51, 52) and Bedbrook (96) and more recently Wilmot and Hall (55) and Marshall et al (73) have warned against surgery, especially early surgery in these critically ill patients. However, modern methods of respiratory and hemodynamic resuscitation (31, 97–99) have allowed these patients to undergo surgery with minimal differences in complication rates between operative and non-operative cases (55, 92). Indeed, Wilberger's recent study showed that those operated on in the first 24 hours had a lower rate of complications than those operated on at later times (55). In the study from our center referred to above, the only difference in morbidity between the surgical and non-surgical cases was a slight increase in the incidence of deep venous thrombosis in the operated group (92). The length of stay in the two groups did not differ (92). In the randomized trial of the timing of surgery by Vaccaro et al (93), there was no significant difference in length of acute postoperative intensive care stay or length of inpatient rehabilitation between the early and late groups. This was reiterated by Mirza et al (65) and Chen et al (80). Thus, with respect to complications, there is no compelling evidence that early surgery increases the rate of complications (55, 92, 93). The issue of early decompression is reviewed in detail by Fehlings and Tator (100) and the reader is referred to this publication for more in depth perusal. Clearly, to better define the role of surgery in the management of acute SCI, randomized, controlled prospective trials are required.

CONCLUSIONS

Although the ultimate aim of clinicians is complete restoration of both motor and sensory function after acute SCI, at the start of the new millennium, our main therapeutic interventions are still prevention and primary resuscitation, as well as the modest gains of pharmacotherapy with corticosteroids. The role of decompression and its timing are still being evaluated. Our understanding of primary and secondary SCI has improved, and limitation of the acute injury and amelioration of these early cascades is being intensively targeted, however recovery of the intermediate and chronic injury still remains elusive. It seems likely that combination therapies addressing multiple mechanisms will be required to have meaningful clinical impact. Definitive recommendations of therapies with significant impact on functional outcome are still a hope for the future. Our knowledge base at a cellular level is rapidly advancing, but as of yet, direct translations to clinical care are still for the most part, elusive.

REFERENCES

1. Sandler AN, Tator CH: Effect of acute spinal cord compression injury on regional spinal cord blood flow in primates. **J Neurosurg** 45: 660–676, 1976.
2. Collins WF: A review and update of experiment and clinical studies of spinal cord injury. **Paraplegia** 21: 204–219, 1983.
3. Hall ED: Pathophysiology of spinal cord injury. Current and future therapies. **Minerva Anestesiol** 55: 63–66, 1989.
4. Tator CH, Fehlings MG: Review of the secondary injury theory of acute spinal cord trauma with emphasis on vascular mechanisms. **J Neurosurg** 75: 15–26, 1991.
5. Allen AR: Surgery for experimental lesions of spinal cord equivalent to crush injury of fracture dislocation of spinal column. A preliminary report. **J Am Med Assoc** 57: 878–880, 1911.
6. Allen AR: Remarks on the histopathological changes in spinal cord due to impact. An experimental study. **J Nerv Ment Dis** 31: 141–147, 1914.
7. Tator CH: Update on the pathophysiology and pathology of acute spinal cord injury. **Brain Pathol** 5: 407–413, 1995.
8. Demopoulos HB, Flamm ES, Seligman ML, Mitamura JA, Ransohoff J: Membrane perturbations in central nervous system injury: theoretical basis for free radical damage and a review of the experimental data, in Popp AJ, et al (eds): *Neural Trauma.* New York, Raven Press, 1979, pp 63–78.
9. Harvey C, Rothschild BB, Asmann AJ, Stripling T: New estimates of traumatic SCI prevalence: a survey-based approach. **Paraplegia** 28: 537–544, 1990.
10. Tator CH: Review of experimental spinal cord injury with emphasis on the local and systemic circulatory effects. **Neurochirurgie** 37: 291–302, 1991.
11. Agrawal SK, Fehlings MG: Mechanisms of secondary injury to spinal cord axons in vitro: role of Na^+, $Na(^+)$-$K(^+)$-ATPase, the $Na(^+)$-H^+ exchanger, and the $Na(^+)$-Ca^{2+} exchanger. **J Neurosci** 16: 545–552, 1996.
12. Young W, Koreh I: Potassium and calcium changes in injured spinal cords. **Brain Res** 365: 42–53, 1986.
13. Osterholm JL, Mathews GJ: Altered norepinephrine metabolism, following experimental spinal cord injury. 2. Protection against traumatic spinal cord hemorrhagic necrosis by norepinephrine synthesis blockade with alpha methyl tyrosine. **J Neurosurg** 36: 395–401, 1972.
14. Agrawal SK, Fehlings MG: The role of NMDA and non-NMDA ionotropic glutamate receptors in traumatic spinal cord axonal injury. **J Neurosci** 17: 1055–1063, 1997.
15. Faden AI, Simon RP: A potential role for excitotoxins in the pathophysiology of spinal cord injury. **Ann Neurol** 23: 623–626, 1988.
16. Demopoulos HB, Flamm ES, Pietronigro DD, Seligman ML: The free radical pathology and the microcirculation in the major central nervous system disorders. **Acta Physiol Scand Suppl** 492: 91–119, 1980.
17. Hall ED, Yonkers PA, Horan KL, Braughler JM: Correlation between attenuation of posttraumatic spinal cord ischemia and preservation of tissue vitamin E by the 21-aminosteroid U74006F: evidence for an in vivo antioxidant mechanism. **J Neurotrauma** 6: 169–176, 1989.

18. Hung TK, Albin MS, Brown TD, Bunegin L, Albin R, Jannetta PJ: Biomechanical responses to open experimental spinal cord injury. **Surg Neurol** 4: 271–276, 1975.

19. Faden AI, Jacobs TP, Holaday JW: Comparison of early and late naloxone treatment in experimental spinal injury. **Neurology** 32: 677–681, 1982.

20. Faden AI, Jacobs TP, Smith MT: Evaluation of calcium channel antagonist nimodipine in experimental spinal cord ischemia. **J Neurosurg** 60: 796–799, 1984.

21. Wagner FC Jr, Stewart WB: Effect of trauma dose on spinal cord edema. **J Neurosurg** 54: 802–806, 1981.

22. Anderson DK, Means ED, Waters TR, Spears CJ: Spinal cord energy metabolism following compression trauma to the feline spinal cord. **J Neurosurg** 53: 375–380, 1980.

23. Anderson DK, Hall ED: Pathophysiology of spinal cord trauma. **Ann Emerg Med** 22: 987–992, 1993.

24. Eismont FJ, Clifford S, Goldberg M, Green B: Cervical sagittal spinal canal size in spine injury. **Spine** 9: 663–666, 1982.

25. Young WHPP, Kume-Kick J: Cellular, ionic and biomolecular mechanisms of the injury process, in Benzel EC, Tator CH (eds): Contemporary Management of Spinal Cord Injury. Park Ridge: American Assoc. **Neurolg. Surg.,** 1995, pp 27–42.

26. Blahd WH Jr, Iserson KV, Bjelland JC: Efficacy of the posttraumatic cross table lateral views of the cervical spine. **J Emerg Med** 2: 243–249, 1985.

27. McDonald RL, Schwartz ML, Mirich D, et al: Diagnosis of cervical spine injury in motor vehicle crash victims-how many xrays are enough? **J Trauma** 30: 392–397, 1990.

28. Miller MD, Gehweiler JA, Martinez S, Charlton OP, Daffner RH: Significant new observations on cervical spine trauma. **Am J Roentgenol** 130: 659–663, 1978.

29. Cohen WA, Blake MJ, Maravilla KR, et al: Identification of an MR imaging protocol to evaluate injury to spinal ligaments, intervertebral discs, and facets. (Abstract). Proceeds of the Annual Meeting of the American Society of Neuro Radiology.Nashville, Tenn., U.S.A.; May, 1994.

30. Rao SC, Fehlings MG: The optimal radiologic method for assessing spinal canal compromise and cord compression in patients with cervical spinal cord injury. Part I: An evidence-based analysis of the published literature. **Spine** 24: 598–604, 1999.

31. Vale FL, Burns J, Jackson AB, Hadley MN: Combined medical and surgical treatment after acute spinal cord injury: results of a prospective pilot study to assess the merits of aggressive medical resuscitation and blood pressure management. **J Neurosurg** 87: 239–246, 1997.

32. Bracken MB, Shepard MJ, Collins WF, et al: A randomized, controlled trial of methylprednisolone or naloxone in the treatment of acute spinal-cord injury. Results of the Second National Acute Spinal Cord Injury Study. **N Engl J Med** 322: 1405–1411, 1990.

33. Bracken MB, Shepard MJ, Collins WF Jr, et al: Methylprednisolone or naloxone treatment after acute spinal cord injury: 1-year follow-up data. Results of the Second National Acute Spinal Cord Injury Study. **J Neurosurg** 76: 23–31, 1992.

34. Bracken MB, Shepard MJ, Holford TR, et al: Administration of methylprednisolone for 24 or 48 hours or tirilazad mesylate for 48 hours in the treatment of acute spinal cord injury. Results of the Third National Acute Spinal Cord Injury Randomized Controlled Trial. National Acute Spinal Cord Injury Study. **JAMA** 277: 1597–1604, 1997.

35. Bracken MB, Shepard MJ, Holford TR, et al: Methylprednisolone or tirilazad mesylate administration after acute spinal cord injury: 1-year follow up. Results of the third National Acute Spinal Cord Injury randomized controlled trial. **J Neurosurg** 89: 699–706, 1998.

36. Bracken MB, Collins WF, Freeman DF, et al: Efficacy of methylprednisolone in acute spinal cord injury. **JAMA** 251: 45–52, 1984.
37. Bracken MB, Shepard MJ, Hellenbrand KG, et al: Methylprednisolone and neurological function 1 year after spinal cord injury. Results of the National Acute Spinal Cord Injury Study. **J Neurosurg** 63: 704–713, 1985.
38. Matsumoto T, Tamaki T, Kawakami M, et al: Complications of methylprednisolone sodium succinate in the treatment of acute spinal cord injury (Abstract). American Academy of Orthopaedic Surgeons, 2000 Annual Meeting, Orlando, FL, U.S.A., 2000;
39. Pointillard V, Petitjean ME, Wiart L, et al: Pharmacological therapy of spinal cord injury during the acute phase. **Spinal Cord** 38: 71–76, 2000.
40. Tator CH, Fehlings MG: Review of clinical trials of neuroprotection in acute spinal cord injury. **Neurosurgery Focus** 6(1): Article 8, 1999.
41. Geisler FH, Dorsey FC, Coleman WP: Past and current clinical studies with GM-1 ganglioside in acute spinal cord injury. **Ann Emerg Med** 22: 1041–1047, 1993.
42. Dolan EJ, Tator CH, Endrenyi L: The value of decompression for acute experimental spinal cord compression injury. **J Neurosurg** 53: 749–755, 1980.
43. Kobrine AI, Evans DE, Rizzoli HV: Experimental acute balloon compression of the spinal cord. Factors affecting disappearance and return of the spinal evoked response. **J Neurosurg** 51: 841–845, 1979.
44. Rivlin AS, Tator CH: Objective clinical assessment of motor function after experimental spinal cord injury in the rat. **J Neurosurg** 47: 577–581, 1977.
45. Nystrom B, Berglund JE: Spinal cord restitution following compression injuries in rats. **Acta Neurol Scand** 78: 467–472, 1988.
46. Tarlov IM: Spinal cord compression studies. III Time limits for recovery after gradual compression in dogs. **Arch Neurol Psychiat** 71: 588–597, 1954.
47. Dimar JR, Glassman SD, Raque GH, Zhang YP, Shields CB: The influence of spinal canal narrowing and timing of decompression on neurologic recovery after spinal cord contusion in a rat model. **Spine** 24: 1623–1633, 1999.
48. Bedbrook GM: Spinal injuries with tetraplegia and paraplegia. **J Bone Joint Surg [Br]** 61: 267–284, 1979.
49. Bedbrook GM, Sedgley GI: The management of spinal injuries—past and present. **Int Rehabil Med** 2: 45–61, 1980.
50. Comarr AE, Kaufman AA: A Survey of the neurological results of 858 spinal cord injuries. A comparison of patients treated with and without laminectomy. **J Neurosurg** 13: 95–106, 1956.
51. Guttman L: Initial treatment of traumatic paraplegia and tetraplegia, in Harris P (ed): *Spinal injuries symposium.* Edinburgh: Morrison & Gibb, Ltd., Royal College of Surgeons, 1963, pp 80–92.
52. Guttman L: *Spinal cord injuries. Comprehensive management and research,* 2nd ed., Blackwell Scientific Publications, Oxford, 1976.
53. Ditunno JF, Sipski ML, Posaniak EA, Saas WE, Herbison GJ: Wrist extensor recovery in traumatic quadriplegia. **Arch Phys Med Rehabil** 68: 287–290, 1987.
54. Tator CH, Duncan EG, Edmonds VE, Lapczak LI, Andrews DF: Neurological recovery, mortality and length of stay after acute spinal cord injury associated with changes in management. **Paraplegia** 33: 254–262, 1995.
55. Wilmot CB, Hall KM: Evaluation of the acute management of tetraplegia: conservative versus surgical treatment. **Paraplegia** 24: 148–153, 1986.
56. Wu L, Marino RJ, Herbison GJ, Ditunno JF Jr: Recovery of zero-grade muscles in the zone of partial preservation in motor complete quadriplegia. **Arch Phys Med Rehabil** 73: 40–43, 1992.

57. Dall DM: Injuries of the cervical spine. II. Does anatomical reduction of the bony injuries improve the prognosis for spinal cord recovery? **S Afr Med J** 46: 1083–1090, 1972.

58. Harris P, Karmi MZ, McClemont E, Matlhoko D, Paul KS: The prognosis of patients sustaining severe cervical spine injury (C2-C7 inclusive). **Paraplegia** 18: 324–330, 1980.

59. Katoh S, El Masry WS, Jaffray D, et al: Neurologic outcome in conservatively treated patients with incomplete closed traumatic cervical spinal cord injuries. **Spine** 21: 2345–2351, 1996.

60. Aebi M, Mohler J, Zach GA, Morscher E: Indication, surgical technique and results of 100 surgically-treated fractures and fracture-dislocation of the cervical spine. **Clin Orthop** 203: 244–257, 1986.

61. Wiberg J, Hauge HN: Neurological outcome after surgery for thoracic and lumbar spine injuries. **Acta Neurochir (Wien)** 91: 106–112, 1988.

62. Haldey M, Fitzpatrick B, Sonntag V, Browner C: Facet fracture-dislocation injuries of the cervical spine. **Neurosurgery** 30: 661–666, 1992.

63. Wolf A, Levi L, Mirvis S, et al: Operative management of bilateral facet dislocation. **J Neurosurg** 75: 883–890, 1991.

64. Frankel H, Hancock D, Hyslop G, et al: The value of postural reduction in the initial management of closed injuries of the spine with paraplegia and tetraplegia Part 1. **Paraplegia** 7: 179–182, 1969.

65. Mirza SK, Krengel WF 3rd, Chapman JR, et al: Early versus delayed surgery for acute cervical spinal cord injury. **Clin Orthop** (359) 104–114, Feb. 1999.

66. Brunette DD, Rockswold GL: Neurologic recovery following rapid spinal realignment for complete cervical spinal cord injury. **J Trauma** 27: 445–447, 1987.

67. Cotler JM, Herbison GJ, Nasuti JF, Ditunno JF Jr, An H, Wolff BE: Closed reduction of traumatic cervical spine dislocation using traction weights up to 140 pounds. **Spine** 18: 386–390, 1993.

68. Gillingham J. Letter to the editor. Early management of spinal cord trauma. **J Neurosurg** 44: 766–767, 1976.

69. Waters RL, Adkins RH, Yakura JS, Sie I: Effect of surgery on motor recovery following traumatic spinal cord injury. **Spinal Cord** 34: 188–192, 1996.

70. Burke DC, Berryman D: The place of closed manipulation in the management of flexion-rotation dislocations of the cervical spine. **J Bone Joint Surg [Br]** 53: 165–182, 1971.

71. Miller LS, Cotler HB, DeLucia FA, Cotler JM, Hume EL: Biomechanical analysis of cervical distraction. **Spine** 12: 831–837, 1987.

72. Larson SJ, Holst RA, Hemmy DC, Sances A Jr: Lateral extracavitary approach to traumatic lesions of the thoracic and lumbar spine. **J Neurosurg** 45: 628–637, 1976.

73. Marshall LF, Knowlton S, Garfin SR, et al: Deterioration following spinal cord injury. A multicenter study. **J Neurosurg** 66: 400–404, 1987.

74. Anderson PA, Bohlman HH: Anterior decompression and arthrodesis of the cervical spine: long-term motor improvement. Part II. Improvement in complete traumatic quadriplegia. **J Bone Joint Surg [Am]** 74: 683–692, 1992.

75. Bohlman HH, Anderson PA: Anterior decompression and arthrodesis of the cervical spine: long-term motor improvement. Part 1. Improvement in incomplete traumatic quadriparesis. **J Bone Joint Surg [Am]** 74: 671–682, 1992.

76. Bohlman HH, Freehafer A: Late anterior decompression of spinal cord injuries. **J Bone Joint Surg [Am]** 57: 1025, 1979.

77. Bohlman, H. H., Kirkpatrick, J. S., Delamarter, R. B., and Leventhal, M. Anterior de-

compression for late pain and paralysis after fractures of the thoracolumbar spine. **Clin Orthop** 24–29, 1994.

78. Brodkey JS, Miller CF Jr, Harmody RM: The syndrome of acute central cervical spinal cord injury revisited. **Surg Neurol** 14: 251–257, 1980.

79. Transfeldt EE, White D, Bradford DS, Roche B: Delayed anterior decompression in patients with spinal cord and cauda equina injuries of the thoracolumbar spine. **Spine**15: 953–957, 1990.

80. Chen TY, Dickman CA, Eleraky M, Sonntag VK: The role of decompression for acute incomplete cervical spinal cord injury in cervical spondylosis. **Spine** 23: 2398–2403, 1998.

81. Benzel EC, Larson SJ: Functional recovery after decompressive spine operation for cervical spine fractures. **Neurosurgery** 20: 742–746, 1987.

82. Benzel EC, Larson SJ: Recovery of nerve root function after complete quadriplegia from cervical spine fractures. **Neurosurgery** 19: 809–812, 1986.

83. Bohlman HH, Freehafer A, Dejak J: The results of treatment of acute injuries of the upper thoracic spine with paralysis. **J Bone Joint Surg [Am]** 67: 360–369, 1985.

84. Botel U, Glaser E, Niedeggen A: The surgical treatment of acute spinal paralysed patients. **Spinal Cord** 35: 420–428, 1997.

85. Donovan WH, Kopaniky D, Stolzmann E, Carter RE: The neurological and skeletal outcome in patients with closed cervical spinal cord injury. **J Neurosurg** 66: 690–694, 1987.

86. Duh MS, Shepard MJ, Wilberger JE, Bracken MB: The effectiveness of surgery on the treatment of acute spinal cord injury and its relation to pharmacological treatment. **Neurosurgery** 35: 240–248, 1994.

87. Krengel WF 3d, Anderson PA, Henley MB: Early stabilization and decompression for incomplete paraplegia due to a thoracic-level spinal cord injury. **Spine** 18: 2080–2087, 1993.

88. Levi L, Wolf A, Rigamonti D, Ragheb J, Mirvis S, Robinson WL: Anterior decompression in cervical spine trauma: does the timing of surgery affect the outcome? **Neurosurgery** 29: 216–222, 1991.

89. Maynard FM, Reynolds GG, Fountain S, Wilmot C, Hamilton R: Neurological prognosis after traumatic quadriplegia. Three-year experience of California Regional Spinal Cord Injury Care System. **J Neurosurg** 50: 611–616, 1979.

90. Murphy KP, Opitz JL, Cabanela ME, Ebersold MJ: Cervical fractures and spinal cord injury: outcome of surgical and nonsurgical management. **Mayo Clin Proc** 65: 949–959, 1990.

91. Pointillart V, Petitjean ME, Wart L, Vital JM, Lassie P, Thicoipe M, Dabadie P: Pharmacological therapy of spinal cord injury during the acute phase: **Spinal Cord** 2000; 38(2):71-6.

92. Tator CH, Duncan EG, Edmonds VE, Lapczak LI, Andrews DF: Comparison of surgical and conservative management in 208 patients with acute spinal cord injury. **Can Neurol Sci** 14: 60–69, 1987.

93. Vaccaro AR, Daugherty RJ, Sheehan TP, et al: Neurologic outcome of early versus late surgery for cervical spinal cord injury. **Spine** 22: 2609–2613, 1997.

94. Wagner FC Jr, Chehrazi B: Early decompression and neurological outcome in acute cervical spinal cord injuries. **J Neurosurg** 56: 699–705, 1982.

95. Weinshel SS, Maiman DJ, Baek P, Scales L: Neurologic recovery in quadriplegia following operative treatment. **J Spinal Disord** 3: 244–249, 1990.

96. Bedbrook GM, Sakae T: A review of cervical spine injuries with neurological dysfunction. **Paraplegia** 20: 321–333, 1980.

97. Kiss ZHT: Neurogenic shock, in Geller ER (ed): Shock and Resuscitation. New York, McGraw-Hill, 1993, pp 421–440.
98. Levi L, Wolf A, Belzberg H: Hemodynamic parameters in patients with acute cervical cord trauma: description, intervention, and prediction of outcome. **Neurosurgery** 33: 1007–1016; discussion 1016, 1993.
99. Rosner MJ, Elias Z,Coley I: New principles of resuscitation for brain and spinal injury. **NC Med J** 45: 701–708, 1984.
100. Fehlings MG, Tator CH: An evidence-based review of decompressive surgery in acute spinal cord injury: rationale, indications, and timing based on experimental and clinical studies. **J Neurosurg** 91: 1–11, 1999.

CHAPTER

18

Surgical Management of Patients with Sports-Related Spinal Injuries

JULIAN E. BAILES, JR., M.D., AND CRAIG A. VAN DER VEER, M.D.

The diagnosis and management of spinal injury in the athlete is complicated by several issues beyond that seen in other patients. Chief among these is the desire in many athletes to return to active participation in contact sports. Although the catastrophic spinal cord injury with or without vertebral column involvement is important to understand and consider in the clinical setting, it is fortunately uncommon. More often, we are attending to young athletes with muscular, ligamentous, and intervertebral disc injuries, and occasionally patients with spinal stenosis in whom surgery poses a difficult dilemma. The least invasive and most effective surgical treatment is advantageous, allowing the resumption of athletic activities as soon as safely possible. There are no large series of prospective, randomized studies of spinal surgery in athletes to guide us in treatment recommendations. Rather, experience has been gathered and our philosophy remains dynamic in order to offer the athlete the best possible choice for resumption of activities without further spinal-related symptoms. This article will describe our experience with management of spinal injuries in athletes and will attempt to formulate recommendations for surgical treatment based on known predictors of best outcome and ability to return to athletic competition.

There are approximately 1,000 cases of sports-related spinal cord injury in the United States annually. This figure represents about 10% of the total number of spinal cord injuries seen from all causes, with motor vehicle crashes and falls as the usual etiology. In football participation, we believe that roughly 40 players annually sustain a fracture or fracture-dislocation of the spine, almost always located in the cervical region (1, 2). Annually about one-fourth of this number (10 players) suffer permanent spinal cord injury in football, which represents the largest risk in organized sports. The majority of sports-related spinal injuries, however, occur in unsupervised or recreational activities, such as diving, skiing, surfing, and "sand lot" games (3).

CLASSIFICATION OF INJURIES

The study of spinal injuries in athletes may be facilitated by dividing the injuries into two broad categories. The first consists of injuries that occur during participation in unsupervised, recreational sports such as diving, skiing, surfing, and other miscellaneous activities. Because of the limited degree of training, supervision, and obligated rules in such activities, it is difficult to achieve any improvement in injury patterns. There is also a limited ability to enforce safety guidelines and manufacturing standards for equipment in unsupervised, recreational activities. The second category of sports injuries involves those that occur in supervised, organized sports with higher incidence of bodily contact, velocity or torque forces, competition, and team participation. This type of injury is seen primarily in athletes participating in football, wrestling, ice hockey, and gymnastics. Among the recreational sports, diving accounts for the largest number of cervical spine injuries (4).

Athletic injuries to the cervical vertebral column and spinal cord have similar biomechanics but vary somewhat with the sport involved (1). Diving and water sports such as surfing may result in cervical fractures and/or spinal cord injury if the forehead of the participant strikes the bottom of the swimming pool, lake, or ocean. This usually results in a hyperflexion mechanism injury (4). Skiers and surfers also are susceptible to a variety of impact positions because they are propelled by falls or tidal action, which initiates different mechanisms of injury to the vertebral column. Among football players, neck injuries occur most commonly by axial loading, frequently combined with hyperflexion forces. Hyperextension, lateral flexion, compressive, and rotational mechanisms, however, may all be involved (5). Gymnasts sustain neck injuries as a result of missed maneuvers or landing askew during dismounts, which produces a mechanism of injury consistent with an uncontrolled fall. Wrestling participants sustain injuries that usually consist of hyperflexion and may simulate the biomechanics of a fall. They are also subjected to tremendous axial, rotational, and horizontal shearing forces that place great stress on the facet joints, intervertebral discs, and ligaments.

CERVICAL SPINE

Types of Injuries

The authors have designed and prospectively applied a classification system for the management of athletic spinal injuries (1) *(Table 18.1)*. This classification consists of three types of athletic cervical spine in-

TABLE 18.1
Classification of Athletic Spinal Injuries

Type 1—Permanent Spinal Cord Injury
  Complete paralysis
  Anterior cord syndrome
  Brown-Séquard syndrome
  Central cord syndrome
  Mixed incomplete syndrome
Type II—Transient Spinal Cord Injury
  Spinal concussion
  Neurapraxia
  Burning hands syndrome
Type III—Radiologic Abnormality Without Neurologic Deficit
  Congenital spinal stenosis
  Acquired spinal stenosis
  Herniated cervical disc
  Unstable fracture or fracture and dislocation
  Stable spinal fracture (lamina, spinous process, minor portion of vertebral body)
  Ligamentous injury (unstable)
  Spear tackler's spine

juries. Each type may cause difficulty in diagnosis and management, including the potential for being a career-ending malady.

TYPE I

Type I injuries are those that cause permanent spinal cord damage, which may vary from immediate and complete paralysis below the level of injury to various patterns of incomplete spinal cord injury syndromes *(Fig. 18.1)*. In patients with anterior spinal cord syndrome, there is preservation of only posterior column function. Patients with central cord injury syndrome experience selective weakness of the upper extremities with relative preservation of lower extremity function. We often see an overlap of spinal cord injury syndromes, however, rather than the classic anatomical presentation. A central cord/Brown-Sequard combination, which consists of motor/sensory deficit on different sides of the body with a relatively greater weakness in the upper extremities, often is found.

At times the athlete may have symptoms that are minor but are associated with radiologic evidence of spinal cord injury. Typically the latter is documented by a magnetic resonance imaging (MRI) scan or a myelogram suggestive of intrinsic spinal cord contusion, which is seen most clearly on intermediate MRI images as a high-intensity lesion within the spinal cord. Usually there is little argument that documen-

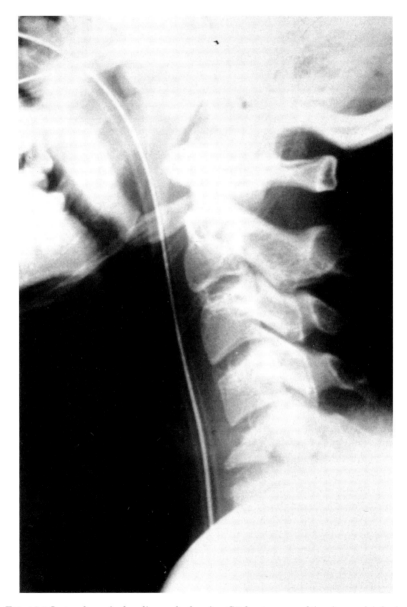

FIG. 18.1 Lateral cervical radiograph showing C5 fracture resulting in quadriplegia.

vice for stenosis; however, there are two major pitfalls in relying on such a ratio. Athletes have been shown to have significantly larger vertebral bodies than those of control individuals, which gives an abnormal ratio in at least one cervical level (18). Secondly, a bone measurement does not elucidate the relative size and accommodation of the cervical spinal cord. A "functional" MRI is relied on to clarify the spinal canal to cord relationship.

Additional Type III injuries are herniated intervertebral cervical discs, which are frequently difficult to manage in the athlete. The symptoms of a herniated intervertebral cervical disc are usually radiculopathy, cervical pain, and occasional myelopathic signs, regardless of whether the injury occurs spontaneously or traumatically *(Fig. 18.3)*. There is little controversy about treatment because most intractable herniated

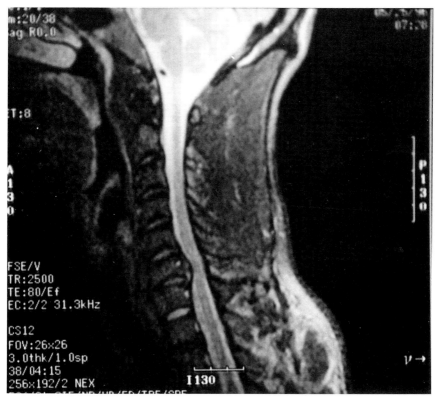

FIG. 18.3 Lateral MRI scan in a wrestler with a large C6-7 disc herniation, which was managed successfully conservatively.

cervical discs are surgically removed, either by an anterior approach if they are central or a posterior or anterior approach if they are lateral. There are no absolute guidelines that indicate whether a bone fusion should be performed. It has been suggested, however, that healed anterior interbody fusion results in a preservation of strength in the cervical spine when tested in flexion and extension (19). A posterior surgical approach may be advantageous by maintaining the integrity of the anterior and posterior longitudinal ligaments. In either case, it may be possible for the patient to return to contact sports after recuperation and demonstration of stability on flexion-extension radiographs. If the patient has congenital spinal fusion, some increase in movement at the motion segments above and below the fused level would be expected. Unless congenital spinal fusion is associated with more widespread abnormalities consistent with Klippel-Feil syndrome, a narrowed spinal canal, multilevel fusion, motion on flexion-extension radiographs, or recurrent neurological symptoms, this entity alone should not preclude engagement by the patient in contact sports.

Recently, Torg et al (8) described a group of athletes who are high risk for cervical quadriplegic injury with the clinical term "spear tackler's spine." Spear tackler's spine is thought to be a contraindication for participation in contact sports activities. Torg et al found that football players with (1) developmental cervical canal stenosis, (2) persistent straightening or reversal of the normal cervical spine lordotic curve, (3) evidence of preexisting, posttraumatic radiographic abnormalities of the cervical spine and, (4) documentation of having previously used spear tackling techniques are predisposed to injury from cervical spine axial energy forces. When a spine with a congenitally narrowed canal is straightened, impact at the top or crown of the helmet causes buckling of the neck because the movement of the head is momentarily stopped while the trunk continues to accelerate forward. Radiographic documentation of prior traumatic cervical spine injuries, such as healed cervical compression fractures, ligamentous instability, and intervertebral cervical disc bulge or herniation, indicates that athletes with these injuries are habitual users of spear tackling techniques. In their study, Torg et al (8) reported a series of 15 athletes whose playing techniques were examined because the athletes had cervical spine or brachial plexus symptoms; four of these athletes sustained permanent neurologic injuries. It was concluded that axial loading impact to the persistently straightened cervical spine, which occurs when athletes deliberately engage in frequent head impact, resulted in permanent spinal cord injury in these athletes. Occasionally, if no significant bone or ligamentous instability is present, the cervical lordosis is restored through physiotherapy. If the player can be coached against using head vertex impact, a return to competition may be allowed. Otherwise it is recommended that individuals with symptoms of tackler's spine be withheld from participation in contact sports.

Once the patient has undergone initial evaluation and cervical traction to reduce the fracture, a decision can be made concerning the optimal method of spinal stabilization. Bone healing is often satisfactory after 12 weeks of halo orthosis immobilization (14). Surgical treatment usually still is required for severe comminuted fractures of the vertebral body, fractures of posterior elements with extreme instability, Type II odontoid fractures, incomplete spinal cord injuries with canal or cord compromise, and in patients who have neurologic deterioration with loss of higher spinal cord levels of function.

In summary, the management of most spinal injuries in the athlete follows accepted principles as applied in the general population. The achievement of structural stability, restoration of mechanical and neurological function, and the pain-free state are the primary goals of surgical treatment of spinal surgery. Under most circumstances, once either a surgical stabilization or halo orthosis immobilization has been prescribed for the athlete with major bony and/or spinal cord injury, he or she is not allowed to return to contact sports participation. A notable exception may exist where a vertebral column injury has been internally stabilized in an athlete in a relatively non-contact sport or team position.

Surgical Decision Making for the Cervical Spine

If the athlete's symptoms are monoradicular and stability is assured by adequate testing, consideration of an anterior approach with fusion would be less advantageous to the athlete. A microinvasive approach with decompression of the anterior border of the foramen does not compromise flexibility, range of motion, sagittal balance, or the inherent strength of the facet, as long as greater than 50% of the facet surface is intact (20). If the radiographic pathology demonstrates neural compression located medial such that a posterior lateral approach is inadequate, an anterior fusion may be the best option. This raises other controversies including the use of autograft versus allograft and the use of instrumentation to augment the strength and rigidity of the fusion.

In the decision-making process, a simple construct called "the law of thirds" is utilized. The anterior border of the spinal canal is divided into thirds from lateral foramen to lateral foramen Abnormalities limited to a lateral one-third of the spinal canal should be approached posteriorly if the spine is stable. Disease processes of two adjacent thirds or of all three should be approached anteriorly. Two nonadjacent thirds pathology may be treated either anteriorly, or by a bilateral posterior lateral approach. A "tongue" of soft disc material which extends medially beyond this medial and middle third border, can usually be removed posteriorly. This makes the distinction between hard and soft disc of critical importance. The best test remains a thin cut contrast enhanced CT scan, as MRI can be misleading and is poorly predictive of the density of material anterior to the nerve root in the proximal foramen.

If an anterior fusion is planned, consideration of autograft vs. allograft and the use of instrumentation must be made. While both have been touted acceptable alternatives, the match of bone density of structural tri-cortical autograft with the vertebral body is clearly superior, the rate of uninstrumented fusion higher (21–24) and the rate of late pseudoarthrosis is lower. With microsurgical techniques applied to harvesting autologous bone graft, pain from an autograft is not a limiting factor in the patient's recovery. Allograft may be less desirable due to slower bone formation, delayed vascular ingrowth, delayed incorporation, and rejection (25).

A healed fusion is often considered in more anatomical terms of a natural segmentation defect (Klippel-Feil) as long as the spinal canal dimensions are adequate. Multiple level fusions are usually considered to disqualify the athlete from major contact sports participation at any level of competition.

When operating posteriorly, there are two serviceable and complimentary procedures to weigh: the microscopic laminotomy/foramenotomy (ML), and microendoscopic laminotomy/foramenotomy (MED). They are both based upon the original key hole laminotomy procedure for cervical spine pathology popularized by neurosurgeons in the 1940s until the Smith Robinson anterior approach predominated treatment (26). The addition of modern microscopic microinvasive techniques and today's ever shrinking endoscopic fiberoptic cameras provide unique advantages for each procedure. These procedures should not be viewed as alternative techniques, but as complimentary solutions to the myriad of individual variations in cervical spine pathology.

Lumbar Spine

In the lumbar spine, experience has shown that microdiscectomy, with a small, 2.0 to 2.5 cm midline incision, minimal bony resection of the hemilamina and gentle retraction of the paraspinal musculature, is capable of producing excellent results in the athletic population. A microscopic discectomy, with minimal disruption of the remaining nuclear disc material, once the offending fragment has been excised, seems to offer the best chance for a good outcome. A rapid rehabilitation program, facilitated by the superior physical conditioning of the athlete, will often allow the return to contact sports participation within 6 weeks postoperatively. Certainly, every effort can be made to avoid surgical intervention in the athlete with only a pain syndrome from a herniated lumbar disc, and the authors have been impressed with the ability of many muscular, well-conditioned, and motivated athletes to return to play following conservative rehabilitative measures for a herniated lumbar disc syndrome. Another common source of problems seen in the lumbar spine is facet joint or lumbar spondylolysis causing low back pain. Both of those entities are commonly seen in athletes with repetitive movements entailing lumbar hyperextension. For example, gymnasts, football lineman, and wrestlers often make lumbar extension techniques under weight loaded conditions. These areas respond well to injections of combination local anesthetic and steroid combination under fluoroscopic guidance, thus avoiding surgical therapy in most instances *(Fig. 18.4)*.

The surgical treatment of the athlete with a lumbar injury or degenerative condition represents a unique set of circumstances: the patient is generally youthful and healthy, has a short window of opportunity for surgical intervention, and tends to stress the surgical repair to extremes not seen in the general population. Because of these stresses, the athlete's needs for early stability of the vertebral column predominates even the durability of the surgical repair. Special consideration must be given to the age of the athlete, the rigors of the sport involved, the athlete/patient's chronology in their sport, and even the time of the year relative to the athlete's season of competition. Microinvasive spine surgery, whether cervical, thoracic, or lumbar involves the same principles: (1) less is more, or at least as much; (2) avoid fusion when possible, and (3) preserve the internal tendons of the paraspinous muscles, the long and short rotators.

Although both MED and ML are microinvasive, the approach of the MED is less so because no muscle fibers or internal tendons are cut, but compressed and stretched by a series of dilators. The MED is best suited to soft disc ruptures and proximal foraminal disease because of a smaller arc of dissection and a lack of depth perception. The smaller arc of dissection is limited by the length of the endoscopic tube, which requires a fixed focal length and therefore, a fixed tube length. The endoscopic technique has no depth of field because there is no stereoscopic image source, but a single 20 degree angled fiberoptic camera 1.5 mm in diameter. The ML, because of the additional advantage of depth of field and a greater arc of motion is better suited to work anteriorly to

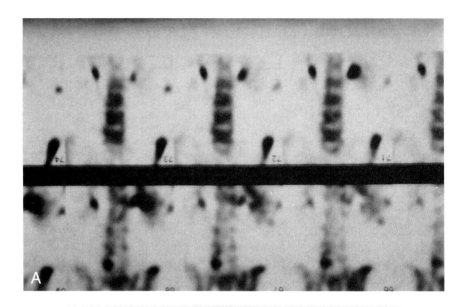

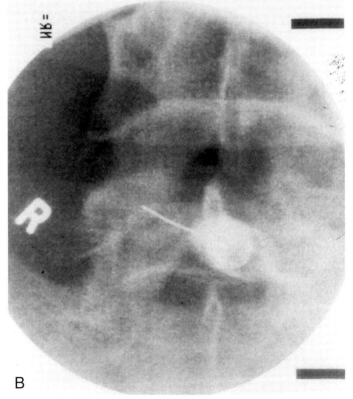

FIG. 18.4 (A) Radionuclide scan showing symptomatic pars defect in a football player, (B) treated by local injections and without surgery.

the nerve root for spondylitic disease and far lateral foraminal nerve root compression. Both are performed as outpatient procedures with a minimal complication rate and a high degree of success. The MED averages less than a 5-hour stay, and the microdiscectomy a 12 to 24 hour observation.

The Thoracic Spine

Thoracic disc rupture is especially difficult for the athlete, both from the standpoint of the loss of function and the potentially highly invasive surgery. Thoracic discs represent a small percentage of the disc ruptures, but because of the limited space in the spinal canal, a disproportionate risk of postoperative spinal cord dysfunction. A thoracotomy for lateral approach to the disc rupture may be a season or career ending treatment. Microinvasive procedures offer a low risk, short rehabilitation alternative. Thoracoscopic procedures offer the advantage of an intercostal trochar approach with three working channels of 4 to 8 mm and completely avoid an assault on either the erector spinae musculature or the accessory respiratory muscles like the serratus posterior inferior the injury of which hamper a rapid recovery. They offer a time course of recovery similar to the endoscopic cervical discectomy of 6 to 8 weeks and a return to noncontact conditioning in as little as 2 to 3 weeks.

Another minimally invasive option providing better steroscopic vision and tactile feedback is a microscopic transpedicular approach through a microscopic transpedicular laminotomy. With the patient in the supine position, preferably on an Andrews frame for rotational stability, the location of the disc level is confirmed with a spinal needle confirmed by x-ray. The path of the needle is marked with Indigo carmine vital dye as the needle is removed. Meticulous attention is needed to assume that the needle is perpendicular to the floor, especially with larger patients as the needle guides the trajectory to the affected level. A 2 cm incision is then made 2 cm off the midline and carried down to the thorocodorsal fascia. The facet can be easily palpated beneath the muscle, and working gently with small periosteal dissectors, the muscle fibers are split but not detached, exposing the interlaminar space. Retraction with a small thin Williams or Aesculap microlaminotomy retractor is adequate. A high power microscope and drill with a diamond 2 to 2 1/2 mm burr is then used to form a small laminotomy defect descending into the floor of the spinal canal via the superior medial pedicle margin. Access to the disc space is then easily acquired, and with the angle of vision provided, the surgeon can easily see to midline with a minimal or no retraction of the thecal sac. The thoracic disc ruptures in the youthful tend to be soft and cheese-like in their consistency, and easily removed. The degenerative disc can then be removed, more extensively or not, according to the surgeon's preference much like a lumbar discectomy with cervical downpushing currettes and micropituitary rongeurs. Great care must be exercised to limit the depth of disc removal to less than three-quarters the depth of the disc space, especially when working toward the left side of the disc space. The closure is simple, in layers, with subcutaneous sutures and medical adhesive, the musculature injected with long acting anesthetic and discharge in 12 hours after bowel and bladder function and ambulation are assumed.

Minimally invasive spinal procedures offer great promise for the return of not only high level athletes, but also for middle aged and beyond "weekend warrior." Their applications are highly applicable to the elderly as they offer a surgical solution with a minimum of recumbent recovery. The early mobilization not only prevents deconditioning and quadriceps atrophy, but should be very effective in prevention of deep venous thrombosis and pulmonary embolic phenomena.

The role of microscopic and minimally invasive spinal surgery is clearly expanding, driven by both physician expectations and patient/consumer demands. With the rapid expansion of technology, surgeons must continue to expand the limits of small incisions; continue to innovate with new versions of traditional procedures. The consensus of outcome analysis indicates that microsurgical techniques, combined with accurate preoperative radiographic diagnosis, offer the athlete the best chance of return to full competition and to remain functional and pain free.

REFERENCES

1. Bailes JE, Hadley MN, Quigley MR, Sonntag VKH, Cerullo LJ: Management of athletic injuries of the cervical spine and spinal cord. **Neurosurgery** 29:491–497, 1991.
2. Cantu RC, Mueller FO: Catastrophic spine injuries in football. **J Spinal Disord** 3:227–231, 1990.
3. Bailes JE, Maroon JC: Neurosurgical injuries in athletes, in Tindall GT, Cooper PR, Barrow DL, eds: *The practice of neurosurgery*. Baltimore, Williams & Wilkins, 1996, pp 1649–1672.
4. Bailes JE, Herman JM, Quigley MR, Cerullo LJ, Meyer PR Jr: Diving injuries of the cervical spine. **Surg Neurol** 4:155–158, 1990.
5. Bailes JE, Maroon JC: Management of cervical spine injuries in athletes. **Sports Med Clin North Am** 8:43–58, 1989.
6. Zwimpfer TJ, Bernstein M: Spinal cord concussion. **J Neurosurg** 72:894–900, 1990.
7. Torg JS, Pavlov H, Genuario SE, Sennett B, Wisneski RJ, Robie BH, Jahre C: Neurapraxia of the cervical spinal cord with transient quadriplegia. **J Bone Joint Surg [Am]** 68:1354–1370, 1986.

8. Torg JS, Sennett B, Pavlov H, Leventhal MR, Glasgon SG: Spear tackler's spine. **Am J Sports Med** 21:640–649, 1993.
9. Clancy WG, Brand RL, Bergfield JA: Upper trunk brachial plexus injuries in contact sports. **Am J Sports Med** 5:209–216, 1977.
10. Poindexter DP, Johnson EW: Football shoulder and neck injury: A study of the "stinger." **Arch Phys Med Rehabil** 65:601–602, 1984.
11. Maroon JC: "Burning hands" in football spinal cord injuries. **JAMA** 238:2049–2051, 1977.
12. Wilberger JE, Abla A, Maroon JC: Burning hands syndrome revisited. **Neurosurgery** 19:1038–1040, 1986.
13. Kline DG, Hudson AR: Acute injuries of peripheral nerves, in Youmans, ed: *Neurological surgery*. Philadelphia, WB Saunders Co., 1990, pp 2423–2510.
14. Sonntag VKH, Hadley MN: Nonoperative management of cervical spine injuries. **Clin Neurosurg** 34:630–649, 1988.
15. White AA, Johnson RM, Panjabi MM, Southwick WO: Biomechanical analysis of chemical stability in the cervical spine. **Clin Orthop Relat Res** 109:85–96, 1975.
16. Meyer PR Jr, Heim S: Surgical stabilization of the cervical spine, in Meyer PR Jr, ed: *Surgery of spine trauma*. New York, Churchill Livingstone, 1989, pp 397–523.
17. Torg JS. *Athletic injuries to head, neck and face*. St. Louis, MO, Mosby Year Book, 1991.
18. Herzog RJ, Wiens JJ, Dillingham MF, Sontag MJ: Normal cervical spine morphometry and cervical spinal stenosis in asymptomatic professional football players. **Spine** 16:5178–5186, 1991.
19. Johnson RM, Wolf JW Jr: Stability, in Bailey RW, ed: *The cervical spine*. Philadelphia: JB Lippincott Co., 1983, pp 35–53.
20. Zdeblick TA, Ducker TB: The use of freeze dried allograft bone for anterior cervical fusions. **Spine** 16:726–729, 1991.
21. Brown MD, Malinin TL, Davis PB: A roentgenographic evaluation of frozen allografts versus autograft in anterior cervical spine fusions. **Clinical Orthopaedics** 119:231–236, 1976.
22. Fernyhough JC, White JL, LaRocca H: Fusion rates in multilevel cervical spondylosis comparing allograft fibula with autograft fibula. **Spine** 16:726–729, 1991.
23. Kaufman HH, Jones E: The principles of bony spinal fusion. **Neurosurgery** 24:264–270, 1989.
24. Raynor RB, Pugh J, Shapiro I: Cervical facetectomy and its effect on spine strength. **J Neurosurg** 63:278, 1985.
25. Dickman CA, Maric Z: The biology of bone healing and techniques of spinal fusion. **Barrow Neurological Institute Quarterly** 10:2–12, 1994.
26. Robinson RA, Smith GW: Anterolateral cervical disc removal and fusion for cervical disc syndrome. **Bull Johns Hopkins Hospital** 96:223–224, 1955.

19

Decision Making in Degenerative Cervical Spine Surgery

NICHOLAS THEODORE, M.D., AND VOLKER K. H. SONNTAG, M.D.

To practicing neurological surgeons, nothing may seem more mundane than the evaluation and treatment of patients with degenerative cervical spine disease. Few areas of neurosurgical management, however, lead to more heated debates and dogmatic diatribe and are as controversial as the treatment of patients with cervical degenerative disease, whether for a herniated disk or multilevel disease causing spondylotic myelopathy. Anterior, posterior, and combined approaches all have their disciples. Part of the problem is the lack of a well-established natural history of disease progression or randomized controlled clinical trials to establish treatment standards for this heterogeneous disorder.

In this discussion, degenerative cervical disease and spondylosis are used as catch-all terms that encompass progressive senescent changes in the intervertebral disk, the vertebral body and uncovertebral joints anteriorly, and the zygapophyseal joints and ligamentum flavum posteriorly. All of these structures that form the spinal canal can contribute to the development of compressive syndromes. These changes, which can be assessed radiographically, can be expected to affect 25% to 50% of the population by the age of 50 years and 75% to 85% by the age of 65 years (1, 5, 9). An algorithmic approach to the treatment of this heterogeneous group of patients, which depends on the location of compression and the patient's neurological condition, is presented.

HISTORY OF CERVICAL SPINE SURGERY

After Virchow described a ruptured lumbar disk associated with trauma (51), the delay in establishing the intervertebral disk as a definable pathologic entity was considerable. In 1905 Walton and Paul performed a posterior exploration for a neoplasm, which, on autopsy, was most likely a herniated disk (52). In his 1925 book *Tumors of the Spinal Cord* (14). Charles Elsberg reported the first posterior diskectomy. Stookey is credited with first describing cervical stenosis and expounded upon Elsberg's experience in his report of a series of cervical extradural "chondromas" approached through a hemilaminectomy (49). Sentinel works by Semmes and Murphey(42) and by Spurling and Scoville (48) helped to define cervical disk herniations as the responsible agents for radiculopathy and to establish the posterior "key-hole" approach as the procedure of choice for removing a lateral herniated disk. In 1952 Brain and Northfield recognized that myelopathy and radiculopathy were distinct clinical disorders directly attributable to cervical spondylosis (6).

With Robinson's and Smith's 1955 report, anterior cervical disk removal and fusion became viable options for the treatment of cervical disk herniations (34). In 1960 Hirsch described his experience with anterior cervical diskectomy without fusion (24). Other major improvements in anterior cervical surgery included the addition of the surgical microscope (20, 33) and the use of cervical plates for stabilization (32, 40).

Although posterior cervical surgery was the first surgical option for the treatment of degenerative diseases, the principles of posterior fusion after trauma were not formulated until 1942.(35) Various wiring techniques and, ultimately, lateral mass fusion techniques, as described by Roy-Camille and coworkers (37) and Magerl (29) followed. Another lasting addition to the posterior approach for degenerative cervical disorders was laminoplasty as first described by Hattori in 1973 (21).

In addition to refinements in surgical techniques, innovations in imaging have been extremely helpful in the treatment of degenerative disorders of the cervical spine. Both computed tomography (CT, with and without myelography) and magnetic resonance (MR) imaging have greatly enhanced the treatment of degenerative spinal disorders.

DIAGNOSIS

In broad terms, patients with symptomatic cervical spondylosis can be placed into one of three categories: (1) those with neck pain only but no clinical or symptomatic evidence of radiculopathy or myelopathy, (2) those with radiculopathic signs and symptoms (at one or multiple levels) with or without neck pain, and (3) those with clinical or symptomatic evidence of myelopathy with or without concomitant radiculopathy and neck pain. Assigning patients to one of these three groups allows a rational approach to the treatment of most patients with symptomatic cervical spondylosis.

Patients with only neck pain are probably least frequently seen by practicing neurological surgeons. Abnormal findings on examination can include decreased mobility, tenderness, and muscle spasms. Neck pain can be the harbinger of multiple disease processes, and cervical spondylosis is only one on a long list of possibilities. Therefore, patients who seek treatment for neck pain alone should undergo a thorough history and physical examination to rule out subtle signs and symptoms of radiculopathy or myelopathy. Plain and dynamic radiographs of the cervical spine should be obtained in all cases to rule out degenerative instability, which can be an indication for fusion across the unstable motion segment. If patients have severe or long-standing pain, MR imaging of the cervical spine is needed to rule out other disease processes and to assess the degree of spondylosis.

Patients in the second group are the most commonly encountered instance of degenerative cervical spine disease. They can exhibit any or all of the following symptoms: neck and arm pain, paresthesias, or weakness. Pain can also radiate to the scapula or chest. Physical examination reveals weakness, sensory loss, and hyporeflexia. Specific neurological tests such as the Spurling's maneuver can be used to elicit radicular symptoms and to confirm the diagnosis. Evaluation of these patients consists of plain cervical radiography and MR imaging of the cervical spine. Patients with foraminal stenosis sometimes require an additional imaging study to confirm a suspected source of radiculopathy that may not be evident on MR imaging. If so, myelography with postmyelography CT is the study of choice. Studies of nerve conduction velocities can help rule out concomitant peripheral nerve entrapment syndromes.

Unless there is evidence of motor dysfunction, patients with acute radiculopathy should all undergo conservative therapy for at least 6 weeks. Therapeutic modalities used with varying success include cervical orthosis, nonsteroidal anti-inflammatory medications, muscle relaxants, analgesics, physical therapy, traction, epidural steroid injections, and selective nerve root blocks (46). The level of improvement associated with conservative therapy is controversial and ranges between 29% and 75%. Surgery-based studies tend to report lower rates of improvement with conservative treatment than with surgery (30). Surgery is reserved for patients who have failed a reasonable trial of conservative therapy, those who have a neurological deficit, or those who have a medically intractable pain syndrome (25, 38, 54).

Management for patients in the last group is the most controversial. These myelopathic patients can exhibit symptoms that range from numb, clumsy hands to spastic quadriparesis. With upper level degenerative lesions (C3 to C5), common symptoms are loss of manual dexterity, nonspecific arm weakness, and paresthesias. With lower lesions (C5 to C8), symptoms usually include spasticity and proprioceptive loss in the legs with gait dysfunction and feelings of unsteadiness as well as symptoms of radiculopathy in the arms. Findings on physical examination include motor weakness, sensory loss, spasticity with exaggerated reflexes, gait instability, extensor plantar responses, and lower motoneuron findings in the upper extremities. Lhermitte's sign can be produced with neck flexion and extension. Myelopathic syndromes can also include a Brown-Séquard type of presentation or central cord-type syndromes. Cervical spondylotic changes are almost ubiquitous as patients reach middle age and must be diagnosed accurately in those thought to be suffering from this common disorder. Other causes of spastic paraparesis in midlife include multiple sclerosis (MS), amyotrophic lateral sclerosis (ALS), primary lateral sclerosis, and syringomyelia. Although MS and syringomyelia can be diagnosed on MR imaging, motoneuron disease cannot. This diagnosis can be difficult to make: In one series of patients with ALS, 5% had undergone cervical laminectomy (36). Diagnostic studies include plain cervical radiography with dynamic views and MR imaging. Myelography with postmyelography CT is a useful adjunct, especially in patients with multilevel disease. The ability to visualize the bony anatomy accurately is essential in patients with significant disease posterior to the vertebral body. This information is needed to plan the levels and extent of surgical decompression. Although not indicated in all cases, the persistent utility of CT-myelography cannot be underestimated (25, 38, 45, 54).

The difficulty in deciding upon the treatment for myelopathic patient derives from the controversy surrounding the natural history of patients with spondylotic myelopathy and reflects the lack of randomized or even large long-term retrospective studies of this heterogeneous group of patients (2, 19, 25, 27, 30, 36, 39, 54). Although available studies suggest that not all patients with symptomatic cervical spondylosis deteriorate, it seems to be impossible to determine which symptomatic patients are at risk for deterioration, a low threshold for decompression exists in most surgical practices today. Some have called for randomized trials to demonstrate the efficacy of surgery compared to conservative therapy for the treatment of symptomatic spondylosis, but this plea is unlikely to be widely embraced (36). In today's litigious society, it is hard to imagine conducting such a study, which would relegate patients exhibiting symptoms from spinal cord compression to a nonsurgical treatment pathway. This concern is especially worrisome because neurological deterioration in these patients can be insidious over months to years or it can occur instantaneously after even a trivial trauma.

Notwithstanding, short-term improvement with nonoperative therapy occurs in 30% to 50% of patients, depending on the defining criteria (27). Conservative therapy for these patients is designed to decrease symptoms and to increase function. It includes but is not limited to the following: cervical orthosis, nonsteroidal anti-inflammatory medications, muscle relaxants, analgesics, physical therapy, and epidural steroid injections. Ultimately, most patients with cervical spondylotic myelopathy should be considered to undergo surgical decompression.

SELECTION OF SURGICAL APPROACH

Once the decision has been made to operate, which operation is best for each individual patient needs to be determined. No irrefutable evidence is available to help make this decision. The surgeon's experience, the patient's wishes, and the experience of other surgeons as detailed in the literature are all important factors to be considered. As an aid in the decision-making process, an algorithmic approach has been established based on the primary neurological diagnosis of either radiculopathy or myelopathy *(Figs. 19.1 and 19.2)*.

Radiculopathy

Surgical candidates include patients who have failed conservative therapy or who have a neurological deficit and a corresponding resectable lesion on a recent (within 6 months) imaging study. The first

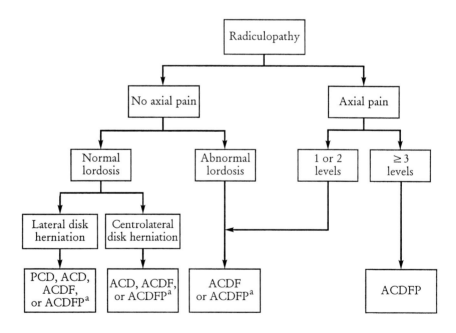

FIG. 19.1 Algorithm for the treatment of radiculopathy. PCD=posterior cervical decompression, ACD=anterior cervical diskectomy, ACDF=anterior cervical diskectomy with fusion (bone graft), and ACDFP=anterior cervical diskectomy with fusion (plating) [a]Choice of procedure depends on the surgeon's and patient's preference.

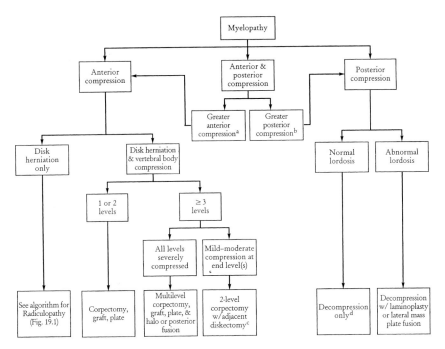

FIG. 19.2 Algorithm for the treatment of myelopathy. [a]If no postoperative improvement, reimage and consider posterior decompression. [b]If no postoperative improvement, reimage and consider anterior decompression. [c]Diskectomy above, below, or both as needed. [d]In young patients, consider adjunct fusion.

issue is whether patients complain of axial pain. Some degree of neck pain, which can even be severe at times, is associated with cervical disk herniation. However, the presence of axial neck pain as a constant symptom is a clear criterion for cervical fusion. In cases of one- or two-level disk herniation associated with axial pain, anterior cervical diskectomy with fusion is indicated (Fig. 19.1).

The next decision is whether to use allo- or autograft bone for fusion. No strong evidence suggests that autograft bone is associated with statistically superior outcomes compared to allograft (4, 7, 16) When allograft and autograft are compared, factors such as the complication rate associated with graft harvest, the potential for transmission of an infectious disease with allograft, and the rate of fusion of the two types of bone need to be considered (4, 41, 43) Consequently, the choice of allo- or autograft bone is a joint decision of the patient and surgeon.

The addition of a cervical plate to treat patients with radiculopathy is controversial. Some evidence suggests that its use may decrease the length of recovery (10, 18, 43, 44). Placing a cervical plate after fusion may also obviate the need for a cervical orthosis—another factor to consider. Despite the lack of prospective data, the number of cervical plates placed after diskectomy with fusion continues to increase. As with the choice of bone grafting material, the decision to add a cervical plate after an uncomplicated diskectomy should be based on the surgeon's personal experience and the patient's wishes.

In surgical candidates with radiculopathy but without axial neck pain, the next most important issue concerns the lordosis of the spine *(Fig. 19.1)*. In patients with abnormal lordosis, anterior cervical diskectomy with fusion should be undertaken. Fusion helps to re-establish normal lordosis, which otherwise can worsen after diskectomy without fusion (3). Again, the choice of grafting material and the decision to place a plate should be based on the patient's and surgeon's joint decision. No strong evidence suggests that the addition of a cervical plate in this subset of patients improves outcome for single-level disease. Some evidence, however, suggests that a cervical plate may decrease the rates of pseudarthrosis and graft collapse in patients undergoing multiple-level diskectomies with fusion (10).

Perhaps the most troubling but most commonly seen patients are those with no axial neck pain and normal cervical lordosis. In these patients, the location of the disk herniation—whether it is lateral only or centrolateral—must be considered. For patients with a lateral disk herniation, a posterior approach via a laminoforaminotomy is an option. This approach offers the ability to decompress the nerve root directly and obviates the need for fusion or plating because there is no significant structural damage to the spine. The procedure, however, is painful compared to the anterior approach, and this factor is an important consideration for some patients. A posterior approach also eliminates the risk of recurrent laryngeal nerve injury, an especially important concern in patients who depend on their voices for their livelihood.

If an anterior approach is entertained, patients without axial pain and with normal lordosis are candidates for anterior cervical diskectomy without fusion *(Fig. 19.1)*. One prospective, randomized study that compared anterior cervical diskectomy with diskectomy and fusion found no difference in patient satisfaction or return to preoperative activity (11). This technique is now being performed less frequently than it once was, but it avoids all the complications associated with grafting and plating and eliminates the need for a postoperative orthosis (47). Opponents of this surgery argue that the failure to reconstruct the foraminal height sets patients up to develop recurrent stenosis. Cervical diskectomy without fusion may also be associated with a longer recovery time compared to patients undergoing fusion. Available studies, however, do not seem to support this notion (11, 47). If an anterior approach is chosen and fusion is preferred, the choice of grafting material and whether to add a plate are best decided jointly by the surgeon and patient.

Myelopathy

Because of the heterogeneity and complexity of patients with myelopathy, treatment must be individualized. For patients with symptomatic spondylotic myelopathy, the question is seldom when to operate but what approach to use. First, however, the available imaging studies must be scrutinized. Often, some degree of compression is present both anteriorly at the level of the disk space and posterior to the vertebral body and ligamentum flavum *(Fig. 19.2)*. The region of maximal compression is the site that should be addressed first.

When the greatest compression is located anteriorly rather than posteriorly, whether this compression largely reflects disk herniation or whether compression exists behind the vertebral body is next determined. If the spinal canal is compressed at the disk space, the algorithm for radiculopathy can be followed *(Fig. 19.3)*. For patients who have anterior compression both at the level of the disk space and adjacent to the vertebral body, a corpectomy is indicated *(Fig. 19.4)*. What was once a formidable operation is now performed routinely with excellent outcomes (8, 12, 13, 15, 17, 28, 31).

Surgical decision making, however, can become problematic when the disease involves more than two adjacent levels *(Fig. 19.2)*. Corpectomies involving three or more levels can be performed, but the incidence of complications tends to increase as well (13). When possible, strong consideration should be given to performing a two-level corpectomy with an adjacent diskectomy. Whether the diskectomy is performed above or below the level of the corpectomy again depends upon the location of the compression. The level (superior or inferior) that seems to be the least compressed should be addressed through a wide diskectomy; the adjacent vertebral body is undercut to relieve compression *(Fig. 19.2)*. Bone grafts placed within the corpectomy defect and disk space provide three points of fixation because screws can be placed at either end of the corpectomy and at the vertebral body level adjacent to the diskectomy. If this strategy is technically impossible or the compression is adjacent to all three (or more) levels, a multilevel corpectomy with fusion and plating should be considered. Postoperatively, these patients should be placed in a halo brace or a posterior fusion should be considered because these constructs tend to fail more often than shorter ones.

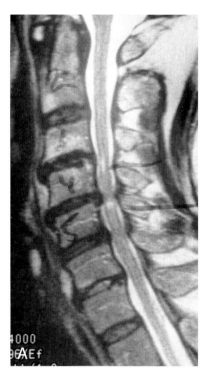

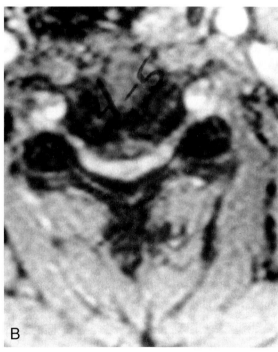

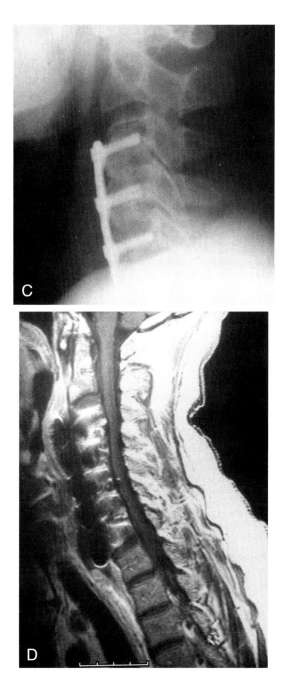

FIG. 19.3 A 63-year-old male with myeloradiculopathy. (*A*) T2-weighted sagittal magnetic resonance (MR) image of the cervical spine demonstrating compression at the disk spaces at multiple levels. (*B*) T2-weighted axial MR image demonstrating marked spinal canal compromise at the level of the disk space. (*C*) Postoperative radiograph after a multilevel diskectomy with allograft fusion and plating. (*D*) Postoperative T1-weighted sagittal MR image demonstrating excellent decompression of the spinal canal. Minimal artifact is produced by the titanium plate and screw system.

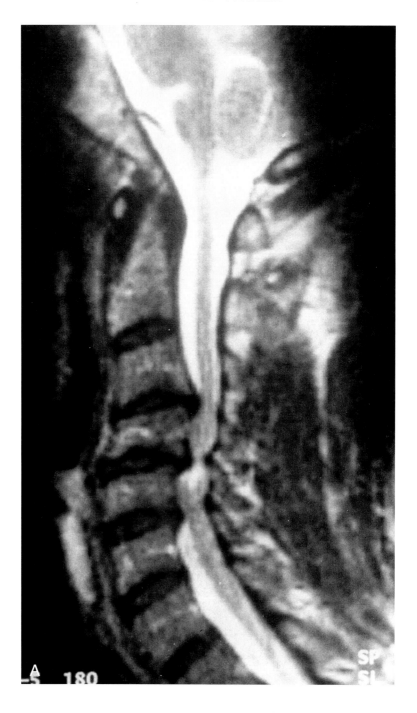

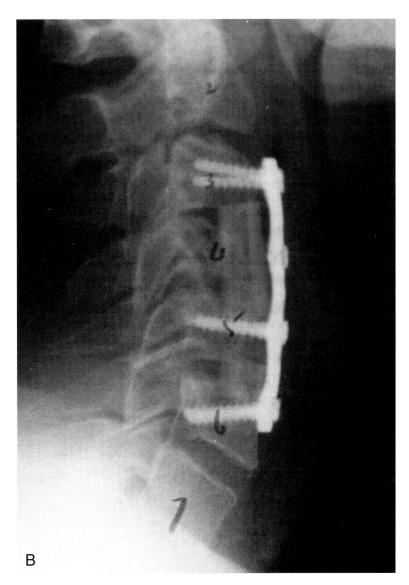

B

FIG. 19.4 A 58-year-old female with severe myelopathy. (A) T2-weighted sagittal magnetic resonance image of the cervical spine demonstrating compression at multiple levels. The spinal canal is compressed by the vertebral body of C4 and at the level of the
C5–6 disk space. (B) Postoperative radiograph after corpectomy with adjacent diskectomy. When possible, this type of construct can obviate the need for a multilevel corpectomy. Biomechanically, it is superior to a construct with screws placed only at the top and
bottom of the corpectomy.

In patients with greater posterior than anterior compression, lordosis is assessed *(Fig. 19.2)*. For patients with normal lordosis, laminectomy alone should be considered. This procedure quickly and effectively alleviates posterior compression. In young patients, however, a laminoplasty or augmentation of a laminectomy with lateral mass fusion should be considered. Theoretically, these procedures decrease the possibility of post-laminectomy kyphosis (23, 26, 50). The true incidence of this complication is unknown, but the effects can be devastating. Many techniques for laminoplasty and posterior fusion have been described, and which method offers the safest and most durable method for decompressing the spinal cord and nerve roots while preventing latent kyphosis is unclear.

In patients with abnormal lordosis and posterior compression, decompression with laminoplasty or lateral mass plate fusion is indicated to restore lordosis or to prevent the curvature from worsening *(Fig. 19.5)*(21,50).

The most complicated cases of myelopathy arise in patients with circumferential compression from both anterior and posterior sources. In these patients the initial decompression should be directed toward the site of greatest compression, following the algorithm as described *(Fig. 19.2)*. If patients fail to improve or stabilize, they should be re-imaged with MR imaging or CT myelography, and decompression of the opposite side should be considered.

Adjacent Level Disease

A caveat must be made concerning the evaluation of spondylotic patients with disease involving multiple levels. Purists would argue that surgery should be confined to the symptomatic levels, but this strategy is not always wise. Given the natural progression of degenerative cervical spine disease, regions of congenital stenosis or near-compressive lesions adjacent to regions of true compression should probably be decompressed during the primary surgery. This approach is especially valid now that strong evidence suggests that anterior cervical diskectomy with fusion accelerates degenerative changes above and below the level of the fused segments (53). Recently, a large retrospective study confirmed this phenomenon, reporting that the incidence of adjacent level disease was a 2.9%/year(22). Within 10 years of surgery, 25% of the patients developed symptomatic radiculopathy or myelopathy at segments adjacent to the site of a previous anterior cervical arthrodesis. More than two-thirds of these patients required another surgical procedure. Consequently, close attention should be paid to the levels adjacent to the planned level(s) of decompression and their early decompression should be considered.

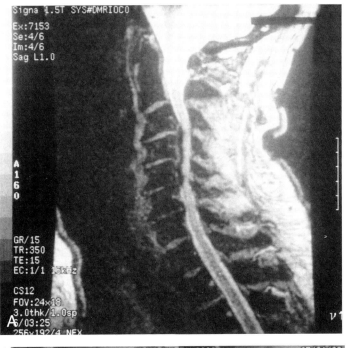

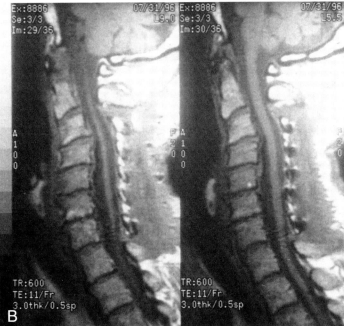

FIG. 19.5 A 65-year-old male with myeloradiculopathy. (*A*) T2-weighted sagittal magnetic resonance (MR) image of the cervical spine demonstrating marked stenosis of the spinal canal at multiple levels. In this case, a laminoplasty was chosen because the compression was distributed equally. (*B*) Postoperative T1-weighted sagittal MR image showing marked expansion of the cervical spinal canal without evidence of increasing kyphosis.

CONCLUSION

The treatment of degenerative cervical spine disease requires a standardized approach that begins with an extensive history and physical examination. Appropriate imaging studies, including plain radiography and MR imaging, follow. Conservative therapy should be employed in all patients with radiculopathy but without a severe neurological deficit. An algorithmic approach based on the neurological symptoms can help determine the best course of action for a given patient. The possibility of adjacent segment disease should be considered during surgical planning.

REFERENCES

1. Adams CBT, Logue V: Studies in cervical spondylitic myelopathy: I-III. **Brain** 94:557–594, 1971.
2. Arnasson O, Carlsson CA, Pellettieri L: Surgical and conservative treatment of cervical spondylotic radiculopathy and myelopathy. **Acta Neurochir (Wien)** 84:48–53, 1987.
3. Bayley JC, Yoo JU, Kruger DM, et al: The role of distraction in improving the space available for the cord in cervical spondylosis. **Spine** 20:771–775, 1995.
4. Bishop RC, Moore KA, Hadley MN: Anterior cervical interbody fusion using autogeneic and allogeneic bone graft substrate: A prospective comparative analysis. **J Neurosurg** 85:206–210, 1996.
5. Bohlman HH, Emery SE: The pathophysiology of cervical spondylosis and myelopathy. **Spine** 13:843–846, 1988.
6. Brain WR, Northfield D: The neurological manifestations of cervical spondylosis. **Brain** 75:187–225, 1952.
7. Brown MD, Malinin TI, Davis PB: A roentgenographic evaluation of frozen allografts versus autografts in anterior cervical spine fusions. **Clin Orthop** 119:231–236, 1976.
8. Chiles BW 3rd, Leonard MA, Choudhri HF, et al: Cervical spondylotic myelopathy: Patterns of neurological deficit and recovery after anterior cervical decompression. **Neurosurgery** 44:762–770, 1999.
9. Connell MD, Wiesel SW: Natural history and pathogenesis of cervical disc disease. **Orthop Clin North Am** 23:369–380, 1992.
10. Connolly PJ, Esses SI, Kostuik JP: Anterior cervical fusion: Outcome analysis of patients fused with and without anterior cervical plates. **J Spinal Disord** 9:202–206, 1996.
11. Dowd GC, Wirth FP: Anterior cervical discectomy: Is fusion necessary? **J Neurosurg** 90:8–12, 1999.
12. Ebersold MJ, Pare MC, Quast LM: Surgical treatment for cervical spondylitic myelopathy. **J Neurosurg** 82:745–751, 1995.
13. Eleraky MA, Llanos C, Sonntag VKH: Cervical corpectomy: Report of 185 cases and review of the literature. **J Neurosurg** 90:35–41, 1999.
14. Elsberg CA: *Tumors of the Spinal Cord and the Symptoms of Irritation and Compression of the Spinal Cord and Nerve Roots. Pathology. Symptomatology. Diagnosis and Treatment.* New York, Paul B Hoeber, 1925.
15. Emery SE, Bohlman HH, Bolesta MJ, et al: Anterior cervical decompression and

arthrodesis for the treatment of cervical spondylotic myelopathy. Two to seventeen-year follow-up. **J Bone Joint Surg [Am]** 80:941–951, 1998.

16. Fernyhough JC, White JI, LaRocca H: Fusion rates in multilevel cervical spondylosis comparing allograft fibula with autograft fibula in 126 patients. **Spine** 16:S561–S564, 1991.

17. Fessler RG, Steck JC, Giovanini MA: Anterior cervical corpectomy for cervical spondylotic myelopathy. **Neurosurgery** 43:257–267, 1998.

18. Geer CP, Papadopoulos SM: The argument for single-level anterior cervical discectomy and fusion with anterior plate fixation. **Clin Neurosurg** 45:25–29, 1999.

19. Gregorius FK, Estrin T, Crandall PH: Cervical spondylotic radiculopathy and myelopathy. A long-term follow-up study. **Arch Neurol** 33:618–625, 1976.

20. Hankinson HL, Wilson CB: Use of the operating microscope in anterior cervical discectomy without fusion. **J Neurosurg** 43:452–456, 1975.

21. Hattori S: A new method of cervical laminectomy. **Central Jpn J Orthop Traumatic Surg** 16:792–794, 1973.

22. Hilibrand AS, Carlson GD, Palumbo MA, et al: Radiculopathy and myelopathy at segments adjacent to the site of a previous anterior cervical arthrodesis. **J Bone Joint Surg [Am]** 81:519–528, 1999.

23. Hirabayashi K, Bohlman HH: Multilevel cervical spondylosis. Laminoplasty versus anterior decompression. **Spine** 20:1732–1734, 1995.

24. Hirsch C: Cervical disc rupture. Diagnosis and therapy. **Acta Orthop Scand** 30:172–186, 1960.

25. Hunt WE: Cervical spondylosis: Natural history and rare indications for surgical decompression. **Clin Neurosurg** 27:466–480, 1980.

26. Kimura I, Shingu H, Nasu Y: Long-term follow-up of cervical spondylotic myelopathy treated by canal-expansive laminoplasty. **J Bone Joint Surg [Br]** 77:956–961, 1995.

27. LaRocca H: Cervical spondylotic myelopathy: Natural history. **Spine** 13:854–855, 1988.

28. Macdonald RL, Fehlings MG, Tator CH, et al: Multilevel anterior cervical corpectomy and fibular allograft fusion for cervical myelopathy. **J Neurosurg** 86:990–997, 1997.

29. Magerl F: External skeletal fixation of the lower thoracic and lumbar spine, in Uhthoff HK, Stahl E (eds): *Current Concepts of External Fixation of Fractures.* Berlin, Springer-Verlag, 1982, p 353.

30. McCormack BM, Weinstein PR: Cervical spondylosis. An update. **West J Med** 165:43–51, 1996.

31. Naderi S, Özgen S, Pamir MN, et al: Cervical spondylotic myelopathy: Surgical results and factors affecting prognosis. **Neurosurgery** 43:43–50, 1998.

32. Orozco R, Llovet J: Osteosinterior en las fracturas del raquir cervical. **Rev Ortop Traumatol** 14:285–288, 1970.

33. Robertson JT: Anterior removal of cervical disc without fusion. **Clin Neurosurg** 20:259–261, 1973.

34. Robinson RA, Smith GW: Anterolateral cervical disc removal and interbody fusion for cervical disc syndrome. **Bull Johns Hopkins Hosp** 96:223, 1955.

35. Rogers WA: Treatment of fracture-dislocation of the cervical spine. **J Bone Joint Surg** 24:245–258, 1942.

36. Rowland LP: Surgical treatment of cervical spondylotic myelopathy: Time for a controlled trial. **Neurology** 42:5–13, 1992.

37. Roy-Camille R, Saillant G, Bertaux D, et al: Early management of spinal injuries, in McKibbin B (ed): *Recent Advances in Orthopaedics.* Edinburgh, Churchill Livingstone, 1979, p 57.

38. Rushton SA, Albert TJ: Cervical degenerative disease. Rationale for selecting the appropriate fusion technique (anterior, posterior, and 360 degree). **Orthop Clin North Am** 29:756–777, 1998.

39. Sadasivan KK, Reddy RP, Albright JA: The natural history of cervical spondylotic myelopathy. **Yale J Biol Med** 66:235–242, 1993.

40. Saunders RL: Anterior reconstructive procedures in cervical spondylotic myelopathy. **Clin Neurosurg** 37:682–721, 1991.

41. Schnee CL, Freese A, Weil RJ, et al: Analysis of harvest morbidity and radiographic outcome using autograft for anterior cervical fusion. **Spine** 22:2222–2227, 1997.

42. Semmes RE, Murphey F: The syndrome of unilateral rupture of the sixth cervical intervertebral disk with compression of the seventh cervical nerve root. Report of four cases with symptoms simulating coronary disease. **JAMA** 121:1209–1214, 1943.

43. Shapiro S: Banked fibula and the locking anterior cervical plate in anterior cervical fusions following cervical discectomy. **J Neurosurg** 84:161–165, 1996.

44. Shapiro SA, Snyder W: Spinal instrumentation with a low complication rate. **Surg Neurol** 48:566–574, 1997.

45. Singh A, Crockard HA: Quantitative assessment of cervical spondylotic myelopathy by a simple walking test. **Lancet** 354:370–373, 1999.

46. Slipman CW, Lipetz JS, Jackson HB, et al: Therapeutic selective nerve root block in the nonsurgical treatment of atraumatic cervical spondylotic radicular pain: A retrospective analysis with independent clinical review. **Arch Phys Med Rehabil** 81:741–746, 2000.

47. Sonntag VKH, Klara P: Controversy in spine care. Is fusion necessary after anterior cervical discectomy? **Spine** 21:1111–1113, 1996.

48. Spurling RG, Scoville WB: Lateral rupture of the cervical intervertebral discs. A common cause of shoulder and arm pain. **Surg Gynecol Obstet** 78:350–358, 1944.

49. Stookey B: Compression of the spinal cord due to ventral extradural cervical chondromas. Diagnosis and surgical treatment. **Arch Neurol Psychiatry** 20:275–291, 1928.

50. Tanaka J, Seki N, Tokimura F, et al: Operative results of canal-expansive laminoplasty for cervical spondylotic myelopathy in elderly patients. **Spine** 24:2308–2312, 1999.

51. Virchow RLK: *Untersuchungen uber die Entwickelung des Schadelgrundes im Gesunden und krankhaften Zustande.* Berlin, Reimber, 1857.

52. Walton GL, Paul WE: Contribution to the study of spinal surgery: One successful and one unsuccessful operation for the removal of tumor. **Bost Med Surg J** 153:114–117, 1905.

53. Wu W, Thuomas KA, Hedlund R, et al: Degenerative changes following anterior cervical discectomy and fusion evaluated by fast spin-echo MR imaging. **Acta Radiol** 37:614–617, 1996.

54. Yonenobu K: Cervical radiculopathy and myelopathy: When and what can surgery contribute to treatment? **Eur Spine J** 9:1–7, 2000.

20

Congress of International Surgeons—International Committee

RICHARD G. PERRIN, M.D., AND H. HUNT BATJER, M.D.

Concern with the human predicament is a fundamental preoccupation for all of us as physicians. This concern is expressed, first and foremost, in our day-to-day work, and, directly or indirectly, through contribution to and participation in altruistic efforts. In this regard the Congress of Neurological Surgeons (CNS) has been providing aid and education for developing parts of the world during the past four decades.

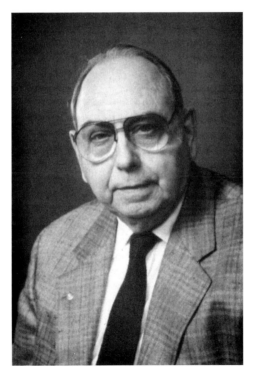

FIG. 20.1 Dr. Roy Tyrer—Past President, CNS.

Pioneers in this effort have included former CNS Presidents Dr. Roy Tyrer *(Fig. 20.1)* and Dr. William Mosberg *(Fig. 20.2)*. Dr. Tyrer served on the second Hope Mission to Peru and in West Africa, and (while President of the CNS) established ties with the Christian Medical College in Vellore, India *(Fig. 20.3)*. Dr. Mosberg served as the CNS representative to CARE-MEDICO and (when he became President of the CNS) established the Congress of Neurological Surgeons International Committee (CNS-IC), chaired by Dr. Tyrer. During the early days of the CNS-IC, efforts were directed to Egypt, Malaysia, Pakistan, Thailand, and Vietnam.

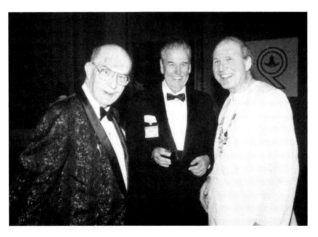

FIG. 20.2 Dr. William Mosberg, flanked by Dr. George Ablin (L) and Dr. Merwyn Bagan (R).

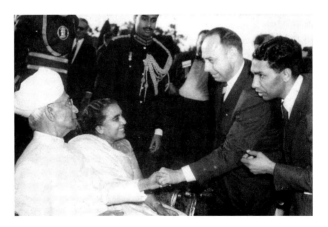

FIG. 20.3 Dr. Tyrer meeting with the Prime Minister of India, in 1963.

Rejuvenation of the CNS-IC became a priority when Dr. Arthur Day was Congress President in 1993. Dr. Steve Gianotta was appointment CNS-IC Chair and stimulated renewed interest in international initiatives. Successive CNS-IC Chairs—Dr. Hunt Batjer (1995), Dr. Richard Perrin (1997), and Dr. Nelson Oyesiku (2000)—implemented a subcommittee structure to encourage International Membership, to enhance the Programme of education and exchange, and to develop foreign assistance *(Fig. 20.4)*. Steps have been taken to promote cooperation and collaboration with other organizations engaged in international neurosurgical education, including the Foundation for International Education in Neurological Surgery (FIENS) and the World Federation of Neurosurgical Societies (WFNS).

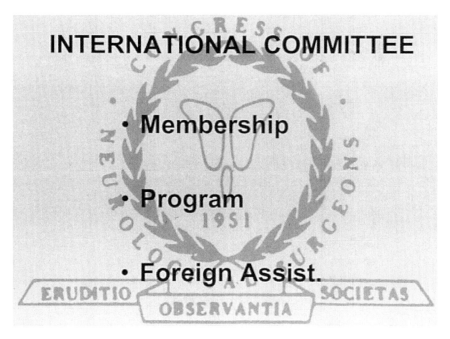

FIG. 20.4 Subcommittee structure of the CSN-IC.

During the interim, the international membership has more than doubled *(Fig. 20.5).* The International Luncheon Seminar—featuring keynote speakers and topical issues—has become a popular part of the CNS Annual Meeting, under the direction of Dr. Russell Andrews.

Foreign assistance has evolved to include the Bookstore, the Foundation for International Neurosurgical Development (FIND), the International Fellowship Programme, and the Volunteer Service Programme *(Fig. 20.6).*

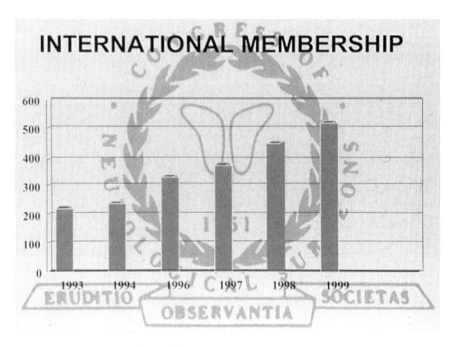

FIG. 20.5 International membership.

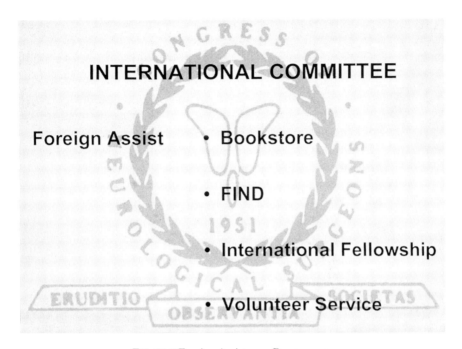

FIG. 20.6 Foreign Assistance Programmes.

The Bookstore receives and distributes donated books and periodicals. Lippincott, Williams & Wilkins—represented by Mr. Tim Grayson—has been a consistent and major supporter, with contributions of textbooks and journals. Recent private donors have included Dr. Gerald Haines and Dr. Ronald Tasker. Books and periodicals have been shipped (or transported by International Committee Faculty for educational courses) to Ecuador, Honduras, India, Peru, and Zimbabwe.

The Foundation for International Neurosurgical Development (FIND) was conceived by Drs. Steve Giannotta and Dan Kelly. FIND collects, collates, and distributes equipment and supplies, ranging from microsurgical instruments to operating microscopes. Dr. Kelly secured from Zeiss a commitment to provide one or two reconditioned contraves operating microscopes per year; deliveries to date have been made to Honduras, India, Nepal, Peru, and Zimbabwe.

The International Fellowship Programme provides training opportunities for recently graduated foreign neurosurgeons at a North American site for periods of 3 to 6 months. This programme has been exceedingly popular. The time-consuming administration of this programme has been energetically conducted by Dr. Gail Rosseau.

The Volunteer Service Programme provides opportunities for North American neurosurgeons to serve abroad.

The CNS-IC aims to encourage, facilitate and promote international neurosurgical assistance and education—with the goal to foster excellent, independent, self-sustaining Neurosurgical facilities abroad. Target sites for foreign assistance currently supported by the CNS-IC include Ghana, Honduras, India, Nepal, Peru and Zimbabwe.

Dr. Lee Finney has established a charitable foundation to provide aid to Honduras. Dr. Finney, with the assistance of various neurosurgical volunteers *(Figs. 20.7, 20.8)*, has developed, encouraged, and supported an evolving neurosurgical programme. The CNS-IC has contributed instruments and an operating microscope to this effort.

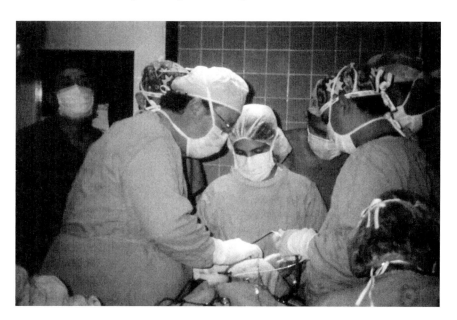

FIG. 20.7 Dr. Marion Walker operating in Honduras.

Drs. Ab Guha and Robin Sengupta have established a Neurosurgical Institute in Calcutta, India. The CNS-IC has provided support in the form of instruments, books, an operating microscope, and educational courses. Faculty includes Drs. Andrews, Chakravarti, Kelly, Perrin, and Sriharan.

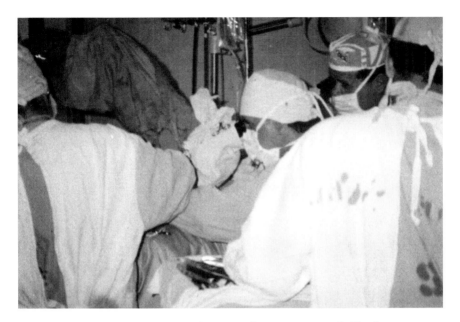

FIG. 20.8 Dr. Roberto Heros demonstrating neurosurgery in Honduras.

Dr. Merwyn Bagan has lived the commitment—practicing and teaching neurosurgery in Nepal for several years. The CNS-IC has assisted with instruments, an operating microscope, and periodicals.

Dr. Anselmo Piñeda is the energetic, enthusiastic, and irrepressible force behind a substantial programme in Peru. A number of CNS volunteers have participated in this endeavour, including Drs. Branch, Brockmeyer, Dempsey, Hardy, and Teo (among others) *(Fig. 20.9)*.

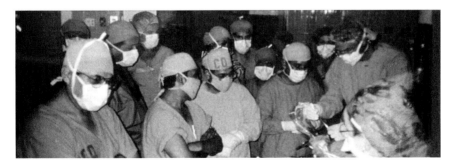

FIG. 20.9 Dr. Doug Brockmeyer teaching neurosurgical technique in Peru.

The Zimbabwe Project, conceived by Dr. Nozipo Maraire has received books, periodicals, instruments (including an operating microscope), as well as Faculty participation in educational courses *(Fig. 20.10)*. This effort has been bolstered by a WFNS Neurosurgical course held during the Spring, 1999. Neurosurgical residents from UCLA (Dr. Philip Theodopoulos) and the University of Toronto (Dr. J. Riva-Camrin) have spent 3 month blocks in Harare as part of this project.

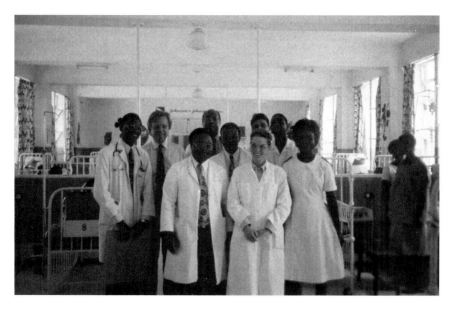

FIG. 20.10 Dr. Kalangu, Professor of Neurosurgery in Harare, and Dr. Perrin with house-staff on ward rounds.

A number of organizations including FIENS, FIND, WFNS, and others, have as their focus the advancement of neurosurgical education and services in the developing world. There is a need to consolidate and coordinate the various energies and resources to avoid duplication of efforts and to focus and concentrate on sustainable endeavours. The challenges are great, and the rewards are even greater.

IV

General Scientific Session IV Controversies in Sellar and Skull Base Surgery: Indications, Outcomes, and Costs

21

The Expanding Role of Endoscopy in Skull-Base Surgery

Indications and Instruments

HAE-DONG JHO, M.D., PH.D.

INTRODUCTION

Since modern neurosurgery was developed a century ago, its evolution can be divided into three stages based on how neurosurgical operations have been performed. The first stage of neurosurgery is naked-eye direct-vision surgery. Although ancillary visualizing surgical tools such as magnifying glasses were explored sporadically, the vast number of neurosurgical operations were performed under the direct vision of the surgeons' naked eye until 1960s. Transsphenoidal surgery was performed under naked-eye vision with the use of a head mirror. Cranial and spinal surgeries were performed under direct naked-eye visualization.

The second stage of neurosurgery is microscopic neurosurgery, which was developed in 1960s. Following a half century, microscopic neurosurgery has established a solid ground as the classic method of performing neurosurgical operations in the cranial cavity, spine, and peripheral nerves. The progressive development of microscopic optics, microscope mounting systems, microsurgical equipment, and ancillary tools have been followed in parallel with improved surgical skills and surgical outcomes. The development of microscopic neurosurgery enabled neurosurgeons to perform the anastomosis of blood vessels as small as 1 millimeter in diameter.

While microscopic neurosurgery has been at its acme in recent years, the third stage of neurosurgery—image neurosurgery—has been in a developmental stage. Views of the surgical anatomy are brought into monitored images under the guidance of which neurosurgeons perform various surgical procedures. An endoscope conveys the image of surgical anatomy onto the video monitor via electronic devices. Intraoperative monitoring devices such as a magnetic resonance (MR) scan, computed tomographic (CT) scan, computer-assisted image-guided system, fluoroscopic image-guidance, image-guiding robotic arm, etc. can depict the anatomical information on monitors in addition to real-time operating scenes on the main monitor in the operating room. When the technology of 1 or 2-millimeter wireless videocameras is available, it would not be long before small wireless videocameras would be deployed in the small surgical anatomic cavity to display the surgical anatomy on the image monitors. Although the endoscopic optical system is a practically available image-conveying tool at this time, various other image-generating tools may be developed in the future. Telesurgery is one of the other examples in the advent of image neurosurgery. The author will present his view and experience in the surgical treatments of skull-base pathology with the use of an endoscope as a tool for image neurosurgery.

RISK REDUCTION IN NEUROSURGERY

During the early stage of modern neurosurgery, neurosurgical morbidities and mortality were inconceivably higher than those of now when judged with the current standard. During the Cushing-Dandy period, mortality after acoustic neuroma surgery was approximately in the 20% range. Microscopic neurosurgery has lowered this to a 1% range. Despite a significant reduction of surgical risk in neurosurgery with the adoption of microscopic surgery, morbidities related to neurosurgery are still significant. For example, achieving better results in hearing loss and facial paralysis after acoustic neuroma surgery continues to be a challenge for the neurosurgeon. As a way to reduce surgical risks in acoustic neuroma treatments, radiosurgery treatment has been introduced. This is not a surgical treatment in a true sense, but radiation treatment with the adoption of stereotactic techniques. However, this alternative treatment, which has very minimal short-term risks, has made neurosurgeons set higher goals in their surgical results more so than in the past. Instead of mortality, postoperative hearing preservation and normal facial function have been a main concern to neurosurgeons who presently operate on acoustic neuromas.

The current microsurgical treatment in acoustic neuroma surgery still requires the use of brain retractors, a stay in a monitored room or intensive care unit postoperatively, several days of hospitalization, and a few weeks of recuperation. Presently, the risk following microsurgical removal of acoustic neuromas is definitely higher than that following radiosurgery. Most often, the surgical risk of microsurgical treatments is related to surgical procedure and techniques. Major morbidities after microsurgical treatment are related to the use of brain retraction, which can be avoidable. It is not uncommon to note changes in the signal intensity at the cerebellum in MR scans in patients after acoustic neuroma surgery. It is the result of brain retraction during tumor removal. Regardless of the patient's tolerance to the cerebellar damages, it should have been avoided in the first place. The brain tissue, which is unable to tolerate a few minutes of anoxia, would not tolerate metallic retraction directly applied to the cerebellum. Although neurosurgeons believe that a brain retractor is a brain protector that prevents inadvertent damage to the brain during an operation, neurosurgeons may have to learn how to operate without the use of brain retractors in order to avoid retractor-induced brain damage. Conventional skull-base surgery has made a contribution in intracranial surgery in a way that avoids unnecessary brain retraction by applying various basal approaches made away from the brain itself. This protective surgical concept has to be maintained in order to avoid damage to the brain. In addition, precise minimally invasive surgical approaches may enhance quick postoperative recovery as well as lessen surgical trauma to the patient contrary to maximally invasive approaches. Subsequently, the patient's stay in a monitored room or intensive care unit may be eliminated, and the hospital stay as well as the postoperative recovery period may be shortened. Minimal precise surgical exposure can be better served when an improved visualizing optical tool is introduced into the surgical anatomy other than the operating microscope. Such a visualizing tool can be an endoscope. However, endoscopic neurosurgery is still in a fledgling stage because appropriate neurosurgical endoscopes are not yet developed and adequate surgical tools are not yet available. Although it remains to be proven, the author's experience has been promising that minimalism in neurosurgical approaches with the adoption of image neurosurgery can reduce surgical risk and improve surgical outcomes in skull-base surgery.

INDICATIONS OF ENDOSCOPY IN SKULL-BASE SURGERY

In skull-base surgery, endoscopy can be used for endoscope-assisted microsurgery, combined surgery with microscopic surgery, or sole endoscopic surgery. An endoscope can be utilized as an ancillary visualizing tool during microscopic surgery. Its use during aneurysm surgery or tumor surgery has been advocated by others. An endoscope can disclose hidden corners of the anatomy that cannot be seen with the operating microscope. The operation is primarily performed under the operating microscope, and when endoscopic inspection is desired at the surgical site, an endoscope is inserted into the surgical anatomy under the visual guidance of the operating microscope. A simultaneous videodisplay system has been introduced for this purpose. Endoscopic images can be displayed at the corner of microscopic images, or vice versa. In order to facilitate the application of an endoscope for this purpose, bent endoscopes are introduced. These bent endoscopes carry their camera and ancillary attachments away from the microscopic view.

Combined surgery can be performed by two surgeons: one surgeon performs microscopic transcranial surgery and another surgeon performs endoscopic transnasal surgery for complex skull-base pathology at the anterior cranial base. This combined surgery is also performed for pituitary adenomas with one surgeon performing endoscopic surgery for the nasal part of the surgery followed by another surgeon performing microscopic tumor surgery. This combined surgery can be useful when a neurosurgeon is not familiar with the use of an endoscope but has an endoscopic rhinologist who can assist in skull-base surgery.

When a neurosurgeon is well trained in the use of an endoscope, endoscopic skull-base neurosurgery can performed solely under endoscopic visualization. Although significant advances have been made in endoscopic spinal surgery, endoscopic skull-base surgery is at a very early stage of development. Endoscopic endonasal surgery can be performed for midline skull-base pathology arising from the crista galli at the anterior cranial fossa to the foramen magnum. Surgical procedures are performed through a nostril without a skin incision. The skull base is reconstructed through a nostril when the surgical mission is accomplished intracranially. Endoscopic transcranial skull-base surgery has been developing through a precise miniature cranial opening at the nasion, eyebrow, temple, or retromastoid area. Instead of conventional extensive skull-base approaches, these miniature exposures have an advantage of a shortcut direct approach to the surgical target while employing the advantages of a brain protective strategy of the conventional skull-base surgery. The use of an endoscope enhances the visualizations of the surgical anatomy through a miniature surgical exposure.

ENDOSCOPES AS NEUROSURGICAL TOOLS

Endoscopes have been used in neurosurgery for a century. However, their use has been limited to ventricular procedures because a hollow cavity in the neurosurgical target organs is a cavity containing cerebrospinal fluid, the cerebral ventricles. Only in recent years have endoscopic neurosurgeons started to apply endoscopic techniques in neurosurgical treatments outside the cerebral ventricles. Improvements in endoscopic optics, camera systems, electronic equipment, and computer technology have brought neuroendoscopy to reality. Endoscopic-assisted microsurgery has been popularized in recent years. With this technique, optical advantage of an endoscope is utilized during microscopic neurosurgery. Microscopic visualization of a surgical target requires a certain minimal diameter of the width relative to the depth of a surgical corridor. Although scientific data is lacking in ratios between the depth and width of a surgical corridor for an optimal surgical exposure, a 2-inch depth surgical corridor requires at least a 0.5-inch di-

ameter of width in order to adequately visualize the surgical target with
a currently available operating microscope. This four-to-one ratio between
the depth and the width of a surgical corridor is an approximate ratio for
a minimal surgical exposure when the operating microscope is used. An
additional increase in width may be required depending on surgical tools
that surgeons are going to use for the completion of the surgical mission
because the use of two-bladed microsurgical tools such as bipolar forceps
are required in microsurgical procedures. This four-to-one ratio in surgical exposure is not required when an endoscope is utilized for surgical visualization. The minimal diameter of the surgical corridor for endoscopic
surgery is only intrinsic to the diameter of an endoscope and ancillary surgical tools, but not to the depth of the surgical corridor itself. While the objective lens of the operating microscope is located remotely for the surgical target, the tip of an endoscopic optical lens is placed in very close
proximity to the surgical target. This optical close proximity of an endoscope allows endoscopic neurosurgery to adopt a minimal surgical exposure. Another advantage of the use of an endoscope is the optical characteristics of an endoscope such as a wide-angle view, close-up magnification
view, and angled view to different directions. An endoscope provides a
wide angle view when it is compared to the operating microscope. It can
visualize a wider perimeter of the surgical target than the operating microscope. When an endoscope is advanced close to the surgical target, it
magnifies the focused subject. When visualization is required in different
directions from the straight surgical trajectory, an angled lens endoscope
allows direct visualization by directing the angled lens toward the particular direction. These optical characteristics of an endoscope allow endoscopic neurosurgeons to adopt a minimalistic surgical strategy.

INSTRUMENTAL IMPROVEMENT

The endoscopes earlier neurosurgeons adopted in ventricular endoscopy were urological endoscopes. In recent years, endoscopes that
are made for other specialities have been utilized in neurosurgical procedures, especially those made for rhinological purposes. Although some
neurosurgical endoscopes, either rigid rod-lens endoscopes or flexible
endoscopes, have been developed, these endoscopes are mostly for ventricular procedures. Other neurosurgical endoscopes for spinal or cranial use are in the process of development, however, those endoscopes
will require a period of testing before being accepted as adequate neurosurgical endoscopes. In other words, neurosurgical endoscopes are
now in the process of development in many different directions. Ideal endoscopes for particular neurosurgical procedures have to be developed
with an ergonomic design. Some of the recent developments are angled

shaft endoscopes such as Perneczky-designed microscope-assisting endoscopes and Tamaki-endoscopes, angled-lens endoscopes to a reverse-direction, spinal endoscopes, etc. The next few years will bring further development in neurosurgical endoscopes. Until now, ideal endoscopes for transcranial or endonasal skull-base surgery are not yet available.

Endoscope holders also require further development. Two different types of endoscope holders are currently available. One type is a nitrogen-gas-powered endoscope holder. As a mounting system of the operating microscope does, an endoscope power holder should provide point-to-point rigid fixation upon the release of the power button. Instead, its holding arm drips a significant distance from the fixation point where the holder is fixed. Two currently available power holders have this sagging problem. The second type is a manual holder that is inexpensive and rigid. However, its endoscope-holding terminal has to be further refined in order to provide an optimal operating area. These endoscope holders will continually evolve to become an adequate endoscope-holding device for neurosurgical use. An endoscope lens cleansing device is a valuable tool when an endoscopic operation is to be performed without interruption. Although only one product is available currently, others are in the process of development. This lens cleansing device functions with an irrigation of saline onto the endoscope lens followed by brief suctioning of water drops from the lens by a reverse flow of saline. By pressing a foot pedal, a battery-powered motor pumps saline forward for irrigation, and by releasing it, a brief moment of reverse flow of saline follows aspirating drops of saline at the tip of an endoscope by the reverse rotation of the motor. It is useful, but a better system is still desirable.

An endoscope holder and an image-guided system will be combined in the future. A currently available image-guided system can be used as a separate tool when image-guided technique is required for an operation. An image-guided robotic arm is in the process of development. It will serve as a combined function of an endoscope holder, an image-guided stereotaxis, and possible automation of certain simple surgical motions. Surgical instruments for endoscopic neurosurgery have to be developed step-by-step as microsurgical instruments have been developed in the past. Physical characteristics of an endoscope require completely different shapes of surgical tools for various neurosurgical procedures. The tips of surgical instruments need to be bent in a way that allows those instruments maneuverable under an endoscopic view. The handles as well as the shafts of those instruments have to be shaped differently from those of current microsurgical instruments. Operating rooms for neuroendoscopy also require changes in design and arrangement of ancillary equipment. Endoscopic surgery is performed under monitored images that often require deploy of multiple monitors in the operating room depending on the operating room setting with nursing staff, assistants, and a surgeon. Web monitors that may be valuable tools for in situ surgical consultation in the future can be installed as well. Thus, the operating room has to be designed to accommodate the needs of endoscopic image surgery. Image-guided robotic systems as well as real time imaging systems such as an intraoperative MR unit or CT unit can also be valuable equipment to be installed with the pre-planned room design (5).

SURGICAL TECHNIQUES FOR ENDOSCOPIC SKULL BASE SURGERY

1. TRANSCRANIAL SKULL BASE ENDOSCOPY

As mentioned earlier, the optical and physical characteristics of an endoscope make minimalism in neurosurgery more practical. Extensive surgical exposure required for the conventional microscopic skull-base surgery is not necessary when an endoscope is applied as a sole visualizing tool. Although lack of adequate surgical instruments makes an endoscopic surgical mission technically difficult, progressive advances have been made for sole endoscopic surgery. The following surgical exposures are examples of surgical approaches adopted for skull-base surgery. The main advantage of these skull-base approaches is that an essential surgical corridor is created at the extracranial area or at the extraaxial area so that brain retractors are not necessary for conducting the surgical mission. All of the following transcranial skull-base surgeries have been performed without the use of brain retractors.

A. Glabellar approach via 1-inch skin incision at the nasion is used as a midline subfrontal approach to the anterior fossa skull base (9). This technique involves a 1-inch curvilinear skin incision at the nasion, transfronto-nasal exposure at the cranial and nasal cavity, further transethmoidal exposure at the cranionasal skull base up to sellar region. This is a minimal approach alternative to a conventional or-bitofrontal skull-base approach via a bicoronal skin incision. The midline anterior cranial base can be approached with this glabellar approach. Although olfactory groove meningiomas are common pathology dealt with this approach, any pathology involving the midline anterior cranial base can be operated on with this technique. When this operation was changed from microscopic surgery to endoscopic surgery, a surgical incision and bony exposure at the skull base become much smaller. When the width of a tumor is medial to the medial orbit, an endoscopic endonasal approach is used instead.

B. Orbitofrontal approach via an eyebrow incision has been used as an alternative for a conventional unilateral orbitofrontal approach via a bicoronal skin incision (10). The essence of this approach is that only the essential operating area is involved in the surgical exposure. The unnecessary portion of the surgical area that is involved in a conventional bicoronal orbitofrontozygomatic approach is eliminated from the surgical exposure with this eyebrow incision, orbitofrontal approach. The surgical incision is a 2-inch long incision at the upper margin of the eyebrow with or without section of the supraorbital nerve. An approximate 2 by 3-cm orbitofrontal craniotomy is performed. The bone flap involved is the superior orbital rim and orbital roof. The remaining bone at the orbital apex is further removed in order to have maximal advantage of using the orbital cavity as a surgical corridor. This surgical exposure discloses the orbital surface of the frontal dura mater in a rostral half, and the globe at a caudal half. When the dura mater is opened, the dura flap, the base of which is made at the globe side, is tacked up with stitches in a way that displaces the adipose tissue at the orbit further away from the frontal brain. This allows an ample surgical corridor inferior to the frontal lobe. Drainage of the cerebrospinal fluid at the sylvian cistern will further widen this surgical corridor. This surgical exposure has been used for pathology at the subfrontal, suprasellar, and parasellar areas. Craniopharyngiomas, meningiomas, and other suprasellar tumors are treated with this approach *(Fig. 21.1)*. Cerebral aneurysms can be taken care of via this approach as well. Whenever an operation was performed under an endoscope, the surgical visualization was superior to that of the operating microscope through this exposure. One concern has been radiating heat generated from the tip of the endoscope when an endoscope is focused on the optic system. Frequent intermittent irrigation has been performed to the endoscope lens in order to cool off any heat generated by the light source. When neurosurgical endoscopes are produced in the future, a cool light source has to be developed. Although no details are available regarding the degree of heat generated by the currently available endoscopes, this potential heat injury needs to be considered when an endoscope is focused on the optic or acoustic nerve for a prolonged time. The cosmetic outcome at the surgical incision site and the configuration of the orbit has been satisfactory.

C. Basal pterional approach via a lateral eyebrow incision has been utilized as an alternative to a conventional orbitofrontozygomatic skull-base approach or conventional pterional approach. The frontalis branch of the facial nerve is mapped out with electromyography (EMG) in the operating room. Surgical incision is made at the upper margin of

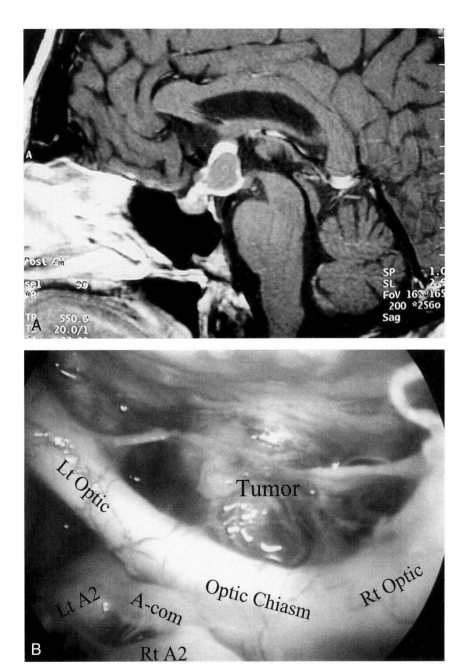

Fig. 21.1 An MR scan, T-1 weighted contrast-enhanced sagittal view, reveals a suprasellar tumor with contrast enhancement along the tumor wall in a 53-year-old woman who had a visual disorder (*A*). Right-sided orbital roof craniotomy was performed via a 4-centimeter eyebrow incision. The entire operation was performed under endoscopic visualization. An intraoperative photograph under an 0-degree-lens endoscope demonstrates a tumor (craniopharyngioma) under the optic chiasm (*B*). (*continues*)

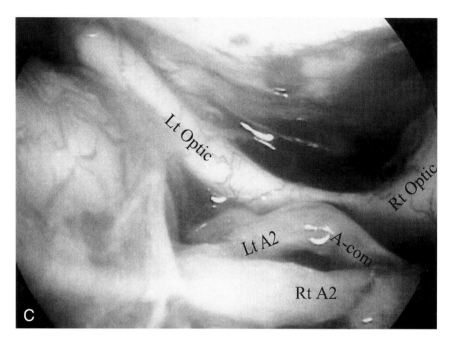

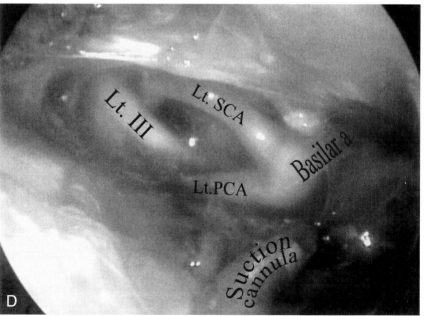

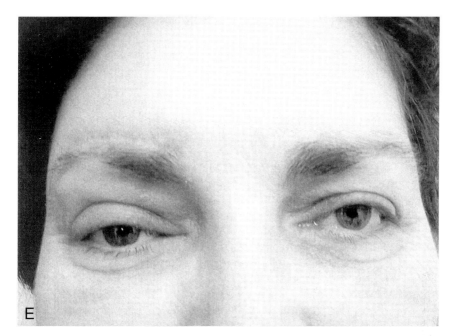

E

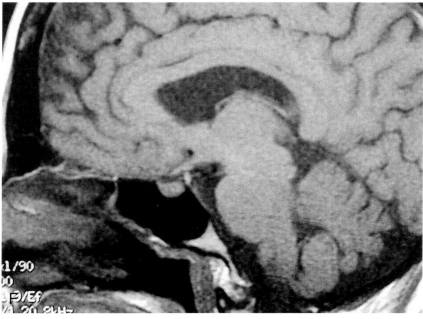

Fig. 21.1 (*Continued*) Another photograph shows the surrounding anatomy after complete tumor removal. (*C*). When an endoscope was inserted under the optic chiasm, the basilar artery, left superior cerebellar artery, left posterior cerebral artery, and left third cranial nerve were visualized (*D*). The surgical incisional line is noticeable with the residual swelling of the right eyelid 2 weeks postoperatively (*E*). The postoperative MR scan, T-1 weighted sagittal view, taken 6 weeks postoperatively demonstrates complete tumor removal (*E*).

the lateral one-half of the eyebrow and extended laterally, further avoiding the frontalis branch of the facial nerve. The length of the surgical incision is approximately 2 inches. The bone at the frontoorbitozygomatic area is exposed. Orbitofrontozygomatic craniotomy is performed as a single piece bone flap. This bone flap contains three facets of cavities—the orbital, frontal cranial, and temporal cranial cavity. The bone flap is shaped like a pyramid with a wide base and tapering tip that contains three cavity surfaces. When the bone flap is lifted, the orbit, frontal dura, and temporal dura are exposed with a natural operating corridor shaped like a pyramid standing on its tip. The remaining bone at the lesser sphenoid wing is excised up to the optic canal. The dura mater is opened with the base of the dural flap at the orbit. The dura is tacked up with stitches and the orbital content is further retracted with the dural flap. This technique has been used for pathology at the cavernous sinus, parasellar, and suprasellar region when an oblique entry to the area is desired rather than a midline entry. Aneurysm surgery has been performed with this approach. This minimal approach provides a maximal basal exposure similar to a conventional orbitofrontozygomatic skull-base approach via a bicoronal incision.

D. Subtemporal basal approach has been used as an alternative to a conventional subtemporal approach. A linear incision is made at the temporal area starting from one centimeter inferior to the zygomatic arch close to the tragus to the frontotemporal area approximately 2 inches in length. A temporal craniotomy is made with a bone flap of 2 centimeters in height by 3 centimeters in width. The caudal margin of the bone flap is made just at the edge of the temporomandibular joint in order to have a maximal basal temporal exposure. When the bottom of the middle cranial fossa is not well exposed by lifting a bone flap, the caudal margin of the craniotomy opening is further drilled until the flat middle cranial fossa is well exposed. Despite this maximal basal exposure at the middle cranial fossa, the operating corridor is somewhat limited when surgical access is to be made to the medial temporal region or anterior cavernous sinus because the medial wall of the middle cranial fossa is acutely sloped rostrally medial to the temporal lobe. Such an anatomy would not easily allow an unobstructed corridor to the anterior cavernous sinus or the tentorial edge without the use of brain retractors. In order to facilitate surgical access without the use of brain retractors, diuretics are often used for this approach. Unless the temporomandibular joint is sacrificed, direct unobstructed surgical access to the medial temporal region extraaxially is somewhat limited. However, the use of an endoscope allows wider visualization at the surgical target area. In addition, angled lens endoscopes can visualize the infratemporal fossa nicely even without sacrifice of the temporomandibular joint. This surgical approach can be used for pathology at the posterior cavernous sinus, Meckel's cave, tentorium, petrous bone, rostral posterior fossa, and middle cranial fossa.

E. Retromastoid approach is used for pathology at the cerebellopontine angle, infratentorial, pineal, and lateral cerebellar region. With a 2-inch linear skin incision made in an obliquely linear fashion, 2- by 3-centimeter craniotomy or craniectomy is made. The bone opening is extended to the margin of the venous sinus. Once CSF is drained from the cistern, an operating surgical corridor is developed. Endoscopic surgery has been developed for microvascular decompression of the cranial nerves, removal of pineal tumors, and removal of the cerebellopontine angle tumors. As mentioned earlier, radiating heat from the endoscopic lens requires particular attention when an endoscope is focused on the cochlear nerve area.

F. Lateral approach to the craniocervical junction is made via a 2-inch linear incision at the posterolateral craniocervical juncture. It may or may not require section of the greater occipital nerve depending on the degree of exposure at the cervical spine. The lateral portion of the occipital bone and hemilaminectomy of the cervical spine is performed. For operating intradural pathology, the atlantooccipital joint is not required to be sacrificed because a trajectory angle to the surgical target with this technique allows an adequate exposure at the ventral aspect of the cervicomedullary juncture. The only indication requiring resection of the atlantooccipital joint may be bony pathology involving the lower clivus and anterior column of the upper spine. In those cases, a stabilization procedure is necessary. The use of an endoscope with this technique allows wider visualization at the area ventral to the cervicomedullary junction.

2. Endonasal Skull Base Endoscopy

Endoscopic endonasal approaches have been made to the midline skull base from the crista galli to the foramen magnum. These surgical approaches have been made for pathology located at the anterior cranial fossa, optic nerve, pterygoid fossa, caverous sinus, sellar and suprasellar area, and clivus including the posterior cranial fossa. An endonasal approach does not require a skin incision besides a small abdominal incision when an abdominal fat graft harvest is necessary. The surgical approaches used for endoscopic endonasal surgery is a paraseptal approach that is made between the nasal septum and middle turbinate, a middle meatal approach that is made between the middle turbinate and lateral wall of the nasal cavity, and a middle turbinectomy approach. Depending on the trajectory angle of the endoscope, each surgical approach provides access to the skull base ranging from the anterior cranial fossa near the crista galli to the clivus near the foramen magnum. When skull-base reconstruction is required, the dural graft is placed for dural reconstruction, an autogenous bone or titanium mesh is placed for bony reconstruction, and additional fat graft is placed extracranially. Nasal packing is not necessary and is not used. Vasoconstrictors or decongestants are not used at the nasal mucosa during surgical procedures. Postoperative discomfort is very minimal and an average hospital stay has been overnight regardless of pathology or surgical procedure. The following are endoscopic endonasal surgical procedures performed for midline skull base pathology.

   A. Endoscopic endonasal approach to the anterior cranial fossa is used for pathology at the anterior cranial fossa such as olfactory groove meningiomas (15). The lateral margin of a tumor has to be medial to the medial wall of the orbit. If not, transcranial approaches have to be used. Either a paraseptal approach or a middle turbinectomy approach is used for this purpose but a middle meatal approach is occasionally used when a unilateral approach to the anterior cranial fossa is required such as the repair of CSF leakage. As described earlier, skull-base reconstruction is required following tumor resection.

   B. Endoscopic endonasal approach to the optic nerve has been used for removal of meningiomas (13). Although any of the three surgical approaches can expose the optic nerve area, a paraseptal approach is preferably used. Surgical exposure is first made at the rostral sphenoid sinus. Once the optic nerve is identified, further rostral and lateral exposure is made around the optic nerve area. Following tumor removal, skull-base reconstruction is required.

   C. Endoscopic endonasal approach to the sellar and suprasellar region is adopted most commonly for pituitary tumor removal (2–4, 6, 8, 11, 12, 14). Fluoroscopic guidance is not necessary once the distinct nasal anatomy is familiarized with. The inferior margin of the middle turbinate is a surgical landmark. The middle turbinate has to be confirmed in reference to the nasopharynx. A paraseptal approach is most commonly adopted among the three different surgical approaches. When a pituitary tumor is excised, the sella is reconstructed with fat graft placement if CSF leakage is encountered intraoperatively or a tumor resection cavity is large. The anterior wall of the sella is reconstructed with either autogenous bone or titanium mesh placement if autogenous bone is not available. The sphenoidal sinus is left as a normal aerated sinu cavity. Any sort of nasal packing is not used.

D. Endoscopic endonasal approach to the cavernous sinus is adopted when the cavernous sinus is involved by tumor (1, 16). A paraseptal or middle turbinectomy approach will expose the lateral aspect of the cavernous sinus. In cases of pituitary adenomas, a paraseptal approach is commonly adopted. In order to protect the carotid artery, abdominal fat graft is placed in the sphenoid sinus when the carotid artery has been exposed. This endoscopic approach allows entry to the cavernous sinus through the medial wall of the cavernous sinus. As the cranial nerves are located at or near the lateral wall of the cavernous sinus, this medial wall entry prevents injury to the cranial nerves. Pituitary tumors are best suited for this technique. However, when a fibrotic meningioma was encountered in the cavernous sinus, it was difficult to dissect from the carotid artery with this technique.

E. Endoscopic endonasal approach to the clivus and posterior cranial fossa is used for pathology invading the clivus or posterior fossa (7, 17). The most common tumors have been chordomas. The dural defect is reconstructed with abdominal fat graft placement *(Fig. 21.2)*.

SURGICAL RESULTS OF ENDOSCOPIC ENDONASAL SKULL-BASE SURGERY

Endoscopic transsphenoidal surgery has been performed by the author on more than 250 patients. The number of patients with a postoperative follow-up period longer than 12 months was 160. There were 70 men and 90 women. Age ranged from 14 to 88 years (median 43 years). Among the 160 patients, 128 had pituitary adenomas, 9 had anterior fossa meningiomas, 7 had clival chordomas, and 16 patients had other pathologies. Twenty-nine patients had previously undergone conventional transsphenoidal surgery, 4 had previous craniotomy, and 9 received previous radiation treatments. Among the 128 patients with pituitary adenomas, 30 (23%) patients had microadenomas, 24 (19%) patients had sellar macroadenomas, 41 (32%) patients had sellar and suprasellar macroadenomas, and 33 (26%) patients had invasive adenomas involving the cavernous sinuses. Among the 9 patients with anterior cranial fossa meningiomas, 7 had gross total removal and 2 had subtotal removal. One of the patients who had a subtotal removal required a reoperation and the other required radiation treatment. Among the 7 patients with clival chordomas, 5 had total removal and 2 had subtotal removal. All but one underwent postoperative gamma-knife surgery at the tumor resection site. One patient who had a total resection did not receive radiation treatment postoperatively, and has not had tumor recurrence. Among the 68 patients with hormone-non-secreting adenomas, 53 (78%) patients had gross total removal and 15 (22%) had subtotal removal. Among the 35 patients with prolactino-

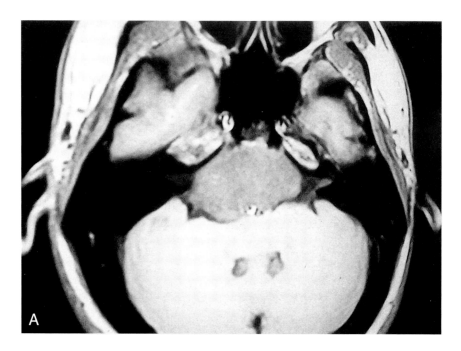

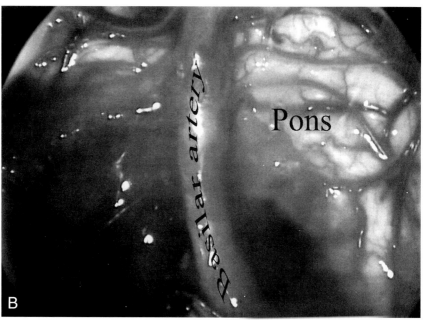

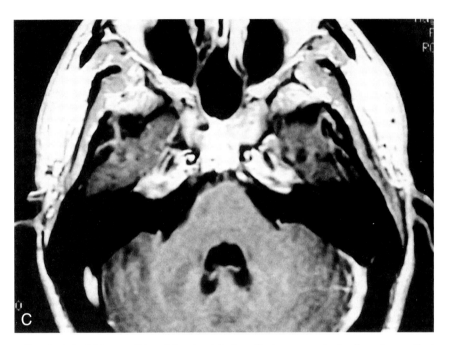

FIG. 21.2 An MR scan, T-1 weighted axial view, discloses a posterior fossa tumor that was encasing the basilar artery, in a 28-year-old man with a bilateral partial sixth cranial nerve palsy (*A*). This clival chordoma was excised with an endoscopic endonasal approach through the right nostril. An intraoperative endoscopic photograph reveals the anterior aspect of the pons and basilar artery (*B*). Gross total tumor removal was accomplished and the clival defect was repaired with abdominal fat graft placement. The tumor resection site was treated with gamma-knife surgery 2 months postoperatively. The postoperative MR scan, T-1 weighted contrasted axial view, taken 1 year postoperatively shows complete tumor removal without any evidence of tumor recurrence (*C*).

mas, 24 (71%) patients had normalized their postoperative prolactin levels. Eleven (70%) patients among the 16 with Cushing's disease had normal postoperative cortisol levels. The remaining 5 patients in this group underwent postoperative gamma-knife surgery. Among the 9 patients with acromegaly, 7 (78%) had postoperative IGF-1 levels within normal limits and with growth hormone levels less than one.

Postoperative complications included deterioration of anterior pituitary function in 11%, CSF leak in 6%, meningitis in 1.2%, temporary diabetes insipidus in 4%, permanent diabetes insipidus in 3%, and sinusitis in 1.2%. One patient who had a large calcified recurrent fibrosarcoma died postoperatively with occlusion of the bilateral internal carotid arteries. Outpatient surgery was performed in two patients with prolactinomas. One hundred and eleven patients (66%) stayed overnight in the hospital, 21 patients (13%) stayed two nights, 19 patients (11%) stayed three nights, and the remaining 14 (8.5%) patients stayed longer than three nights in the hospital.

FUTURE DEVELOPMENT

The optical system of rod-lens endoscopes may change to a wireless microcamera system in the near future. Image display systems have to be improved to a three-dimensional image system, which is being developed. An image-guided robotic system, which is now in a developmental stage, may assist in a precise approach to the surgical target. The robotic arm of this image-guided system may better serve as a holder than the current endoscopic holders. Surgical tools for image neurosurgery have to be developed and refined progressively. Image-conveying systems that are incorporated with the internet may provide instantaneous surgical consultation from remote surgeons. The operating room for this image surgery has to be developed to display simultaneously multiple images conveyed from the actual surgical site, real-time image generators, pre-stored images in computer-assisted image-guided devices and images from the internet. The operating room may resemble a television broadcasting room. This image neurosurgery may enable the surgeon to achieve preplanned surgical goals with precision from the beginning of a surgical approach to the finish of the operation. Ultimately, image neurosurgery may reduce surgical risk and improve outcomes.

CONCLUSIONS

Although it is in an early stage, endoscopic skull-base surgery approaches either transcranial or endonasal has been very promising. With the future development of appropriate surgical tools and adequate training of surgeons, endoscopic neurosurgery in the treatment of skull-base pathology may advance to a higher level of image neurosurgery. The author's experience on endoscopic transcranial and endoscopic endonasal skull-base surgery are reported

ACKNOWLEDGEMENT

Mi-Ja Jho, B.E., and Robin Coret, B.A., assisted in preparation of the manuscript.

REFERENCES

1. Alfieri A, Jho HD: Endoscopic endonasal approach to the cavernous sinus. An anatomical study. **Neurosurgery** 48:1–11, 2001.

2. Carrau RL, Jho HD, Ko Y: Transnasal-transsphenoidal endoscopic surgery of the pituitary gland. **Laryngoscope**– 106:914–918, 1996.
3. Jho HD, Carrau RL, Ko Y: Endoscopic pituitary surgery, in Wilkins RH, Rengachary SS (eds): *Neurosurgical operative atlas.* Baltimore: Williams & Wilkins, 1996, vol 5(1), pp 1–12.
4. Jho HD, Carrau RL: Endoscopy assisted transsphenoidal surgery for pituitary adenoma. Technical note. **Acta Neurochir (Wien)** 138:1416–1425, 1996.
5. Jho HD: Endoscopic endonasal pituitary surgery: Technical aspects. **Contemp Neurosurg** 19(6):1–7, 1997.
6. Jho HD, Carrau RL: Endoscopic endonasal transsphenoidal surgery: Experience with 50 patients. **J Neurosurg** 87:44–51, 1997.
7. Jho HD, Carrau RL, Mclaughlin ML, Somaza SC: Endoscopic transsphenoidal resection of a large chordoma in the posterior fossa: **Acta Neurochir (Wien)** 139:343–348, 1997.
8. Jho HD, Carrau RL, Ko Y, Daily M: Endoscopic pituitary surgery: An early experience. **Surg Neurol** 47:213–223, 1997.
9. Jho HD, Ko Y: Glabellar approach: Midline anterior skull base approach. **Minim Invasive Neurosurg** 40(2):62–69, 1997.
10. Jho HD: Orbital roof craniotomy: Simplified anterior skull approach. **Minim Invasive Neursurg** 40(3):91–97, 1997.
11. Jho HD: Endoscopic pituitary surgery. **Pituitary** 2:139–154, 1999.
12. Jho HD, Alfieri A: Endoscopic endonasal pituitary surgery: Evolution of surgical technique and equipment in 150 operations. **Minim Invasive Neursurg** 44:1–12, 2001.
13. Jho HD: Endoscopic endonasal approach to the optic nerve: A technical note. **Minim Invasive Neurosurg** (in press).
14. Jho HD, Alfieri A: Endoscopic transsphenoidal pituitary surgery: Various surgical techniques and recommended steps for procedural transition. **Br J Neurosurg** 14(5):424–432, 2000.
15. Jho HD, HG Ha: Endoscopic endonasal skull base surgery: Part 1—The anterior cranial fossa skull base. **Minim Invasive Neurosurg** (in press).
16. Jho HD, HG Ha: Endoscopic endonasal skull base surgery: Part 2—The cavernous sinus. **Minim Invasive Neurosurg** (in press).
17. Jho HD, HG Ha: Endoscopic endonasal skull base surgery: Part 3—The clivus and midline posterior fossa. **Minim Invasive Neurosurg** (in press).

22

Pituitary Tumors—Long-Term Outcomes and Expectations

EDWARD R. LAWS, M.D., AND JOHN A. JANE, JR., M.D.

INTRODUCTION

Throughout the history of modern neurosurgery, pituitary tumors have represented one of the more important and challenging areas of neurosurgical management. Most comprehensive neurosurgical reviews list pituitary tumors as the third most common primary brain tumor after gliomas and meningiomas (1, 13, 36, 38, 44, 54, 69). Autopsy studies actually document a higher incidence and suggest that small pituitary tumors may be present in 20% or more of the population (4, 7, 8, 51, 63). Nationally, the transsphenoidal approach to the pituitary region is used in approximately 19% of all operations for primary brain tumors (2, 38, 43, 45, 68).

CLASSIFICATION

Pituitary adenomas are variously categorized *(Table 22.1)* (62). Perhaps the most important distinction is between the nonfunctioning adenoma, which has no endocrine features other than hypopituitarism, and the hyperfunctioning adenoma, which produces an excess of active pituitary hormone. Pituitary adenomas are also classified according to size. By convention microadenomas are 10 mm or less in diameter and macroadenomas are those tumors greater than 10 mm in diameter. Another category of "giant" pituitary adenomas is often added for those lesions that range far beyond the confines of the sella turcica and the suprasellar space. Pituitary adenomas also can be staged. The most useful and widely used staging scheme was proposed by Dr. Jules Hardy *(Fig. 22.1)* (18, 20, 49). In addition to the size of the lesion, this classification takes into account whether the tumor is "enclosed" and noninvasive or whether it has parasellar extension, usually indicating invasion of the structures around the pituitary fossa.

TABLE 22.1
Classification Schemes of Pituitary Adenomas

Classification Scheme	Characteristic Features
Hormonal activity	
Non-Functioning adenoma	Endocrinologically inactive, patient may present with hypopituitarism
Functioning adenoma	Produces excess of active pituitary hormone
	GH adenoma
	PRL adenoma
	GH and PRL adenoma
	ACTH adenoma
	TSH adenoma
	Plurihormonal adenoma
Size	
Microadenoma	≤ 10 mm
Macroadenoma	> 10 mm
Giant	Wide extension beyond sellar and suprasellar space
Growth Characteristics	
Diffuse	Contained within the dura but may extend into suprasellar or parasellar regions
Invasive	Invades dura, bone, or both
Grading of Macroadenomas (Hardy)	
A	Suprasellar extent within 10 mm of planum sphenoidale
B	Suprasellar extent up to 20 mm, elevates the anterior recess of the third ventricle
C (Giant)	Suprasellar extent up to 30 mm, fills the anterior third ventricle
D (Giant)	Suprasellar extent greater than 30 mm, above the level of the foramen of Monro; or, Grade E with asymmetrical lateral or multiple expansions

TREATMENT

General Considerations

A variety of treatments are available for these common, and usually benign, tumors. The various treatment modalities are assessed using outcome measures specific to the patient with pituitary adenoma *(Table 22.2)*. The first of these is survival, measured by the longevity after initial treatment. The second of these is normalization of endocrine function, both in terms of lowering hypersecretion to normal and in terms of restoration of normal pituitary hormonal balance. Another important aspect is freedom from the secondary effects of pituitary disease, particularly pertinent in

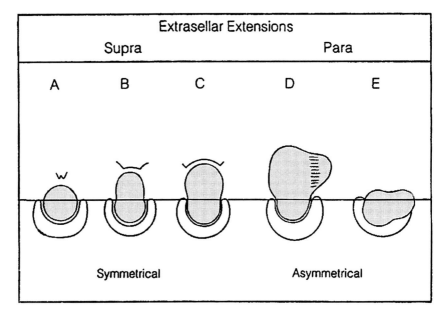

F IG . 22.1 Staging scheme for macroadenomas. Reproduced from Hardy (1979) with permission.

patients who have growth hormone or ACTH secreting pituitary tumors. Finally, freedom from recurrence is an important outcome measure, with major implications for subsequent management of the patient.

Medical Therapy

Effective medical therapy is available for some tumors (53, 59). This is certainly true of most prolactin secreting pituitary adenomas, and is sometimes true for growth hormone secreting tumors (50, 52, 59, 64, 66). The output of cortisol can be blocked with ketoconazole for patients with Cushing's disease, but this treatment has no effect on the underlying pathology (60). The major disadvantage of medical therapy is that

T ABLE 22.2
Therapeutic Goals for Pituitary Adenomas

- Increase survival
- Eliminate mass effect and reverse related signs and symptoms
- Normalize hormone hypersecretion and reverse secondary effects
- Preserve or recover normal pituitary function
- Prevent recurrence
- Provide histological confirmation and characterization

it is suppressive in nature, and the tumors often recur once medical treatment is discontinued. Surgical treatment therefore has long been the mainstay of management for most pituitary tumors.

Radiation Therapy

It has been recognized that many pituitary tumors, although remaining benign, have a tendency to recur. Postoperative radiation therapy has been employed on a fairly regular basis in order to treat residual tumor or to prevent recurrence (71). It has been demonstrated that conventional fractionated external beam radiation therapy is effective, both in lowering excess hormone production and, to a lesser extent, in preventing recurrence of pituitary tumors (55, 65). More recently, techniques of stereotactic radiotherapy and stereotactic radiosurgery (including gamma knife radiosurgery) have been applied to pituitary tumors (27, 28, 40, 48). Evidence is accumulating that these methods are effective in achieving both the goals of normalization of hormonal hypersecretion and prevention of recurrence (26, 32, 41).

Surgery

HISTORICAL PERSPECTIVES

The first successful transsphenoidal approaches in humans were reported in the period from 1907 until 1910 (9, 25, 33, 57, 67). Transsphenoidal surgery began with the direct approach through the nasal and frontal sinuses to the sella turcica. Surgical concepts rapidly evolved, and Kocher's submucosal approach was adopted by Dr. Harvey Cushing. Oskar Hirsch developed an endonasal submucosal approach very similar to what is used by many surgeons today (24). Transcranial approaches, via a subfrontal or pterional route, then became the vogue (10, 14, 23, 56). The transsphenoidal approach was resurrected and modernized beginning in the 1960s with the excellent and pioneering work of Drs. Gerard Guiot and Jules Hardy (15–17, 19, 21). Technical aspects continue to evolve in the 21st century with the introduction of endoscopic techniques and extended skull base approaches, along with various types of computer guided neuronavigation (5, 6, 11, 12, 22, 29–31, 34, 35, 37, 46, 58).

INDICATIONS FOR SURGERY

Surgical indications differ according to the type of tumor, presenting symptoms, and the impact upon the individual patient.

In nonfunctioning pituitary adenomas, most patients present with progressive headache, progressive visual loss, and progressive hypopituitarism. Each symptom is a potential indication for surgical management.

Urgent surgical intervention is indicated for pituitary apoplexy where there is either hemorrhage within a pre-existing nonfunctioning tumor or infarction and swelling of the tumor. Both of these phenomena may cause precipitous and profound adrenal insufficiency and sudden visual loss.

For growth hormone secreting pituitary tumors with acromegaly, surgery remains the first line treatment because it provides prompt relief of excess growth hormone secretion and interrupts the deleterious effects of this hormone on the cardiovascular system, the bones and joints, and upon glucose metabolism. Clearly those growth hormone secreting pituitary adenomas that present with mass effect are treated by surgery with the same indications as one considers for non-functioning tumors. When pituitary apoplexy occurs in the setting of a growth hormone secreting pituitary tumor with acromegaly, the same indication for urgent surgical relief applies.

The majority of prolactin secreting pituitary adenomas are effectively treated by one or another dopamine agonist medical strategies. Some patients with prolactin secreting pituitary tumors present with pituitary apoplexy and may require urgent surgical decompression. There are other categories of patients who are either intolerant of the side effects of dopamine agonist medication or have tumors that lack sufficient receptors to respond to medical treatment, and these individuals are candidates for surgical management.

In patients with ACTH secreting pituitary adenomas producing Cushing's disease, surgery again is a first line form of management. Surgery can immediately lower ACTH levels and normalize cortisol secretion. Some patients have very small lesions that might be treatable with radiation therapy, particularly with focused forms of stereotactic radiosurgery. However, the time period for normalization of ACTH is ordinarily more than 1 year. During this period the patient should continue suppressive medical therapy, usually with ketoconazole.

SURGICAL APPROACHES

Contemporary neurosurgeons use two basic surgical approaches for pituitary tumors, namely the transsphenoidal approach and the craniotomy approach.

Over the years the transsphenoidal approach has become refined and highly developed, and is a versatile and effective method for dealing with pituitary tumors and related lesions involving the sella turcica *(Tables 22.3 and 22.4)*. At the present time the routes of access for the transsphenoidal approach are sublabial transseptal, endonasal submucosal transseptal, direct endonasal with septal pushover, and endonasal endoscopic (6, 12, 29, 39, 42, 47, 70). The endoscope can also be

TABLE 22.3
Transsphenoidal surgery for Pituitary Disorders (1972–2000)

Diagnosis	Number of Patients (%) N=3529
Pituitary Adenoma	3093 (87.6)
Craniopharyngioma, Rathke's Cleft Cyst	132 (3.7)
Arachnoid cysts, Pars intermedia cyst, Colloid cyst	84 (2.4)
CSF Rhinorrhea	76 (2.2)
Hypophysitis	17 (0.5)
Hypophysectomy (Cancer, Diabetic Retinopathy)	22 (0.6)
Miscellaneous Sellar/Sphenoid Lesions	105 (3.0)

used as an adjunct with any of the other transsphenoidal approaches. Neuronavigational techniques using computer-guided systems have been developed and applied to the transsphenoidal approach and are occasionally used in addition to the traditional fluoroscopic guidance (11). Some pituitary tumor surgery has been effectively carried out in the intraoperative MRI scanner (3, 61). Extended transsphenoidal skull base approaches have been utilized for a number of large midline tumors, including pituitary adenomas, meningiomas and craniopharyngiomas (12, 22, 31, 35, 46).

Craniotomy is generally limited to those lesions that have major extension into the frontal or temporal fossa and those lesions wherein the pathology is uncertain. Some giant tumors are best approached using a craniotomy and there are occasional indications for a combined approach using both craniotomy and transsphenoidal routes of access.

Obviously the route of access chosen for craniotomy depends upon the anatomic features of the lesion to be treated, and its effect on the optic nerves and optic chiasm. In general, a subfrontal approach is highly effective for many tumors except for those where the optic chiasm is prefixed. Patients who have parasellar extensions in a lateral direction are

TABLE 22.4
Transsphenoidal Surgery for Adenomas: Case Summary (1972–2000)

Type of Adenoma	Number of Patients (%) N=3093
Functioning adenomas	
GH adenoma (Acromegaly)	537 (17.4)
PRL adenoma	889 (28.7)
ACTH adenoma (Cushing's disease)	490 (15.8)
Post-adrenalectomy ACTH adenoma (Nelson-Salassa syndrome)	65 (2.1)
TSH adenoma	39 (1.3)
Non-functioning adenomas	1073 (34.7)

often best treated by a pterional approach. This is particularly true for those lesions that expand into the cavernous sinus intracranially. A bifrontal interhemispheric approach may be utilized, and in some cases the addition of a transcallosal approach may be useful when tumors invade the third ventricle.

Regardless of the approach the goals of surgery remain the same, and the choice in many cases determines the efficacy of the outcome.

RESULTS AND OUTCOMES IN THE VARIOUS CATEGORIES OF PITUITARY TUMOR

When one considers outcomes for patients with nonfunctioning pituitary adenomas, one must consider relief of visual symptoms, preservation or restoration of normal pituitary function, relief of headache, and recurrence *(Table 22.5)*. Successful surgery for nonfunctioning pituitary adenomas should improve visual loss in approximately 87% of patients and vision should be stabilized in an additional 9%. In about 4% of cases there will be some visual loss as a result of the operation. The operative mortality for nonfunctioning adenomas is higher than most of the other categories because very large and invasive tumors are over-represented among the nonfunctioning lesions. In our experience the operative mortality rate has been less than 2% and is primarily related to intracranial hemorrhage or damage to intracranial structures. Hormonal secretion is normalized in approximately 20 to 30% of patients who have relative hypopituitarism prior to surgery. Hormonal replacement therapy is available for those patients who do not recover normal function.

Recurrence in the clinically nonfunctioning pituitary adenomas remains a significant problem, and increases with the length of follow-up. After about 10 years we have noted a 16% incidence of detectable per-

TABLE 22.5
Results of Surgery in Nonfunctioning Adenomas, 1972–2000

Outcome Measure	Incidence (%)
Vision	
Improved	87
Stabilized	9
Worsened	4
Relief of Headache	95
Operative Mortality	1.05
Normalization of preoperative hypopituitary status	27
Recurrence after 10 years	16
Requiring reoperation	6
Living and well (>10 years)	83

sistence or recurrence of the pituitary tumor. Most of these persistent/recurrent lesions remain relatively dormant, and only 6% of our patients have required additional surgical management for recurrent disease. On long-term (greater than 10 years) follow-up, 83% of our patients are living and well without evidence of disease.

For growth hormone secreting tumors associated with acromegaly, transsphenoidal surgery provides remission, as defined by rigorous endocrine criteria (normalization of IGF-1, random growth hormone less than 2.5 nanograms per milliliter, and nadir growth hormone during an OGTT of less than 1 nanogram per milliliter), in 70% of patients and is more reliably obtained in patients with microadenomas than those with macroadenomas *(Table 22.6)*. Preservation of normal pituitary function occurs in 97% of our patients. The recurrence rate, when one uses rigorous criteria for remission, is between 1 and 2%. On long-term (greater than 10 years) follow-up, when one includes those patients who had adjunctive therapy in the form of radiotherapy, radiosurgery, or octreotide treatment, 72% of patients are living and well without evidence of active disease.

Patients with prolactin secreting pituitary adenomas who are treated surgically represent a very difficult group. Ordinarily these patients have large invasive tumors and are for one reason or another unresponsive to medical management. Normalized prolactin levels occur in as high as 87% of patients with microadenomas, but normalization falls below 50% for those patients with invasive macroadenomas *(Table 22.7)*. The recurrence rate among those patients who are normalized after a transsphenoidal operation is 13% at 10 years. Combining this fact with the generally suboptimal outcome of those patients with giant, large, and invasive tumors, the long-term control rate is 65%. In this group of

TABLE 22.6
Results of Surgery in Growth Hormone Adenomas, 1972–2000

Outcome Measure	Incidence (%)
Disease remission*	
Microadenoma	88
Macroadenoma	65
Improvement in acromegalic symptoms	95
Relief of mass effect	95
Preserved normal pituitary function	97
Recurrence after 10 years	1.3
Living and well (>10 years)	72

*Remission criteria: GH<2.5 ng/ml (basal), nadir GH<1.0 ng/ml during OGTT, normal IGF-1

TABLE 22.7
Results of Surgery in Prolactinomas, 1972–2000

Outcome Measure	Incidence (%)
Disease remission	
Microadenoma	87
Macroadenoma	56
Relief of mass effect	95
Preserved normal pituitary function	97
Recurrence after 10 years	13
Living and well (>10 years) (normal PRL)	65

patients preservation of normal pituitary function has reliably occurred in 97%. Unfortunately, the response to radiation therapy and stereotactic radiosurgery in patients with large invasive prolactin secreting pituitary tumors has been poor.

For the ACTH tumors associated with Cushing's disease, surgery has been highly effective when the lesion treated is a microadenoma *(Table 22.8)*. We have achieved a 91% remission rate when a pituitary microadenoma is detected and removed. Approximately 65% of patients with larger pituitary adenomas secreting ACTH (macroadenomas) are able to achieve initial remission. The 10-year recurrence rate for patients with Cushing's disease has been 12%, and is primarily related to recurrence of tumors that are invasive of dura or the cavernous sinus. Radiosurgery has been an effective adjunct for patients who either fail to obtain remission from transsphenoidal surgery or who develop recurrences; some 68% of patients treated with Gamma Knife radiosurgery in this situation achieve ultimate remission.

For ACTH secreting pituitary tumors in Nelson's syndrome, the outlook is not encouraging. These are usually invasive tumors and often

TABLE 22.8
Results of Surgery in Cushing's Disease, 1972–2000

Outcome Measure	Incidence (%)
Disease remission	
Microadenoma	91
Macroadenoma	65
Relief of mass effect	95
Preserved normal pituitary function	97
Recurrence after 10 years	
Adults	12
Children	42
Living and well (>10 years)	75

are macroadenomas. They have lost the suppressive feedback from adrenal production of cortisol, and are relatively unrestrained. The success rate as measured by initial normalization of serum ACTH levels is approximately 50%. The 10-year recurrence rate for these tumors has been quite high, approaching 24%, and the response to radiation therapy and radiosurgery has likewise been poor.

COMPLICATIONS OF TRANSSPHENOIDAL SURGERY

A discussion of complications should probably focus on the transsphenoidal operation, as craniotomy is done infrequently and for unusually difficult problems. Mortality rates for transsphenoidal surgery have been approximately 0.5 to 1.5% and major morbidity consisting of spinal fluid leak, meningitis, strokes, intracranial hemorrhage, damage to intracranial vessels, and visual loss combined has amounted to approximately 3.5%. Minor complications can occur in the form of sinus disease, nasal septal perforations, epistaxis and wound problems, but these are infrequent and their incidence amounts to no more than 5%. Risk factors for complications include prior surgery or radiation therapy, patients who have a debilitating disease, including cardiovascular disease, cerebrovascular disease, and diabetes mellitus, and patients who have large vascular and invasive tumors. Obviously these categories of patients should be carefully considered, and every adjunct to improve the safety and efficacy of surgical management should be utilized.

CONCLUSION

Significant advances continue to be made in both the scientific and technical aspects of the management of pituitary tumors. Surgery will remain a major form of effective management, and neurosurgeons who treat pituitary tumors will continue to advance our understanding of the intricacies of these fascinating lesions.

REFERENCES

1. Annegers JF, Coulam CB, Abboud CF, Laws ER, Jr., Kurland LT: Pituitary adenoma in Olmsted County, Minnesota, 1935–1977. A report of an increasing incidence of diagnosis in women of childbearing age. **Mayo Clin Proc** 53:641–643, 1978.
2. Black PM: Brain tumors. Part 1 [see comments]. **N Engl J Med** 324:1471–1476, 1991.
3. Black PM, Alexander E, 3rd, Martin C, Moriarty T, Nabavi A, Wong TZ, Schwartz RB, Jolesz F: Craniotomy for tumor treatment in an intraoperative magnetic resonance imaging unit [see comments]. **Neurosurgery** 45:423–431; discussion 431–423, 1999.
4. Burrow GN, Wortzman G, Rewcastle NB, Holgate RC, Kovacs K: Microadenomas of the pituitary and abnormal sellar tomograms in an unselected autopsy series. **N Engl J Med** 304:156–158, 1981.

5. Bushe KA, Halves E: [Modified technique in transsphenoidal operations of pituitary adenomas. Technical note (author's transl)]. **Acta Neurochir (Wien)** 41:163–175, 1978.

6. Carrau RL, Jho HD, Ko Y: Transnasal-transsphenoidal endoscopic surgery of the pituitary gland. **Laryngoscope** 106:914–918, 1996.

7. Clayton RN: Sporadic pituitary tumours: from epidemiology to use of databases. **Best Pract Res Clin Endocrinol Metab** 13:451–460, 1999.

8. Costello RT: Subclinical adenoma of the pituitary gland. **Am J Pathol** 12:205–216, 1936.

9. Cushing H: Partial hypophysectomy for acromegaly. **Ann Surg** 50:1002–1017, 1909.

10. Dandy WE: A new hypophysis operation. **Bull Johns Hopkins Hosp** 29:154, 1918.

11. Elias WJ, Chadduck JB, Alden TD, Laws ER, Jr.: Frameless stereotaxy for transsphenoidal surgery [see comments]. **Neurosurgery** 45:271–275; discussion 275–277, 1999.

12. Fahlbusch R, Thapar K: New developments in pituitary surgical techniques. **Best Pract Res Clin Endocrinol Metab** 13:471–484, 1999.

13. Fan KJ, Pezeshkpour GH: Ethnic distribution of primary central nervous system tumors in Washington, DC, 1971 to 1985. **J Natl Med Assoc** 84:858–863, 1992.

14. Frazier CH: An approach to the hypophysis through the anterior cranial fossa. **Ann Surg** 57, 1913.

15. Guiot G, Bouche J, Oproiu A: [Indications of the trans-sphenoidal approach to pituitary adenomas. Experience with 165 operations]. **Presse Med** 75:1563–1568, 1967.

16. Guiot G, Derome P: [Indications for trans-sphenoid approach in neurosurgery. 521 cases]. **Ann Med Interne (Paris)** 123:703–712, 1972.

17. Hardy J: [Surgery of the pituitary gland, using the trans-sphenoidal approach. Comparative study of 2 technical methods]. **Union Med Can** 96:702–712, 1967.

18. Hardy J: Transphenoidal microsurgery of the normal and pathological pituitary. **Clin Neurosurg** 16:185–217, 1969.

19. Hardy J: Transsphenoidal hypophysectomy. **J Neurosurg** 34:582–594, 1971.

20. Hardy J, Somma M: Acromegaly: Surgical tratment by transsphenoidal microsurgical removal of the pituitary adenoma, in Tindall GT, Collins WF (eds): *Clinical Management of Pituitary Disorders.* New York, Raven Press, 1979, pp 209–217.

21. Hardy J, Wigser SM: Trans-sphenoidal surgery of pituitary fossa tumors with televised radiofluoroscopic control. **J Neurosurg** 23:612–619, 1965.

22. Hashimoto N, Handa H, Yamagami T: Transsphenoidal extracapsular approach to pituitary tumors. **J Neurosurg** 64:16–20, 1986.

23. Heuer GJ: Surgical experiences with an intracranial approach to chiasmal lesions. **Arch Surg** 1:369, 1920.

24. Hirsch O: Endonasal method of removal of hypohyseal tumors. **JAMA** 5:772–774, 1910.

25. Hochenegg J: Operat geheilte Akromegalie bei Hypophysentumor. **Verh Dtsch Ges Chir** 37:80–85, 1908.

26. Inoue HK, Kohga H, Hirato M, Sasaki T, Ishihara J, Shibazaki T, Ohye C, Andou Y: Pituitary adenomas treated by microsurgery with or without Gamma Knife surgery: experience in 122 cases. **Stereotact Funct Neurosurg** 72:125–131, 1999.

27. Jackson IM, Noren G: Gamma knife radiosurgery for pituitary tumours. **Best Pract Res Clin Endocrinol Metab** 13:461–469, 1999.

28. Jackson IM, Noren G: Role of gamma knife therapy in the management of pituitary tumors. **Endocrinol Metab Clin North Am** 28:133 142, 1999.

29. Jankowski R, Auque J, Simon C, Marchal JC, Hepner H, Wayoff M: Endoscopic pituitary tumor surgery. **Laryngoscope** 102:198–202, 1992.

30. Jho HD, Carrau RL: Endoscopic endonasal transsphenoidal surgery: experience with 50 patients. **J Neurosurg** 87:44–51, 1997.

31. Kato T, Sawamura Y, Abe H, Nagashima M: Transsphenoidal-transtuberculum sellae approach for supradiaphragmatic tumours: Technical note. **Acta Neurochir (Wien)** 140:715–718; discussion 719, 1998.

32. Kim MS, Lee SI, Sim JH: Gamma Knife radiosurgery for functioning pituitary microadenoma. **Stereotact Funct Neurosurg** 72:119–124, 1999.

33. Kocher T: Ein Fall von Hypophysis-Tumor mit operativer Heilung. **Dtsch Z Mund Kiefer Gesichtschir** 100:13–37, 1909.

34. Koren I, Hadar T, Rappaport ZH, Yaniv E: Endoscopic transnasal transsphenoidal microsurgery versus the sublabial approach for the treatment of pituitary tumors: endonasal complications. **Laryngoscope** 109:1838–1840, 1999.

35. Kouri JG, Chen MY, Watson JC, Oldfield EH: Resection of suprasellar tumors by using a modified transsphenoidal approach. Report of four cases. **J Neurosurg** 92:1028–1035, 2000.

36. Kuratsu J, Ushio Y: Epidemiological study of primary intracranial tumors: A regional survey in Kumamoto Prefecture in the southern part of Japan. **J Neurosurg** 84:946–950, 1996.

37. Laws ER, Jr.: Transsphenoidal microsurgery in the management of craniopharyngioma. **J Neurosurg** 52:661–666, 1980.

38. Laws ER, Jr., Thapar K: Brain tumors. **CA Cancer J Clin** 43:263–271, 1993.

39. Laws ER, Jr., Thapar K: Pituitary surgery. **Endocrinol Metab Clin North Am** 28:119–131, 1999.

40. Laws ER, Jr., Vance ML: Radiosurgery for pituitary tumors and craniopharyngiomas. **Neurosurg Clin N Am** 10:327–336, 1999.

41. Lillehei KO, Kirschman DL, Kleinschmidt-DeMasters BK, Ridgway EC: Reassessment of the role of radiation therapy in the treatment of endocrine-inactive pituitary macroadenomas. **Neurosurgery** 43:432–438; discussion 438–439, 1998.

42. Liston SL, Siegel LG, Thienprasit P, Gregory R: Nasal endoscopes in hypophysectomy [letter]. **J Neurosurg** 66:155, 1987.

43. Lopez-Gonzalez MA, Sotelo J: Brain tumors in Mexico: Characteristics and prognosis of glioblastoma. **Surg Neurol** 53:157–162, 2000.

44. Lovaste MG, Ferrari G, Rossi G: Epidemiology of primary intracranial neoplasms. Experiment in the Province of Trento, (Italy), 1977–1984. **Neuroepidemiology** 5:220–232, 1986.

45. Mahaley MS, Jr., Mettlin C, Natarajan N, Laws ER, Jr., Peace BB: National survey of patterns of care for brain-tumor patients. **J Neurosurg** 71:826–836, 1989.

46. Mason RB, Nieman LK, Doppman JL, Oldfield EH: Selective excision of adenomas originating in or extending into the pituitary stalk with preservation of pituitary function [see comments]. **J Neurosurg** 87:343–351, 1997.

47. Matula C, Tschabitscher M, Day JD, Reinprecht A, Koos WT: Endoscopically assisted microneurosurgery. **Acta Neurochir (Wien)** 134:190–195, 1995.

48. Mitsumori M, Shrieve DC, Alexander E, 3rd, Kaiser UB, Richardson GE, Black PM, Loeffler JS: Initial clinical results of LINAC-based stereotactic radiosurgery and stereotactic radiotherapy for pituitary adenomas. **Int J Radiat Oncol Biol Phys** 42:573–580, 1998.

49. Mohr G, Hardy J, Comtois R, Beauregard H: Surgical management of giant pituitary adenomas. **Can J Neurol Sci** 17:62–66, 1990.

50. Molitch ME, Thorner MO, Wilson C: Management of prolactinomas. **J Clin Endocrinol Metab** 82:996–1000, 1997.
51. Monson JP: The epidemiology of endocrine tumours. **Endocr Rel Ca** 7:29–36, 2000.
52. Newman CB: Medical therapy for acromegaly. **Endocrinol Metab Clin North Am** 28:171–190, 1999.
53. Orrego JJ, Barkan AL: Pituitary disorders. Drug treatment options. **Drugs** 59:93–106, 2000.
54. Percy AK, Elveback LR, Okazaki H, Kurland LT: Neoplasms of the central nervous system. Epidemiologic considerations. **Neurology** 22:40–48, 1972.
55. Powell JS, Wardlaw SL, Post KD, Freda PU: Outcome of radiotherapy for acromegaly using normalization of insulin-like growth factor I to define cure [comment]. **J Clin Endocrinol Metab** 85:2068–2071, 2000.
56. Ray BS: Hypophysectomy by craniotomy, in Youmans JR (ed): *Neurological Surgery.* Philadelphia, Saunders, Vol 3. 1973, pp 1915–1927.
57. Schloffer H: Erfolgreiche Operationen eines Hypophentamors auf Nasalem Wage. **Wien Klin Wochenschr** 20:621–624, 1907.
58. Sheehan MT, Atkinson JL, Kasperbauer JL, Erickson BJ, Nippoldt TB: Preliminary comparison of the endoscopic transnasal vs the sublabial transseptal approach for clinically nonfunctioning pituitary macroadenomas. **Mayo Clin Proc** 74:661–670, 1999.
59. Shimon I, Melmed S: Management of pituitary tumors. **Ann Intern Med** 129:472–483, 1998.
60. Sonino N, Boscaro M: Medical therapy for Cushing's disease. **Endocrinol Metab Clin North Am** 28:211–222, 1999.
61. Sutherland GR, Louw DF: Intraoperative MRI: A moving magnet. **CMAJ** 161:1293, 1999.
62. Thapar K, Kovacs K, Laws ER: The classification and molecular biology of pituitary adenomas. **Adv Tech Stand Neurosurg** 22:3–53, 1995.
63. Tomita T, Gates E: Pituitary adenomas and granular cell tumors. Incidence, cell type, and location of tumor in 100 pituitary glands at autopsy. **Am J Clin Pathol** 111:817–825, 1999.
64. Trainer PJ, Drake WM, Katznelson L, Freda PU, Herman-Bonert V, van der Lely AJ, Dimaraki EV, Stewart PM, Friend KE, Vance ML, Besser GM, Scarlett JA, Thorner MO, Parkinson C, Klibanski A, Powell JS, Barkan AL, Sheppard MC, Malsonado M, Rose DR, Clemmons DR, Johannsson G, Bengtsson BA, Stavrou S, Kleinberg DL, Cook DM, Phillips LS, Bidlingmaier M, Strasburger CJ, Hackett S, Zib K, Bennett WF, Davis RJ: Treatment of acromegaly with the growth hormone-receptor antagonist pegvisomant [see comments]. **N Engl J Med** 342:1171–1177, 2000.
65. Tsang RW, Brierley JD, Panzarella T, Gospodarowicz MK, Sutcliffe SB, Simpson WJ: Role of radiation therapy in clinical hormonally-active pituitary adenomas. **Radiother Oncol** 41:45–53, 1996.
66. Vance ML, Harris AG: Long-term treatment of 189 acromegalic patients with the somatostatin analog octreotide. Results of the International Multicenter Acromegaly Study Group. **Arch Intern Med** 151:1573–1578, 1991.
67. von Eiselsberg A: The operative cure of acromegaly by removal of a hypophysial tumor. **Ann Surg** 48:781–783, 1908.
68. Walker AE, Robins M, Weinfeld FD: Epidemiology of brain tumors: the national survey of intracranial neoplasms. **Neurology** 35:219–226, 1985.
69. Wen-qing H, Shi-ju Z, Qing-sheng T, Jian-qing H, Yu-xia L, Qing zhong X, Zi-jun L,

Wen-cui Z: Statistical analysis of central nervous system tumors in China. **J Neurosurg** 56:555–564, 1982.
70. Wilson WR, Laws ER, Jr.: Transnasal septal displacement approach for secondary transsphenoidal pituitary surgery. **Laryngoscope** 102:951–953, 1992.
71. Zaugg M, Adaman O, Pescia R, Landolt AM: External irradiation of macroinvasive pituitary adenomas with telecobalt: a retrospective study with long-term follow-up in patients irradiated with doses mostly of between 40–45 Gy. **Int J Radiat Oncol Biol Phys** 32:671–680, 1995.

CHAPTER

23

Small Skull Base Meningiomas

Surgical Management

ROBERT D. STRANG, M.D., AND OSSAMA AL-MEFTY, M.D.

INTRODUCTION

Meningiomas represent 15 to 32% of all primary intracranial neoplasms and have an annual incidence of 2.3 to 3.8 per 100,000 population (19, 24, 26, 28). They are generally benign lesions arising from arachnoidal meningothelial cells (6, 29) and are intimately involved with the dural coverings of the central nervous system. Although they may be found anywhere along these coverings, nearly half of meningiomas are found at the cranial base (11, 29). Ever since the classic monograph by Cushing and Eisenhardt in 1938 describing the classification, clinical behavior, and surgical results of meningiomas, surgical resection has been established as the treatment modality of choice for these neoplasms. The management of skull base meningiomas, however, had been associated with higher morbidity rates in early surgical series, but the advent of advanced cranial base techniques has improved the safety and efficacy of surgical treatment of these lesions.

The cranial base is an intricate region that represents a coalescence of important osseous, vascular, and neurological structures including the carotid artery, the brainstem, and all of the cranial nerves. Because of the region's complexity, even benign and slow growing neoplasms such as meningiomas can cause neurological deficits when they are quite small. Clearly, larger lesions presenting with mass effect, brainstem compression, or progressive neurological deficit should be treated with surgical resection. For small asymptomatic meningiomas, close follow-up with serial neurological assessments and neuroimaging is a valid treatment option, particularly in the older patient or those with significant medical co-morbidities. However, there is considerable controversy regarding the optimal treatment of patients with small, symptomatic skull base meningiomas. Proposed treatment modalities for the latter group include surgical resection, fractionated radiotherapy, radiosurgery, or a combination thereof. For most in this group, the option of careful follow-up is not an attractive one because without some sort of intervention, there is little hope of improving their symptoms or halting the progression of the disease to avoid further, potentially debilitating, deficits. This presentation will focus on the role of surgical resection in the management of small, symptomatic skull base meningiomas.

When discussing skull base meningiomas, the designation of "small" is somewhat relative and arbitrary. By virtue of their location in a place that, neuroanatomically, is not tolerant of even minor volumetric displacements, skull base meningiomas tend to become symptomatic at a much earlier stage than do their convexity counterparts. For this reason, lesions that might be considered small at the convexity, may, in fact, be considered quite large when they occur at the skull base. To be considered small, a skull base meningioma should meet several basic, albeit subjective, criteria. First, the lesion should not be large enough to present with mass effect or brainstem compression. Second, the tumor should not be of such size that, if it were asymptomatic, its size would prohibit conservative management with serial follow-up. Finally, the lesion should be of a size that would not exclude it from radiosurgical treatment on the basis of dimensions alone. We have arbitrarily assigned the designation of "small" to those skull base meningiomas that measure ≤ 2.5 cm in greatest diameter. Most meningiomas meeting this size constraint will also meet the aforementioned criteria.

CLINICAL FEATURES

Some skull base meningiomas may present with a constellation of signs and symptoms that are characteristic, if not, pathognomonic for such lesions based on a particular location. Tuberculum sella meningiomas classically present with the "chiasmal syndrome" which consists of primary optic atrophy and bitemporal visual field deficits. These meningiomas arise from the tuberculum sella, the chiasmatic sulcus or the diaphragma sella and, as such, are intimately involved with the optic nerves and chiasm. This close relationship explains why patients with tuberculum sella meningiomas present with visual loss even early in the disease process. Such immediate proximity to the optic apparatus makes these lesions ideal candidates for microsurgical resection over any other form of treatment, including stereotactic radiosurgery *(Fig. 23.1)*.

Clinoidal meningiomas arise from the region of the anterior clinoid process. Based on their point of origin, three distinct types have been described (1). Type I clinoidal meningiomas originate from the inferomedial aspect of the anterior clinoid process. In this region, as the internal carotid artery emerges from the cavernous sinus, it is devoid of

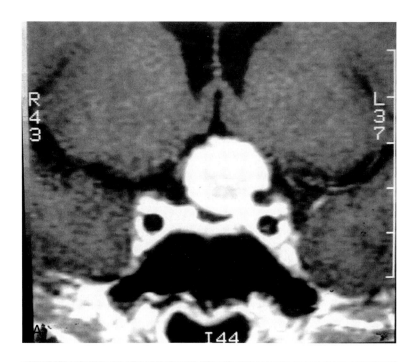

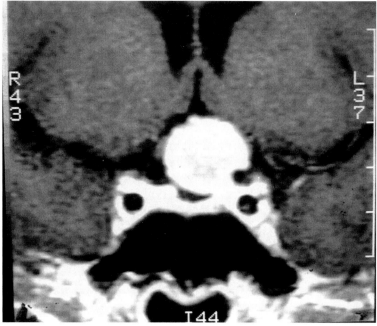

B

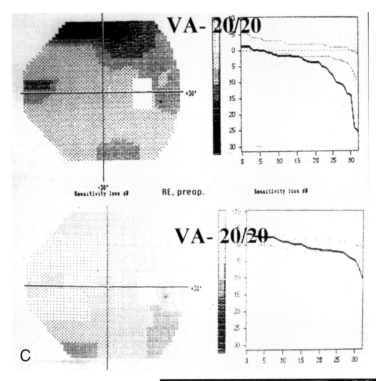

C

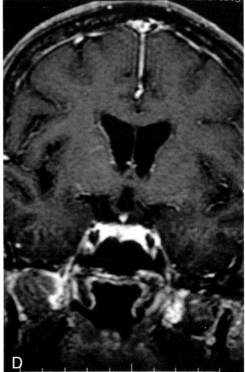

D

FIG. 23.1 (*A*) Enhanced, coronal T1-weighted MRI in a patient with a tuberculum sella meningioma and severely compromised vision. (*B*) Following complete microsurgical resection, there was dramatic improvement in vision. Preoperative (top) and postoperative (bottom) ophthalmologic examinations revealed remarkable improvement of visual field and visual acuity in the left eye. (*C*) Similar changes were also seen on the right. (*D*) Enhanced, coronal T1-weighted MRI demonstrates no evidence of recurrence at 3-year follow-up. Note that the optic chiasm has returned to its normal position and the pituitary stalk has been preserved.

an arachnoidal covering (40). Type I clinoidal meningiomas may, therefore, adhere densely to or even invade the carotid artery, making complete surgical resection complicated. Type II clinoidal meningiomas, on the other hand, do not tend to involve the carotid artery to this degree. They arise from the superior or lateral surface of the anterior clinoid process and do not contact the artery until after it has become invested in the arachnoid of the carotid cistern. An arachnoid plane persists between tumor and artery and complete extirpation becomes quite feasible using microsurgical technique even when the artery is completely encased. Type III clinoidal meningiomas originate at the optic foramen and may extend bi-directionally to involve the optic canal and the anterior clinoid process. In this tumor type, there is usually an arachnoid plane between the tumor and vascular structures, but such a barrier separating the mass from the optic nerve may be absent. The proximity of tumor origin in all three types of clinoidal meningiomas explains why these lesions may present with unilateral visual disturbances even when they are quite small. Additionally, this spatial arrangement makes radiotherapy and radiosurgery unattractive treatment options for these lesions.

Cavernous sinus meningiomas can be quite complex in origin and configuration. They include both tumors that arise from the cavernous sinus directly, and those that grow to secondarily involve it. Although proptosis may be present in larger lesions, smaller meningiomas of the cavernous sinus usually present with some form of oculomotor dysfunction or facial paresthesias (12, 25).

Meningiomas arising in the region of Meckel's cave can vary greatly in their extent. Like meningiomas involving the cavernous sinus, Meckel's cave meningiomas include both tumors that arise from Meckel's cave itself as well as those arising from adjacent structures that grow to secondarily involve it. Although some of these lesions will be confined to Meckel's cave, many will grow to extend into the posterior and/or the middle cranial fossae. Predictably, the most common presentation of these lesions involves trigeminal nerve dysfunction. Trigeminal hypesthesia and neuralgia are seen most frequently, but atypical facial pain and headache are also common (30).

CASE MATERIAL

In a preliminary review of our cases from 1983 to 2000, we have identified 629 cases of skull base meningiomas treated by the senior surgeon (OAM). Of these 629 tumors, 67 (10.7%) were found that measured ≤ 2.5 cm in maximal diameter and were symptomatic. An analysis of these 67 lesions revealed that all met the criteria for "small" as set forth above. By far, the most common presentations were related to cranial neuropathy, although seizure, headaches, and dizziness were also seen. Twenty-eight (42%) of the small, symptomatic skull base meningiomas were treated by surgical resection with gross total removal being the goal at the outset. Complete follow-up information was available for all of the cases. Average follow-up period for operated cases was 44.4 months with a range of 1 to120 months. Thirty-nine lesions (58%) were treated nonoperatively. The average follow-up period for this group was 47.3 months with a range of 1 to84 months. For the purposes of this discussion, we would like to employ the terms "S-knife" for lesions treated by surgical intervention and "N-knife" for lesions managed nonsurgically. This terminology is by no means intended as disparaging nomenclature, but rather it is meant to stress the fact that nonoperative management (N-knife) is, indeed, a treatment modality of its own.

In the S-knife treated group, the location of meningiomas was quite diverse and covered essentially the entire skull base. The locations of the tumors are summarized in *Table 23.1*. Five tumors (18%) involved the petroclival region. The sphenoid wing, cavernous sinus, jugular foramen, and tentorium were each affected by 3 tumors (11%). The cerebellopontine angle, foramen magnum, tuberculum sella, and Meckel's cave were each involved twice (7%), and one meningioma (3.5%) was found at the planum sphenodale, the anterior clinoid process, and the sphenopetroclival region. This distribution is similar to that seen in other surgical and radiosurgical series (8, 13, 15, 17, 18, 23, 36, 38). The most common clinical presentation was related to cranial neuropathy (*Table 23.2*). In all, 36 cranial nerves were affected in 28 patients. There

TABLE 23.1
Tumor location in S-knife series

Tumor Location	No. of Patients
Petroclival	5
Sphenoid wing	3
Cavernous sinus	3
Jugular foramen	3
Tentorium	3
Cerebellopontine angle	2
Foramen magnum	2
Tuberculum sella	2
Meckel's cave	2
Planum sphenoidale	1
Clinoidal	1
Sphenopetroclival	1
Total	28

TABLE 23.2
Clinical Findings in S-knife series

Clinical findings in 28 patients	No. Affected
Cranial Neuropathy	36
Optic	8
Oculomotor	5
Trigeminal	8
Abducens	7
Acoustic	3
Lower cranial neuropathy	5
Headache	4
Dizziness	2
Seizures	1

were 8 visual field or acuity changes (22%); 5 oculomotor nerve palsies (14%); 8 (22%) disturbances of trigeminal nerve function (5 dysesthesias, 3 pain); 7 abducens palsies (19%); 3 hearing loss (8%); and 5 lower cranial neuropathies (14%). In addition to cranial neuropathy, some patients were also affected by headache (4 patients), dizziness (2 patients), and seizures (1 patient).

As in the S-knife treated group, there was diversity of tumor location in the N-knife treated group. These results are summarized in *Table 23.3*. The majority of tumors in this group involved the cavernous sinus (10, 26%), the petroclival region (9, 23%), and the anterior clinoid process (5, 13%). The cerebellopontine angle and the tentorium were each affected by 4 tumors (10% each). There were 3 olfactory groove meningiomas (7.7%) and the sphenoid wing, clivus, orbit, and foramen magnum were each involved once (2.5% each). The clinical findings in

TABLE 23.3
Tumor location in N-Knife series

Tumor Location	No. of Patients
Cavernous sinus	10
Petroclival	9
Clinoidal	5
Cerebellopontine angle	4
Tentorium	4
Olfactory groove	3
Sphenoid wing	1
Clivus	1
Orbit	1
Foramen magnum	1
Total	39

TABLE 23.4
Clinical Findings in N-knife series

Clinical findings in 39 patients	No. Affected
Subjective visual changes	3
Mild ptosis	2
Cranial Neuropathy (total)	16
Trochlear	2
Trigeminal	6
Abducens	3
Acoustic	3
Lower cranial neuropathy	2

this group can be found in *Table 23.4.* There were 3 patients with subjective, intermittent visual changes, and 2 with mild ptosis that was not bothersome. Two patients had trochlear neuropathies, 5 had facial numbness, 1 had facial pain, 3 had abducens palsies, 3 had some hearing loss, and 2 had mild swallowing difficulties.

Serial CT or MRI scans and follow-up neurological exams were performed on all patients in the S-knife and N-knife groups. The median follow-up period after surgery was 44.4 months (ranging from 1 to 120 months) for the S-knife treated group and 47.3 months (ranging from 1 to 84 months) for the N-knife group. There was no mortality or major morbidity in either group. In the S-knife series, complete surgical resection of the tumor was achieved in 21 patients (75%). Of the remaining 7 patients with incomplete resection, 6 had meningiomas arising from either the cavernous sinus or petroclival region. None of the 21 patients in whom complete surgical resection was achieved had signs of clinical or radiographic recurrence during the follow-up period. Five of the 7 patients with residual tumor had evidence of tumor growth at 22 to 108 months. Preoperatively 36 cranial nerves in the S-knife treated group were affected. Following tumor resection, 4 were worse at least temporarily and there were 5 new deficits (2 have resolved). In this group's 28 patients, 10 cranial nerves have demonstrated improved function. In the N-knife series, slight volumetric increases were noted in 4 tumors and the remaining 35 demonstrated no evidence of growth. No patient in this group has either progressed clinically or required subsequent surgical intervention *(Fig. 23.2)*. Based on criteria set forth by Kondziolka et al. (17), this results in a clinical tumor control rate of 100%.

ROLE OF RADIATION TREATMENT IN THE MANAGEMENT OF MENINGIOMAS

Microsurgical resection of meningiomas and their dural attachments has been considered the gold standard for the treatment of these le-

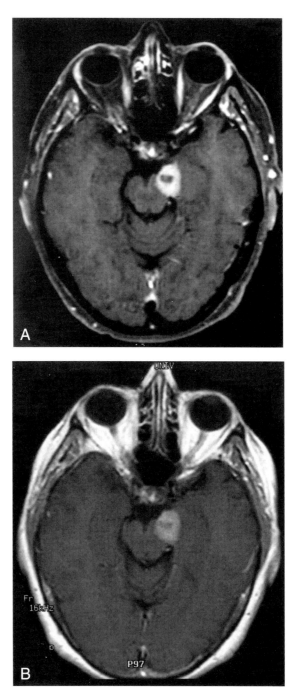

FIG. 23.2 (A) An "N-knife" treated patient with a tentorial meningioma. (B)At 5-year follow-up, there has been no significant change in the size or configuration of the lesion.

sions. This is particularly true in cases of larger lesions where immediate decompression of the neural elements is required. However, some meningiomas, especially those arising from the cranial base, have been considered high risk or inoperable based on location alone. Consequently, several new treatment options, including radiotherapy and radiosurgery, have been introduced. It is important to point out, however, that anatomy-based microneurosurgery (40) and the development of advanced skull base techniques (1, 2, 5, 9, 16, 26, 31, 33, 34, 37) have led not only to a greater understanding of these lesions, but also to increasingly improved outcomes.

Conventional fractionated external-beam radiation therapy has been available on a large scale longer than radiosurgery and, therefore, enjoys longer follow-up in the treatment of benign skull base meningiomas. Its implementation began primarily as an adjunctive treatment to surgical resection in those lesions where complete resection had not been achieved. Nutting et al. have one of the largest series with a 10-year follow-up (24). They found the 5- and 10-year progression free survival (PFS) rates to be 92% and 83% respectively. The only independent prognostic factor for tumor control was location. The most favorable location was the parasellar region with a 90% 10-year PFS compared to only a 69% 10-year PFS for tumors originating along the sphenoid ridge. These results compare favorably with early radiosurgical literature, and therefore, this study may be used as a baseline in evaluating the efficacy of newer treatment modalities. However, the importance of even longer follow-up periods cannot be overstated. Radiation therapy does not result in the cure of skull base meningiomas, but rather it delays their symptomatic recurrence. Mathiesen et al. found that while the 10-year mortality rate was lower in patients treated with radiation therapy, there was no difference in survival at 20-year follow-up (21). They, therefore, concluded that the role of radiation therapy in the management of skull base meningiomas is one of palliation in unresectable tumors.

Although radiotherapy has been reported to result in fewer cranial neuropathies than radiosurgery (24), it has the distinct disadvantage of including nondiseased neural structures in the treatment plan. This may not be as much a concern in the treatment of malignant disease, but the serious long-term side effects of radiation therapy in the treatment of benign brain tumors has been well documented (3, 32). Therefore, stereotactic delivery of high-dose ionizing radiation in single fractions (radiosurgery) has been regarded as an attractive alternative to conventional radiotherapy as an adjunct to or replacement for microsurgical resection. In contrast to surgical resection, the treatment goal of radiosurgery is not eradication of the tumor, but rather "tumor control." The definition of this ideal varies between reports. Some define "progression free survival (PFS)" or "control" as lack of tumor growth (8, 10, 13, 18, 23); others use a measure of "clinical tumor control" as defined by no requirement for surgical resection (17). Based on these definitions, radiosurgical series report control rates ranging from 98 to100% for short-term follow-up of 2 years (8, 13). This control drops to 92 to95% at 35 months and 86.7% at 96 months (23, 36). These results must, however, be interpreted with caution given the natural history and slow growth of meningiomas. During an average follow-up period of 47 months, Olivero et al. found that only 22% of meningiomas demonstrated any detectable growth on neuroimaging (27). The growth rate ranged from 0.2 cm over 180 months to 1 cm over 12 months and all patients remained asymptomatic. This translates to a PFS rate of 78% and a clinical control rate of 100% for these untreated lesions over the 47-month follow-up period. Indeed, our own N-knife series shows similar results with a 90% PFS rate and a 100% clinical control rate over 47.3 months. It, therefore, remains unclear which meningiomas have realistically benefited from radiosurgery and which have merely followed the natural course of a slow-growing, histologically benign lesion. Perhaps for this reason, the radiosurgical literature has begun reporting tumor shrinkage rates with increasing frequency. Depending on the length of follow-up, decreased tumor volume has been reported in 23 to 68% of radiosurgically treated meningiomas (8, 13, 17, 23, 36). However, it remains clear that the goal of radiosurgery is tumor control and not reduction of tumor volume. This is especially relevant since reduction in tumor size does not necessarily correlate with improvement of clinical symptoms; nor does early tumor shrinkage portend long-term tumor control (17, 23, 39). Moreover, the cytoreductive effect of radiosurgery cannot match the outcomes of microsurgery, which, for any S-knife series, will result in tumor volume reduction rates of 100%.

PITFALLS OF RADIOSURGERY

The concept of radiosurgery as a minimally invasive treatment option compared with open microsurgical resection has also been enticing. Certainly, in the short term, the effects of radiosurgery are far less evident than those seen with open surgery; this is true for both its desired results as well as its complications. This philosophy is particularly important to heed when treating meningiomas because extended survivals are reasonable to expect by virtue of their slow-growing, benign nature. Some of the earlier radiosurgical literature reported significant neurological morbidity associated with treatment. Engenhart and colleagues reported delayed brain edema and radiation necrosis in 38% of patients (15). This was probably secondary to considerably higher maximum doses to tumor volume than those that are currently in use today. Over the past decade, significant advances in treatment planning, neuroimaging, and software applications have allowed for safer delivery of radiosurgical doses. In current studies, the rates of brain edema and radiation necrosis have dropped to 6 to7% (8,18). Nevertheless, despite recent advances, the neurological morbidity from radiosurgical treatment of meningiomas remains significant *(Fig. 23.3)*. Present series report treatment related neurological deficits in 8.8 to 19.4% of patients (13, 17, 23, 36, 38). The majority of deficits were related to cranial neuropathy and many patients were affected more than once. Clearly, radiosurgery should not be considered as noninvasive, and patients need to be counseled as to the potential risks and benefits of this and other treatment modalities prior to definitive management.

ADVANTAGES OF MICROSURGERY

It may be argued that microsurgical resection of small symptomatic skull base meningiomas has several distinct advantages over radiosurgery as a primary treatment option. First, microsurgical resection offers the possibility of obtaining tissue for definitive histological diagnosis. Although some have considered meningiomas to have highly characteristic, if not pathognomonic, features on neuroimaging, the literature is replete with reports of various lesions mimicking meningiomas. Cavernous malformations, metastatic lesions, lymphoma, hemangiopericytoma, and inflammatory lesions are among the possible diseases that may resemble skull base meningiomas (4, 14, 25). It is imperative that the correct diagnosis be made because most nonmeningiomatous skull base lesions have better operative outcomes with a greater potential for total resection and cranial nerve recovery when compared to meningiomas (14). Perhaps more importantly, some disease processes, such as sarcoidosis, do not respond to radiosurgery. Treatment with this modality may result in diagnostic delays and, thus, delays in the delivery of definitive care. Even when meningioma is, in fact, the correct diagnosis, it must be remembered that only 90% are considered truly benign (28, 29). The remaining 10% are made up of atypical or frankly malignant variants, both of which may require adjuvant therapy. Moreover, 2% of recurrent meningiomas have dedifferentiated to a more aggressive form (28) so that even prior histological evidence of benignity does not necessarily exclude present aggressive behavior. With these facts in mind, it is surprising that many radiosurgical centers are willing to treat skull base lesions without a tissue diagnosis. Just a decade

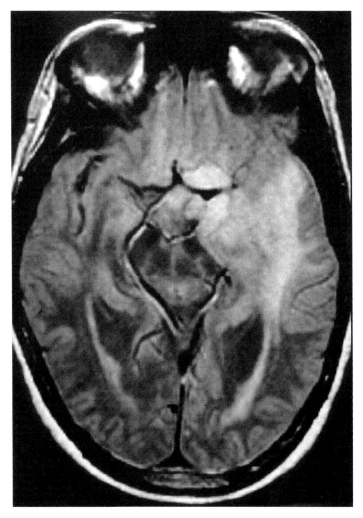

FIG. 23.3 MR image showing severe temporal lobe edema in a patient treated with Gamma-knife radiosurgery. Note the compression of the adjacent mesencephalon.

ago such treatment was a rare occurrence (15). However, there has been an increasing trend to treat based on radiographic criteria alone. During the past 2 years, several of the larger radiosurgical series have reported treating 37 to 44% (17, 23, 36) of patients without histological confirmation of benign meningioma. In the present S-knife series, 2 of 30 patients (7%) were excluded because they were found at surgery to have non-meningiomatous lesions. One patient had a cavernous malformation arising in the cavernous sinus that was completely excised with micro-surgical technique *(Fig.23.4)*. The other was found to have a caseating granuloma involving the petroclival region *(Fig. 23.5)* and appropriate medical therapy was initiated. In neither of these cases would radio-surgery have been considered to be an ideal primary treatment option. At best, misdiagnosis leads to delay in the delivery of definitive care; at worst, it may lead to a detrimental outcome for the patient.

Besides offering tissue for histological diagnosis, open surgery pro-vides immediate decompression of compromised neurovascular struc-tures *(Fig. 23.6)*. Indeed, some failures of radiosurgery have been at-tributed not to tumor growth, but to a failure to provide timely relief of symptoms (17). This is particularly important when pain is the initial presenting symptom. Of all skull base meningiomas, those arising from Meckel's cave and the petroclival region have the highest propensity to present with pain. We have found surgical management for these meningiomas to be most rewarding as it results in rapid and dramatic reduction of pain *(Fig. 23.7)*. Samii et al. have corroborated our obser-vations, and they have reported resolution of facial pain in 100% of pa-tients operated for such lesions (30).

EARLY AND COMPLETE TREATMENT IS OPTIMAL

The importance of addressing skull base meningiomas at an early stage cannot be overstated. Ever since Simpson's landmark paper (35) discussing the significance of the extent of resection for meningiomas in general, it has been known that there is a clear relationship between surgical cure and completeness of resection. This concept holds true for skull base meningiomas as well. In the current S-knife series, there has been no recurrence in any of the small skull base meningiomas that were completely resected. Other authors have demonstrated similar re-sults (25, 30). Mirimanoff and colleagues (22) have shown that there is a significant improvement in the recurrence-free rate after total resec-tion of meningiomas compared to sub-total resections regardless of site (93% 5-year and 80% 10-year vs. 63% and 45% respectively). Levine et al. (20) have shown that smaller, less extensive skull base meningiomas have a better chance for total resection. Although this may seem intu-itive, they were also able to demonstrate with statistical significance that smaller tumors and those with fewer cranial nerves involved were more likely to be completely resected. Moreover, this subgroup of meningiomas had shorter hospital stays and better outcomes as mea-sured by the Karnofsky performance scale. Since ease of surgical re-section and performance outcome are, to some extent, inversely pro-portional to the size and extent of a tumor, it is important to attack

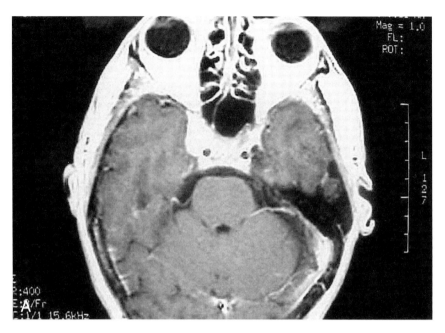

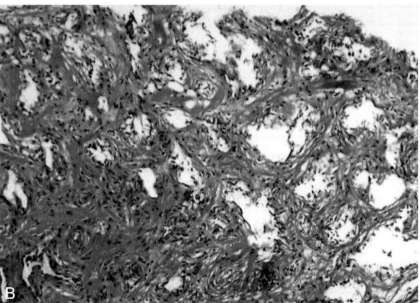

FIG. 23.4 (*A*) Axial postcontrast T1 MRI which demonstrates a homogeneously enhancing right cavernous sinus lesion in a patient presenting with a right sixth nerve palsy. Preoperative diagnosis was meningioma. At surgery the lesion proved to be a cavernous hemangioma of the cavernous sinus. Following complete microsurgical resection, his cranial neuropathy resolved completely. (*B*) H&E preparation shows a compact mass of endothelial-lined sinusoidal spaces devoid of intervening neural tissue.

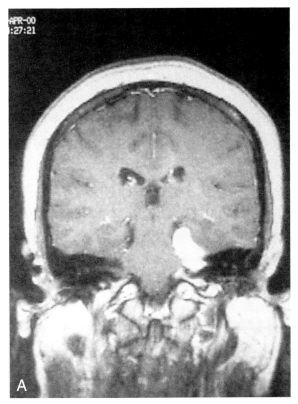

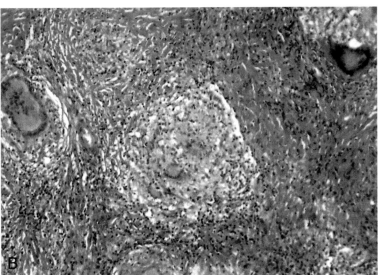

FIG. 23.5 (A) Coronal post contrast T1 MRI revealing a homogeneously enhancing lesion involving the left petrous apex. Preoperative diagnosis was meningioma. Caseating granuloma was found at surgery. (B) H&E preparation demonstrates nodular arrangements of epithelioid histiocytes. Note the formation of giant cells.

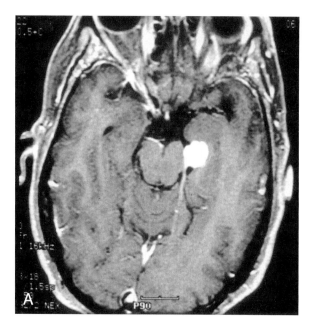

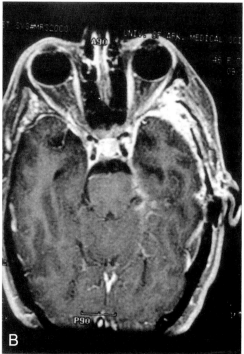

FIG. 23.6 This 46-year-old female presented with seizures referable to the left temporal lobe. (A) Contrast-enhanced, T1 MRI revealed a left tentorial meningioma with compression of the adjacent hippocampal region. (B) Postoperative MRI showing complete
surgical resection. The patient remains seizure free.

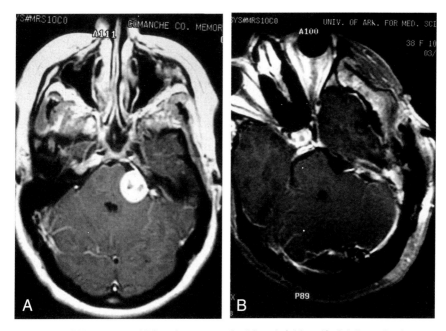

FIG. 23.7 This 38-year-old female presented with painful hemifacial dysesthesias. (*A*) Axial postcontrast T1 MRI which demonstrates a homogeneously enhancing lesion at the ipsilateral petrous apex. (*B*) After complete resection of the lesion, the patient's dysesthesias resolved and she had no new neurological deficits.

these lesions when they are still small and when there is less involvement of neighboring structures.

CONCLUSION

When considering the various treatment options for small symptomatic skull base meningiomas, several salient points exist. Surgical resection of meningiomas remains the gold standard for the treatment of these lesions. Modern microsurgical and skull base techniques have resulted in improved safety and efficacy, reaffirming the role of surgical resection as the primary therapeutic option in the management of skull base meningiomas. Although radiosurgery may be considered for select patients (particularly the elderly or those with significant medical disease), its unproven efficacy in the long-term precludes it from being considered as a primary, first-line treatment standard for small symptomatic skull base meningiomas. Finally, we believe that "N-knife" is a valid treatment option for these lesions in carefully selected patients and its results, to date, are comparable with those of radiosurgery.

REFERENCES

1. Al-Mefty O: Clinoidal meningiomas. **J Neurosurg** 73:840–849, 1990.
2. Al-Mefty O, Fox JL, Smith RR: Petrosal approach for petroclival meningiomas. **Neurosurgery** 22:510–517, 1988.
3. Al-Mefty O, Kersh JE, Routh A, et al.: The long-term side effects of radiation therapy for benign brain tumors in adults. **J Neurosurg** 73:502–512, 1990.
4. Aziz KMA, van Loveren HR: Primary lymphoma of Meckel's cave: Mimicking trigeminal schwannoma: Case report. **Neurosurgery** 44:859–863, 1999.
5. Bricolo AP, Turazzi S, Talacchi A., et al.: Microsurgical removal of petroclival meningiomas: A report of 33 cases. **Neurosurgery** 31:813–828, 1992.
6. Burger PC, Scheithauer BW: *Atlas of Tumor Pathology: Tumors of the Central Nervous System.* Washington, DC, Armed Forces Institute of Pathology, 1994, p 259.
7. Cantore G, Delfini R, Ciappetta P: Surgical treatment of petroclival meningiomas: Experience with 16 cases. **Surg Neurol** 42:105–111, 1994.
8. Chang SD, Adler JR: Treatment of cranial base meningiomas with Linear accelerator radiosurgery. **Neurosurgery** 41:1019–1027, 1997.
9. Day JD: Cranial base surgical technique for large sphenocaverous meningiomas: Technical note. **Neurosurgery** 46:754–759, 2000.
10. Connell PP, Macdonald RL, Mansur DB, et al.: Tumor size predicts control of benign meningiomas treated with radiotherapy. **Neurosurgery** 44:1194–1200, 1994.
11. DeMonte F, Al-Mefty O: Meningiomas, in Kaye AH, Laws ER (eds): *Brain Tumors: An Encyclopedic Approach.* Edinburgh, Churchill Livingstone, 1995, pp 675–704.
12. DeMonte F, Smith HK, Al-Mefty O: Outcome of aggressive removal of cavernous sinus meningiomas. **J Neurosurg** 81:245–251, 1994.
13. Duma CH, Lunsford LD, Kondziolka D, et al.: Stereotactic radiosurgery of cavernous sinus meningiomas as an addition or alternative to microsurgery. **Neurosurgery** 32:699–705, 1993.
14. Eisenberg MB, Al-Mefty O, DeMonte F, et al.: Benign nonmeningeal tumors of the cavernous sinus. **Neurosurgery** 44:949–955, 1999.
15. Engenhart R, Kimmig BN, Hover KH, et al.: Stereotactic single high dose radiation therapy of benign intracranial meningiomas. **Int J Radiat Oncol Biol Phys** 19:1021–1026, 1990.
16. Kawase T, Shiobara R, Toya S: Anterior transpetrosal-transtentorial approach for sphenopetroclival meningiomas: Surgical method and results in 10 patients. **Neurosurgery** 28:869–876, 1991.
17. Kondziolka D, Levy EI, Niranjan A, et al.: Long-term outcomes after meningioma radiosurgery: Physician and patient perspectives. **J Neurosurg** 91:44–50, 1999.
18. Kondziolka D, Lunsford LD, Coffey RJ, et al.: Stereotactic radiosurgery of meningiomas. **J Neurosurg** 74:552–559, 1991.
19. Kuratsu JI, Kocki M, Ushio Y: Incidence and clinical features of asymptomatic meningiomas. **J Neurosurg** 92:766–770, 2000.
20. Levine ZT, Buchanan RI, Sekhar Ln, et al.: Proposed grading system to predict the extent of resection and outcomes for cranial base meningiomas. **Neurosurgery** 45:221–230, 1999.
21. Mathiesen T, Lindquist C, Kihlstrom L, et al.: Proposed grading system to predict the extent of resection and outcomes for cranial base meningiomas. **Neurosurgery** 39:2–9, 1996.
22. Mirimanoff RE, Dosoretz DE, Linggood RM, et al.: Analysis of recurrence and progression following neurosurgical resection. **J Neurosurg** 62:18–24, 1985.
23. Morita A, Coffey RJ, Foote RL, et al.: Risk of injury to cranial nerves after Gamma

Knife radiosurgery for skull base meningiomas: Experience in 88 patients. **J Neurosurg** 90:42–49, 1999.

24. Nutting C, Brada M, Brazil L, et al.: Radiotherapy in the treatment of benign meningioma of the skull base. **J Neurosurg** 90:823–827, 1999.

25. O'Sullivan MG, van Loveren HR, Tew JM: The surgical resectability of meningiomas of the cavernous sinus. **Neurosurgery** 40:238–247, 1997.

26. Pieper DR, Al-Mefty O: Management of intracranial meningiomas secondarily involving the infratemporal fossa: Radiographic characteristics, pattern of tumor invasion, and surgical implications. **Neurosurgery** 45:231–238, 1999.

27. Olivero WC, Lister JR, Elwood PW: The natural history and growth of asymptomatic meningiomas. A review of 60 patients. **J Neurosurg** 83:222–224, 1995.

28. Rohringer M, Sutherland GR, Louw DR, et al.: Incidence and clinicopathological features of meningioma. **J Neurosurg** 71:665–672, 1989.

29. Salazar OM: Ensuring local control in meningiomas. **Int J Radiat Oncol Biol Phys** 15:501–504, 1998.

30. Samii M, Carvalho GA, Tatagiba M, et al.: Surgical management of meningiomas originating in Meckel's cave. **Neurosurgery** 41:767–775, 1997

31. Samii M, Tatagiba M, Carvalho GA: Retrosigmoid intradural suprameatal approach to Meckel's cave and the middle fossa: Surgical technique and outcome. **J Neurosurg** 92:235–241, 2000.

32. Sekhar LN, Patel S, Cusimano M, et al.: Surgical treatment of meningiomas involving the cavernous sinus: Evolving ideas based on a ten year experience. **Acta Neurochir (Suppl)** 65:58–62, 1996.

33. Sekhar LN, Schessel DA, Bucur SD, et al.: Partial labyrinthectomy petrous apicectomy approach to neoplastic and vascular lesions of the petroclival area. **Neurosurgery** 44:537–552, 1999.

34. Seoane E, Rhoto AL: Suprameatal extension of the retrosigmoid approach: Microsurgical anatomy. **Neurosurgery** 44:553–560, 1999.

35. Simpson D: The recurrence of intracranial meningiomas after surgical treatment. **J Neurol Neurosurg Psychiatry** 20:22–39, 1957.

36. Subach BR, Lunsford LD, Kondziolka D, et al.: Management of petroclival meningiomas by stereotactic radiosurgery. **Neurosurgery** 47:437–445, 1998.

37. Tedeshi H, Rhoton AL: Lateral approaches to the petroclival region. **Surg Neurol** 41:180–216, 1994.

38. Tishler RB, Loeffler JS, Lunsford LD, et al.: Tolerace of cranial nerves of the cavernous sinus to radiosurgery. **Int J Radiat Oncol Biol Phys** 27:215–221, 1993.

39. Valentino V, Schinaia G, Raimondi AJ: The results of radiosurgical management of 72 middle fossa meningiomas. **Acta Neurochir** 122:60–70, 1993.

40. Yasargil MG: *Microneurosurgery,* Vol I. New York, Thieme Medical Publishers, 1994, p 26.

24

FUNCTIONAL OUTCOMES IN SKULL BASE SURGERY

What is Acceptable?

FRANCO DEMONTE, M.D., F.R.C.S.C., F.A.C.S.

INTRODUCTION

Great strides have been made over the past several decades in the management of patients with neoplasms involving the base of the skull. The development and widespread use of improved surgical approaches to the skull base, the advances made in diagnostic imaging and surgical navigation and the routine use of multimodality therapy have all resulted in an increasing number of patients who are being cured or who have long remissions from their disease. Identifying the long-term adverse affects of treatment has become increasingly important as patients try to resume previous activities and an independent lifestyle. In 1948 the World Health Organization defined health as not only the absence of disease and infirmity but also the presence of physical, mental, and social well-being (1). Since that time quality-of-life (QOL) issues have become increasingly important as measures of outcome following the treatment of a variety of medical and surgical disorders (2).

WHO DECIDES WHAT IS ACCEPTABLE?

The assessment of outcomes following the treatment of skull base tumors has to date typically focused on technical issues such as the extent of tumor resection, or the incidence of complications, or on oncologic issues such as incidence of and time to tumor recurrence or survival. Only a very few studies are available which assess outcome based on patient-reported quality of life. This concept of health-related quality of life (HRQOL) can be defined as the extent to which one's usual or expected physical, emotional, and social well being are affected by a medical condition or treatment (2). Using this paradigm of outcome assessment, it is the patient who ultimately decides what is an acceptable outcome. What is considered acceptable however may vary by the nature of the neoplastic process, the wishes and expectations of the patient, and the point in the time course of the disease in which the patient finds his or herself. What some patients would consider acceptable might be intolerable for others. This underscores the need to individualize treatments in order to maximize the patient's acceptance of their perceived post-treatment quality of life (2).

HOW IS HRQOL MEASURED?

Although the instruments used for measuring HRQOL differ to some degree, all tend to measure the seven basic dimensions of HRQOL. These include physical concerns (e.g., pain), functional ability (activity), family well-being, emotional well-being, treatment satisfaction, sexuality/intimacy (including body image), and social functioning(2–5). Variation among QOL questionnaires is typically related to the extent to which the above mentioned domains are covered, the emphasis placed on objective or subjective measures, and the format of the questions.

HRQOL measures may be either generic, such as the Medical Outcome Study 36 item shortform health survey (SF-36) (6) or specific such as the Functional Assessment of Cancer Therapy brain subscale (FACT-Brain)(7). Each measure contributes unique information about HRQOL(2–5). Generic measures are most useful when conducting general survey research on health and when making comparisons between disease states. Other advantages of generic measures include established reliability and validity, the ability to detect treatment effects across a broad range of HRQOL domains, and the ability to compare outcomes across a range of different interventions, diseases, and populations. These measures are, however, not as responsive to changes in the clinical status of the patient, nor do they necessarily focus on the most critical health outcomes of interest for a particular disease. Specific measures, on the other hand, are quite responsive to clinical changes. This clinical relevance leads to greater physician acceptability. These measures are not comprehensive and cannot be used to compare across conditions or across different treatment programs. Specific measures are most appropriate for clinical trials in which specific therapeutic interventions are being evaluated (3, 4).

HRQOL IN SKULL BASE SURGERY

There are unique issues that are important to identify when interpreting QOL reports from patients with skull base tumors. The HRQOL in patients with brain injury due to tumor and treatment must be analyzed with the potential effect of neurocognitive impairment in mind (8). Patients with frontal lobe dysfunction, such as those patients with large olfactory groove meningiomas for instance, often have diminished appreciation of their disabilities and limitations, and thus may report a level of function that is not realistic. Reporting of a good QOL may occur in spite of substantial mental impairment due to a lack of insight. Similarly, patients who have previously received radiation therapy to the brain as treatment for their skull base tumors not infrequently evidence neurocognitive effects. Radiation therapy and to some extent systemic chemotherapy tend to affect frontal lobe subcortical white matter tracts. The pattern of deficits is similar to those seen in other subcortical white matter diseases such as multiple sclerosis and AIDS dementia complex (8, 9). Thus, for those patients whose skull base tumors compress or invade the brain, or who have received previous treatments for their tumors, performance-based measures should supplement self-reported information. A three-pronged assessment utilizing measures of (1) functionality and performance, (2) cognition, and (3) self-reported HRQOL is the most telling approach for the evaluation of patients with neurologic involvement (8).

HRQOL Following Surgery for Acoustic Neuroma

The quality of life following surgery of skull base tumors has been studied best for acoustic neuroma. Even -so, few reports are available. These reports are all from the otolaryngological literature and to a large extent from European centers.

Wiegand and Fickel (10) were the first to focus attention on the dichotomy existing between physician and patient-based outcome assessments following the treatment of acoustic neuromas. In 1983 they sent questionnaires to the 832 members of the Acoustic Neuroma Association of which 541 were returned (65% response rate). Ninety percent of the respondents underwent surgery at some point within the decade prior to receiving the questionnaire. Respondents experienced a relatively rapid recovery with 81% managing their own care within 4 months and 70% returning to work in the same period. Despite these encouraging statistics many patients described their experiences in "profoundly negative terms." Depression and anxiety were reported by 38% and 35% of respondents respectively. Sleep disturbance and fatigue were each reported by 26%. Sexual dysfunction troubled 10% of respondents. The surgical removal of an acoustic neuroma in this patient population produced a perception of permanent change in patients' feelings about themselves in 40%, while 15% indicated a severely negative feeling about their post-treatment status. These data were the first to underscore the psychological, social, and functional impact accompanying even successful treatment and the need for a "broader view" of the consequences of treatment of acoustic neuroma. Subsequent studies have confirmed the significant impact that cerebellopontine angle (CPA) surgery for acoustic neuroma has on patient reported QOL *(Table 24.1)* (11–17).

These later reports have also attempted to identify baseline parameters which might predict postoperative HRQOL. Irving et al. found that the functional outcome was better for patients with tumors less than 1.5 cm when compared to those patients with tumors ≥ 1.5 cm (13). This finding, however, was not substantiated in a recent subsequent report from the same group (da Cruz) (12). In fact the study by da Cruz et al. found no difference in reported QOL based on operative approach, tumor size, patient sex, and/or age (12). Both van Leeuwen et al. (17) and Nikolopoulos et al. (14) noted a relatively worse postoperative work or financial status in those patients with larger tumors, but found no impact of operative approach or tumor size respectively. Possibly the most surprising bit of information came from the report by Irving et al. These authors noted that the degree of facial nerve dysfunction did *not* correlate with reported overall QOL. Even when social functioning, the functional measure most likely to be affected by facial nerve weakness, was examined no significant difference between groups could be identified (13).

HRQOL in Other Skull Base Tumors

In 1984, Chan and Thompson reported on 257 patients with intracranial meningiomas, 120 of whom had tumors located at the skull base (18). The average observed survival period in the 112 living patients was 8.2 years with 7.65 of those years being spent with a Karnofsky Performance Score (KPS) of ≥70. Those patients with tumors of the tuberculum sellae and posterior fossa had shorter overall survival (7.9 years and 6.8 years, respectively) and shorter quality survival (6.3 and 5.9 years, respectively). Patients with tumors of the skull base generally had shorter overall survival and quality survival (KPS ≥70) than those patients with tumor away from the base. (mean survival 8.2 years vs. 9.0 years; mean quality survival 7.65 years vs. 8.4 years). Although the KPS is a poor QOL measure this report indicated that patients with skull base tumors, especially those in difficult locations were at risk for a poorer quality of life following treatment. De Jesús et al. noted a 10 point reduction in the mean KPS of patients following removal of cavenous sinus meningiomas. There was no significant improvement over time (19).

Lang et al. using the SF-36 and Glasgow outcome score assessed 17 patients following surgical removal of petroclival meningiomas (20). At one year following surgery 13 patients had made a good to moderate recovery, 3 had severe disability, and 1 had died. In contrast to this rela-

TABLE 24.1

Health-Related QOL Following Surgery for Acoustic Neuroma

Authors + Year of Publication	#Of Respondents/ Total Patients (%)	Time from surgery	HRQOL
Parving et al. 1992 [15]	273/293 (93%)	Median = 6 years Range 6 months–14 yrs	Anxiety 22% Depression 17% Sleep Disturbance 15% Sexual dysfunction 6% 26% reported social consequences are result of surgery 9% never resumed normal activities 10% have been unable to adjust to their postsurgical situation
Irving et al. 1995 [13]	227/257 (88%)	Mean 4.3 years Range 6 months–12 yrs	The group as a whole achieved a return to 80% of ideal QOL 37% of patients reported QOL in excess of 90% of ideal 15% assessed their QOL as less than 50% of ideal
Van Leeuwen et al. 1996 [17]	134/151 (89%)	Range 6 months–13 yrs	~ 45% felt that their general state of health was acceptable (rather than well or excellent) or poor 31% no longer able to work
Anderson et al. 1997 [1]	141/156 (90%)	Mean 3.3 years Median 2 years Range 6 months–7 yrs	24% agreed to some degree that they could not continue work because of their operation 37% reported continued need for medical consultation (mainly because of facial problems + pain)
Nikolopoulos et al. 1998 [14]	53/69 (77%)	1 year–3 yrs	QOL better in 17.4% worse in 53.8% same in 28.8% 50% had fewer social activities 29.4 were worse off financially 21.2% had to change their occupation
De Cruz, et al. 2000 [12]	72/90 (80%)	At least 18 months	For 7 of 8 measured health scales the postoperative QOL was less than a matched population

TABLE 24.2
*The QOL Categories Assessed by the Medical Study 36 Item
Shortform Health Survey (SF-36) [6]*

- Physical Functioning
- Social Functioning
- Role Limitations Due to Physical Problems
- Role Limitations Due to Emotional Problems
- Mental Health
- Energy and Vitality
- Pain
- General Perception of Health

tively good observer-generated outcome data, between 43% and 75% of surviving patients scored themselves below acceptable norms in all eight of the QOL categories measured by the SF-36 *(Table 24.2)*. This study highlights the frequent dichotomy that exists between functionality and self-reported QOL.

Reporting on the long-term results in 36 patients of surgery for temporal bone paragangliomas Briner et al. noted a return to normal social life in 69% of the patients after 6 months and in 97% by 1 to 2 years (21). Approximately one third of patients did, however, report a decreased QOL following surgery. The infratemporal fossa (ITF) type A approach was utilized in 31 patients and the majority of tumors (34 of 36) were large (Fisch class C or C/D). Thirty-six percent of patients reported that difficulty swallowing was the worst postoperative problem, but 97% reported that despite postoperative deterioration in cranial nerve function the deficits were still acceptable.

Trans-sphenoidal removal of nonfunctioning pituitary adenoma was performed in the 48 patients reported by Page et al. and the reported QOL of this group was compared to normative data and to that reported by 42 patients having undergone mastoid surgery (22). Overall, there was no significant difference noted in the HRQOL of the patients with pituitary tumors. Further analysis, however, found that the 18 patients who received radiotherapy following their trans-sphenoidal surgery reported a significantly worse QOL, mainly due to depression and decreased emotional control.

QOL following Anterior Craniofacial Resection

As part of a pilot study 16 patients were assessed one or more years (mean 22 months) following treatment of paranasal sinus tumors requiring anterior-craniofacial resection. Patients harboring paranasal sinus tumors without significant brain or orbital invasion were chosen

TABLE 24.3
Pathology of 16 Patients with Paranasal Sinus Tumors

• Olfactory Neuroblastoma	3
• Adenocarcinoma	3
• Squamous Cell Carcinoma	2
• Basosquamous Carcinoma	1
• Neuroendocrine Carcinoma	1
• Meningioma	1
• Sarcomas	4
• Osteosarcoma, Unclassified, Chondrosarcoma, Teratocarcinosarcoma	

as the simplest tumor-patient paradigm in an attempt to minimize the inhomogeneities inherent in the diverse patient and tumor populations encountered in the field of skull base surgery. Pre- or postoperative radiation therapy was delivered to 14 of 16 patients, and 5 patients received chemotherapy. No attempt was made to separate the various components of the patients' treatment, as all treatments were deemed oncologically necessary.

All 16 patients were alive at follow-up and the encountered pathologies were typical of paranasal malignancies *(Table 24.3)*. The functional assessments used were the Karnofsky Performance Score (KPS) and the Functional Independence Measure (FIM). HRQOL was assessed by patient-generated responses to the Functional Assessment of Cancer Therapy questionnaire (FACT) (23), including its brain and head and neck subscales (7) *(Table 24.4)*.

Not surprisingly, anterior craniofacial resection and other indicated adjunctive therapies for paranasal sinus tumors rarely affected independence. Karnofsky performance scores of 90 or 100 were recorded in 15 of 16 patients (94%). Similarly, 87% of patient had FIM scores >117 *(Table 24.5)*. When the specific measures of QOL were analyzed, all patients reported a good QOL from a neurologic standpoint and 94% also

TABLE 24.4
Functional and QOL Assessments used following Treatment of Paranasal Sinus Tumors

Functional Assessments
    KPS—Karnofsky Performance Scale (0–100)
    FIM—Functional Independence Measure (18–126)
QOL Assessments

FACT—G-	Quality of life including physical, social/family, emotional and functional domains (0–108)
FACT—Brain-	Neurologic subscale of FACT (0–72)
FACT—H/N-	Head and neck subscale of FACT (0–30)

TABLE 24.5
Functional Independence Measure

• 117–126	able to perform most or all ADL's independently
• 108–116	needs supervision of ADL's
• 99–107	needs some assistance with ADL
• 90–98	needs considerable assistance with ADL
• below 90	needs attendant care for many

from a head and neck standpoint. Of note, however, 31% of patients reported a poor quality of life based on their responses to the FACT-general questionnaire.

CASE #1

A 21-year-old female presented with progressive midfacial swelling and hypertelorism Investigation revealed the presence of a massive midfacial tumor with intracranial and intraorbital extension. The patient had a gross total resection performed with reconstruction using free tissue transfers *(Fig. 24.1)*. No adjunct therapy was given for this grade II chondrosarcoma. The patient was assessed 1 year following surgery. She was entirely independent with KPS and FIM of 100 and 124, respectively. A good QOL was reported on both the brain, and head and neck subscales of the FACT despite the significant cosmetic impact of her surgery. She, however, noted her QOL as only fair. The reasons

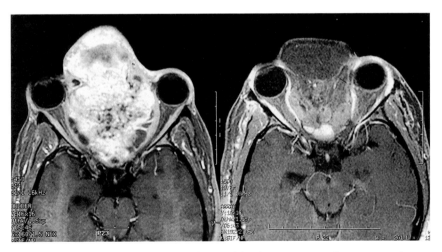

FIG. 24.1 Pre- and postoperative axial T_1-weighted post contrast, fat suppressed magnetic resonance images. Complete excision of this grade II chondrosarcoma and reconstruction by free tissue transfer is illustrated.

were due to her low self-scoring on the family/social well being elements of the FACT-general questionnaire. The patient was subsequently referred to the local cancer support group.

CASE #2

A 55-year-old male physician with nasal obstruction was found to have an upper ethmoidal olfactory neuroblastoma. Gross total resection via transcranial approach was followed by adjuvant radiotherapy with 60 Gy *(Fig. 24.2).* Testing took place 13 months later. The patient had returned to full-time practice with full KPS + FIM scores. Although all QOL scores were still in the "good" range, the patient reported more sadness, poor family communication, and disturbed sleep. Referral to a clinical psychologist and prescription of sleeping aid were beneficial.

CONCLUSIONS AND RECOMMENDATIONS

Review of published data studying the functional outcomes following skull base surgery and our own experiences have consistently identified a substantial population of patients who have a diminished QOL following surgery with or without adjuvant therapies. When both generic

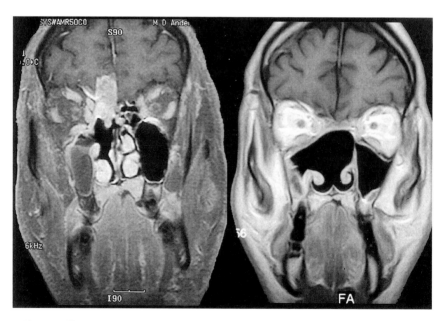

FIG. 24.2 Pre- and postoperative coronal T_1-weighted post contrast MRI. Complete excision of this olfactory neuroblastoma and reconstruction by pedicled pericranial graft is illustrated.

and specific measures are used as part of the assessment, it appears that this diminished QOL is less related to the specifics of the treatment than to the psychosocial changes and adjustments which accompany an illness and its treatment. Notably a patient's perception of their health and QOL is not necessarily related to objectively assessed functionality.

Patient-oriented outcome measures, both generic and specific, should form part of the routine pre- and postoperative assessment of patients with skull base pathologies. Pretreatment and longitudinal assessments are necessary to fully determine the impact of treatment on the patients' well being. This information when compared to similar assessments in nonoperated or alternatively treated patients with similar disease processes may answer questions regarding the timing of therapy or which therapy is, in fact, the best.

ACKNOWLEDGMENTS

The authors would like to thank Raymond Sawaya, M.D., Frederick Lang, M.D., and Paula DeMonte, MA-SLP, for their invaluable suggestions, perspectives, and opinions, and Rosa Lopez for producing the typed manuscript.

REFERENCES

1. World Health Organization Constitution. Geneva: World Health Organization, 1948.
2. Testa MA, Simonson SD: Assessment of quality-of-life. **Curr Concepts** 334(13):835–840, 1996.
3. Cusimano MD: Quality-of-life assessment in patients with lesions of the cranial base. **Skull Base Surg** 9(4):259–264, 1999.
4. Gerszten PC: Outcomes research: A review. **Neurosurgery** 43(5):1146–1156, 1998.
5. Patrick DL, Deyo RA: Generic and disease-specific measures in assessing health status and quality of life. **Med Care** 27(3, suppl):S217-S232, 1989.
6. Ware JE Jr , Sherbourne CD: The MOS 36-item short-form. **Med Care** 30:473–483, 1992.
7. Weitzner MA, Myers CA, Gelke CK, Byrne KS, Cella DF: The functional assessment of cancer therapy (FACT) scale: Development of a brain subscale and revalidation of the FACT-G in the brain tumor population. **Cancer** 75:1151–1161, 1995.
8. Meyers CA: Issues of quality of life in neuro-oncology. **Handbook Clin Neurol** 23(67):389–409, 1997.
9. Meyers CA, Geara F, Wong PF, Morrison W: Neurocognitive effects of therapeutic irradiation for base of skull tumors. **Int J Radiat Oncol Biol Phys** 46(1):51–55, 2000.
10. Wiegand DA, Fickel V: The patient's perspective: Subjective assessment of symptoms, diagnosis, therapy, and outcome in 541 patients. **Laryngoscope** 99:179–187, 1989.
11. Andersson G, Ekvall L, Kinnefors A, Nyberg G, Andersen HR: Evaluation of quality of life and symptoms after translabyrinthine acoustic neuroma surgery. **Am J Otol** 18(4):421–426, 1997.

12. da Cruz MJ, Moffat DA, Hardy DG: Postoperative quality of life in vestibular schwannoma patients measured by the SF36 health questionnaire. **Laryngoscope** 110:151–155, 2000.
13. Irving RM, Beynon GJ, Viani L, Hardy DG, Baguley DM, Moffat DA: The patient's perspective after vestibular schwannoma removal: Quality of life and implications for management. **Am J Otol** 16(3):331–337, 1995.
14. Nikolopoulos TP, Johnson I, O'Donoghue GM: Quality of life after acoustic neuroma surgery. **Laryngoscope** 108:1382–1385, 1998.
15. Parving A, Tos M, Thomsen J, Moller H, Buchwald C: Some aspects of life quality after surgery for acoustic neuroma. **Arch Otolaryngol Head Neck Surg** 118:1061–1064, 1992.
16. Rigby PL, Shah SB, Jackler RK, Chung JH, Cooke DD: Acoustic neuroma surgery: Outcome analysis of patient-perceived disability. **Am J Otol** 18:427–435, 1997.
17. Van Leeuwen JPPM, Meijer H, Braspenning JCC, Cremers CWRJ: Quality of life after acoustic neuroma surgery. **Ann Otol Rhinol Laryngol** 105:423–430, 1996.
18. Chan RC, Thompson GB: Morbidity, mortality, and quality of life following surgery for intracranial meningiomas. **J Neurosurgery** 60:52–60, 1984.
19. De Jesus O, Sekhar LN, Parikh HK, Wright DC, Wagner DP: Longer-term follow-up of patients with meningiomas involving the cavernous sinus: Recurrence, progression, and quality of life. **Neurosurg** 39(5):915–920, 1996.
20. Lang DA, Neil-Dwuer G, Garfield J: Outcome after complex neurosurgery: the caregiver's burden is forgotten. **J Neurosurg** 91:359–363, 1999.
21. Briner HR, Linder TE, Pauw B, Fisch U: Long-term results of surgery for temporal bone paragangliomas. **Laryngoscope** 109:577–583, 1999.
22. Page RCL, Hammersley MS, Burke CW, Wass JAH: An account of the quality of life of patients after treatment for non-functioning pituitary tumours. **Clin Endocrin** 46:401–406, 1997.
23. Cella DF, Tulsky DS, Gray G, et al.: The functional assessment of cancer therapy (FACT) scale: Development and validation of the general version. **J Clin Oncol** 11:570–579, 1993.

25

Surgical Repair of Cranial Nerves

LALIGAM N. SEKHAR, M.D., F.A.C.S., AND CHANDRASEKAR
KALAVAKONDA, M.D.

*"21. And the Lord God caused a deep sleep to fall upon Adam, and he slept: and
he took one of his ribs, and closed up the flesh thereof;*

*22. And the rib, which the Lord God had taken from man, made he a woman,
and brought her unto the man"*

GENESIS, Chapter 2.

INTRODUCTION

Preservation of cranial nerve function is the primary goal during cranial microsurgery. When such preservation is not possible, then cranial nerve reconstruction is attempted. There are several general principles that may help in the preservation of cranial nerve function. A detailed knowledge of microsurgical anatomy is essential. Neurophysiological monitoring during surgery is possible for several cranial nerves, and it is usually helpful. During surgical procedures, the neuroanesthetic technique must be adjusted to allow such monitoring, without muscle relaxation. When the cranial nerve is stretched over a tumor or an aneurysm, the decompression of the nerve from its bony and dural canals (e.g., optic nerve decompression) will relieve the pressure, and reduce the risk of injuries. During the removal of basal tumors involving the cranial nerves, it is prudent to first debulk the tumor (e.g., acoustic neuroma) before starting the cranial nerve dissection. The tumor is then dissected away from the nerve sharply, either parallel or perpendicular to the direction of the cranial nerve fibers, while watching the neurophysiological function of the nerve. Finally, the surgeon should avoid covering cranial nerves with cottonoids, since they stick to the nerve and may tear the nerve when the cottonoid is being removed. If such coverage is desired, pieces of rubber glove (rubber dams) may be used.

PROBLEMS OF CRANIAL NERVE REGENERATION

There are several problems that prevent adequate functional return after cranial nerve repair. Centrally myelinated nerves do not regenerate—

Schwann cells, which produce peripheral myelin, are required for regeneration. Also, the loss of blood supply to a cranial nerve during an operation may impede the regeneration of a nerve or a nerve graft. After the repair of motor cranial nerves, the problem of aberrant regeneration causes disturbances with the optimal return of function. Then regarding sensory nerves, there are problems in addition to their central myelination: ganglion cells, and relay neurons often undergo retrograde degeneration after injuries. Many sensory nerves (e.g., optic nerve, vestibulo-cochlear nerve) have a specialized organization, such that even if there is regeneration, aberrant regeneration may cause poor functional recovery (e.g., tinnitus).

CRANIAL NERVES WHERE REGENERATION IS NOT PRESENTLY POSSIBLE

Because of the presence of central myelin, successful repair of several cranial nerves is not currently possible. These include the olfactory tract, the optic nerve, the trigeminal root (see below), and the vestibulo-cochlear nerve. Experimental studies have shown encouraging results (1–4). Advances in neurosciences will likely allow the repair of these nerves in the near future.

The surgical repair of the remaining nerves, and results of the repair will be discussed subsequently.

GENERAL TECHNIQUES OF CRANIAL NERVE REPAIR

When a cranial nerve is damaged, it should be inspected to see if some fascicles have been preserved. If some fascicles are preserved, they should be kept intact. Both damaged ends of the nerve have to be identified, and this may require further dissection. For example, when the abducens nerve is damaged during the removal of petroclival meningioma, the cavernous sinus may have to be opened in order to find a distal, healthy nerve stump. The two nerve ends can be resutured if it can be done without tension. If such tension is present, or if the nerve ends cannot be approximated, then an interposition graft is necessary (5). The nerves commonly used as grafts are the sural nerve in the leg or the greater auricular nerve in the neck. The cut nerve ends and the graft are stabilized over a small piece of rubber glove or a piece of Gelfoam® (Pharmacia Corporation, Peapack, New Jersey). One or two sutures of 9/0 or 10/0 nylon are used for the suturing. The sutured ends are further reinforced with fibrin glue. In case of intracranial to extracranial grafts, care must be taken during dural and wound closure not to pull out the graft inadvertently.

OCULOMOTOR NERVE

Although initially thought to be impossible, several experimental and clinical studies have shown that the oculomotor nerve regenerates well after resuture or nerve grafting (6–15). However, because of aberrant regeneration (16), recovery of function does not produce binocular vision, which requires a highly coordinated action of the extraocular muscles. The levator palpebrae superioris, the medial rectus, and the sphincter pupillae fibers recover, whereas superior and inferior rectus function do not recover. Oculomotor repair is still important for cosmetic reasons (to prevent a permanent ptosis), and for functional reasons in the event of blindness of the contralateral eye.

In the senior author's experience, fair recovery was observed in two thirds of the nerves resutured, and in three quarters of the nerves after sural nerve graft repair. The oculomotor nerve should always be repaired after inadvertent injury or after intentional resection of nerve segments due to tumor invasion *(Fig. 25.1)*.

TROCHLEAR NERVE

Loss of trochlear nerve function (superior oblique muscle) is compensated spontaneously by many patients. If diplopia is bothersome, superior rectus muscle transposition surgery can easily correct it. However, the trochlear nerve can be repaired if desired, by resuture or with a nerve graft, with good results (14). In the senior author's experience, good recovery was experienced in all four of the patients in whom the nerve was resutured and in one of the two cases where a nerve graft was used after tumor or aneurysm surgery. Grimson et al. reported return of function after intracranial suture of the trochlear nerve that was severed during surgery for a superior cerebellar artery aneurysm (17) *(Fig. 25.2)*.

TRIGEMINAL NERVE

As a mostly sensory nerve that supplies sensation to the face, cheek, tongue, and cornea, the trigeminal nerve has a very important function. The motor division of the nerve is important for chewing. Because of the size of the nerve divisions, and wide area of occupation in the skull base, it is often involved by cranial base tumors, and is often injured during their removal. Reconstruction of the divisions of the nerve (ophthalmic, maxillary, or mandibular) has been performed by the senior author and others (18), with recovery of sensory function (see *Table 25.1*). After resuture of the mandibular nerve (following elective section to facilitate infratemporal approach), only the sensations recovered, but not the motor function. The senior author has performed peripheral nerve graft repair of the damaged trigeminal root in two patients. Recovery of deep sensation (but not light touch) occurred in one patient *(Fig. 25.3)*.

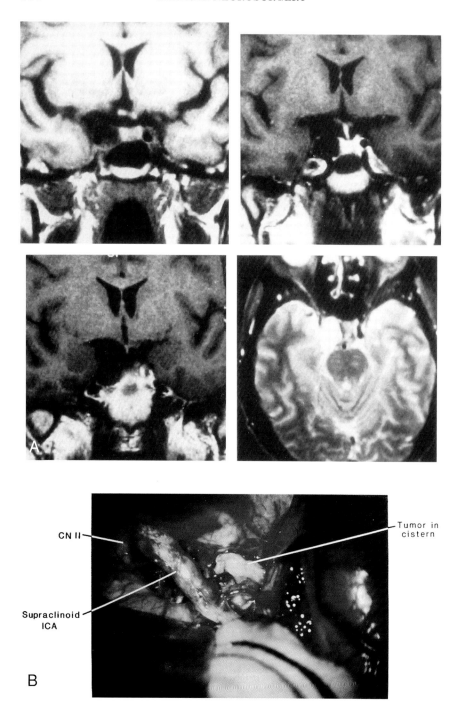

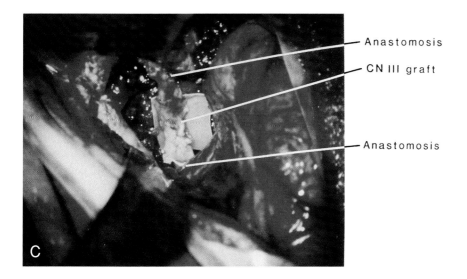

Anastomosis
CN III graft
Anastomosis

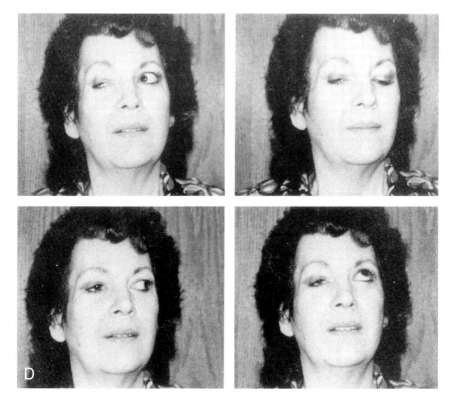

FIG. 25.1 This patient presented with an epidermoid cyst of the cavernous sinus and partial oculomotor palsy (*A*). At surgery, the cyst capsule was found to be invading the oculomotor nerve. It was resected and reconstructed with a sural nerve graft, 3 cm in length (*B, C*). The patient had a partial recovery of medial rotation, but no recovery of the other muscles (*D*).

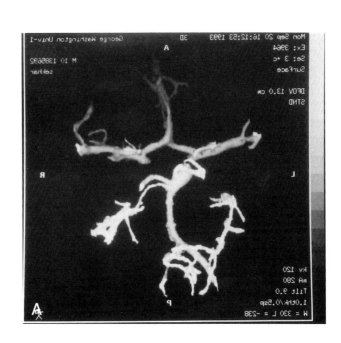

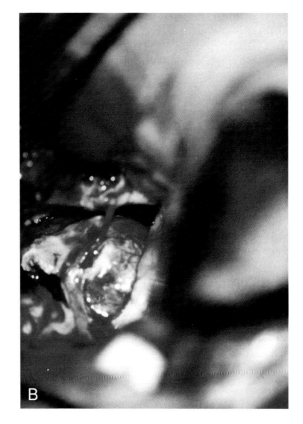

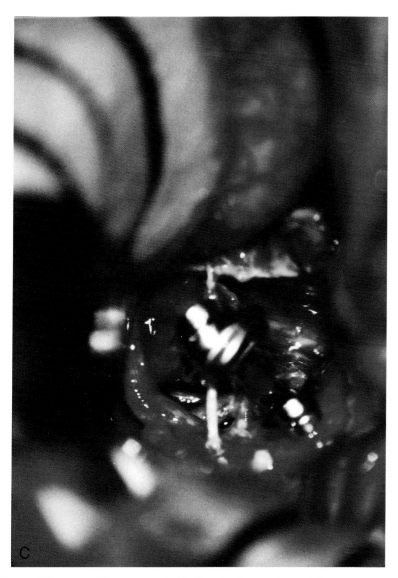

FIG. 25.2 This 10-year-old boy presented with a large basilar-superior cerebellar artery aneurysm (*A*) that required a trans-petrosal approach. Since the trochlear nerve was stretched over the aneurysm (*B*), it was electively divided, and after the aneurysm clipping, it was resutured (*C*). The patient had a complete recovery of trochlear nerve function.

TABLE 25.1
Cranial Nerve Reconstruction: Experience & Results

Cranial Nerve	Procedure	Post-Op Outcome				
		Total	Good	Fair	Poor	Too Early
Oculomotor	Resuture	3	—	2	—	1
	Nerve graft	4	—	3	1	—
Trochlear	Resuture	4	4	—	—	—
	Nerve graft	2	1	—	1	—
Trigeminal						
Ophthalmic	Nerve graft	3	—	1	2	—
Maxillary	Nerve graft	4	—	2	2	—
Mandibular	Resuture	3	1	2	—	—
Nerve root	Nerve graft	2	—	1	1	—
Abducens	Resuture	4	2	1	1	—
	Nerve graft	10	4	2	4	—
Facial	Resuture	4	—	4	—	—
	Nerve graft	28	16	8	4	—
Vagus (sensory)	Nerve graft	5	—	2	3	—
Spinal	Nr Gr-extracr	3	2	1	—	—
	Intra to extracr	2	2	—	—	—
Hypoglossal	Nerve graft	2	—	1	1	—

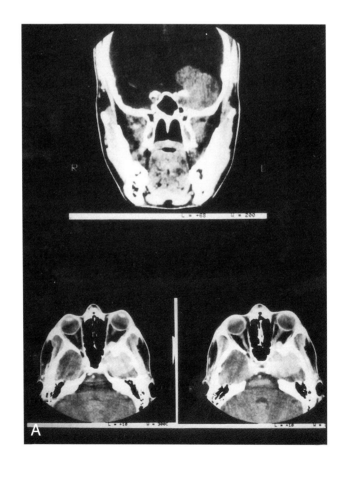

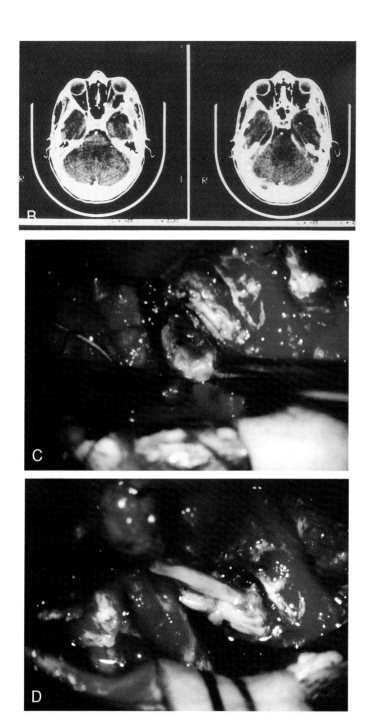

FIG. 25.3 During an operation to completely resect a sphenocavernous meningioma in this young patient (*A, B*), the invaded ophthalmic nerve was excised in the lateral wall of the cavernous sinus, and it was reconstructed with two pieces of sural nerve graft (*C, D*). The patient had recovery of deep sensation in the forehead and partial recovery of the corneal sensation.

ABDUCENS NERVE

Being a motor nerve that supplies a single, but important, extraocular muscle, the abducens nerve is an ideal one for repair. It may be damaged during surgery for basal tumors or aneurysms. Repair is performed by resuture or with a nerve graft interposition (14, 19, 20). It may be difficult to find the distal end of the nerve inside the cavernous sinus, or in the orbital apex medial to the lateral rectus muscle. Even if recovery of lateral rectus function is partial, it is worthwhile, since strabismus surgery can further improve the function. In the senior author's experience, end-to-end repair was performed in four cases (with recovery in all four), and nerve graft repair in 10 patients (six recovered) *(Figs. 25.4, 25.5)*.

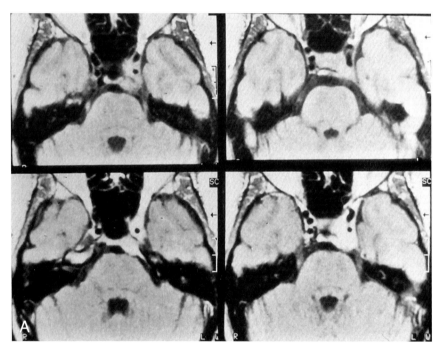

FIG. 25.4 This 33-year-old patient was operated on to remove a growth hormone secreting pituitary adenoma involving the cavernous sinus (*A, B*). At surgery, the tumor-invaded abducens nerve was damaged. However, the nerve was long enough to be reconstructed by resuture (*C*). The patient made a complete recovery of lateral rectus function with gradual disappearance of her diplopia (*D*).

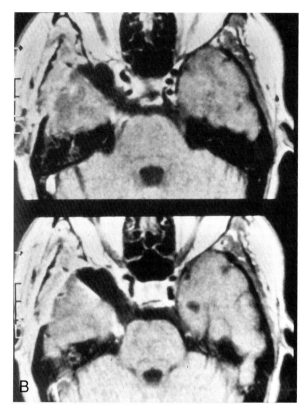

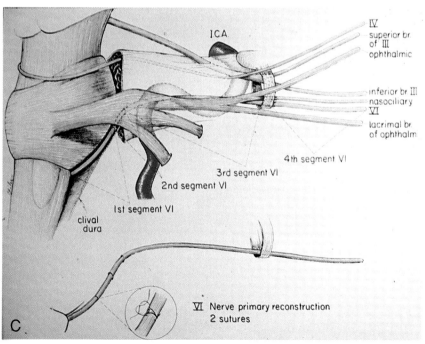

I.C.A.

IV
superior br.
of III
ophthalmic

inferior br III
nasociliary
VI
lacrimal br.
of ophthalm

4th segment VI

3rd segment VI

2nd segment VI

1st segment VI

clival
dura

VI Nerve primary reconstruction
2 sutures

B

C.

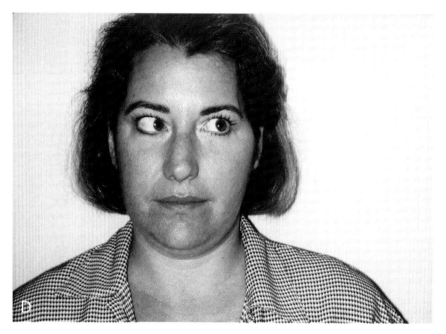

FIG. 25.4 This 33-year-old patient was operated on to remove a growth hormone secreting pituitary adenoma involving the cavernous sinus. The patient made a complete recovery of lateral rectus function with gradual disappearance of her diplopia (D).

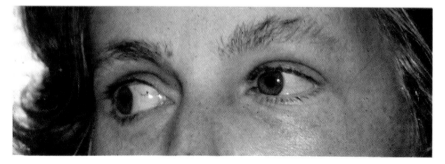

FIG 25.5 This 45-year-old patient was operated to remove a petroclival and cavernous sinus meningioma. The abducens nerve was tumor invaded over a short segment, and had to be resected. It was reconstructed with a sural nerve graft from the cisternal to the cavernous segment. She experienced partial recovery of lateral rectus function. Her diplopia could be further corrected by strabismus surgery, though not completely.

FACIAL NERVE

The facial nerve is the earliest nerve to be repaired, the repair being carried out in the cerebellopontine angle by direct nerve suture, or by intracranial to extracranial interposition grafting (21–24). Since the facial nerve is so important for cosmesis, and for speech and eating, repair of the nerve should be performed whenever it is damaged. The nerve may be damaged in the cerebellopontine angle (CPA) after tumor or aneurysm surgery, in the temporal bone after trauma, surgery, or involvement by tumor, and in the extracranial area under similar circumstances. If the nerve is damaged in the CPA, and there is a gap between the proximal and distal ends, length can be gained by rerouting the intratemporal segment of the facial nerve and performing direct resuture. The nerve can be repaired by sural nerve or greater auricular nerve interposition graft (23) provided a proximal stump is available for anastomosis. After injuries to the nerve in its distal segments, the distal branches need to be identified precisely to allow repair.

The results after facial nerve repair are gratifying (23). When the patient does not have a long-standing paralysis, a House grade III/VI (25) can be achieved. If facial paralysis is long standing, or when the proximal stump cannot be identified, then repair is performed using the technique of partial hypoglossal-to-facial anastomosis (26). The recovery achieved is generally in the order of House grade IV/VI. Recovery after facial nerve repair can be improved further by facial exercises to teach the patient to move the various facial muscles individually. However, such therapy is not available in many centers *(Fig. 25.6)*.

GLOSSOPHARYNGEAL AND VAGUS NERVES

Loss of the function of glossopharyngeal and vagus nerves is disabling due to the impairment of pharyngeal sensation, dysphagia, aspiration pneumonia, and impaired gastrointestinal motility. Unilateral loss of CN IX and X function can be compensated by thyroplasty and arytenoids adduction; and sometimes a jejunostomy is necessary. Bilateral loss of CN IX and X function may occur in patients with fourth ventricular / brainstem tumors, and bilateral glomus vagale / jugulare tumors, and it is very devastating. The best solution for such patients is tracheo-esophageal disconnection, with a permanent tracheostomy.

Because of the problem of aberrant reinnervation, reconstruction of the motor portion of the vagus nerve has not been successful. However, a myoneural graft has been used successfully to treat recurrent laryngeal nerve paralysis. Reconstruction of the ninth and tenth cranial nerves can achieve sensory reinnervation, which itself can be quite valuable. The senior author attempted reconstruction of CN X in five

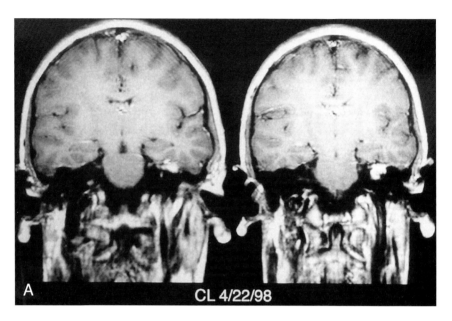

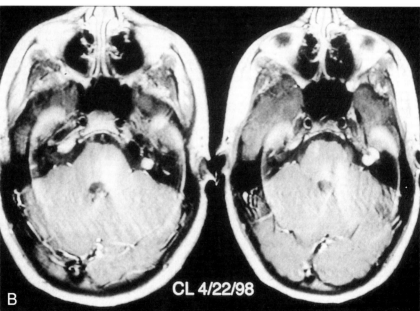

FIG 25.6 This 15-year-old patient presented with complete facial paralysis secondary to a facial nerve schwannoma (A–C). At surgery, her tumor was excised, and the facial nerve was reconstructed with a sural nerve graft from the canalicular to the mastoid segment (D).

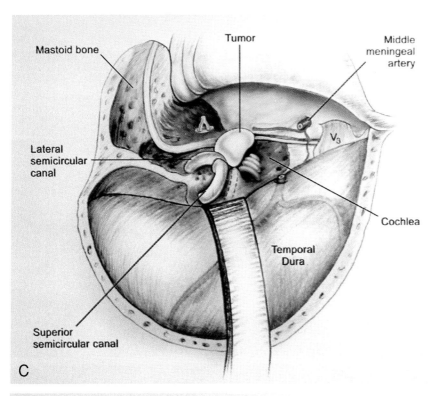

C

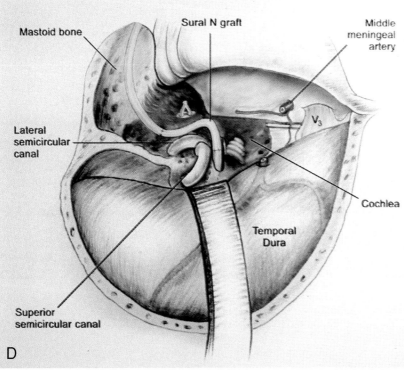

D

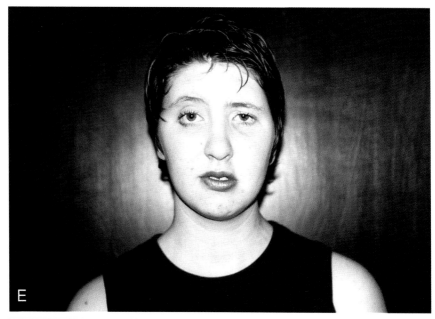

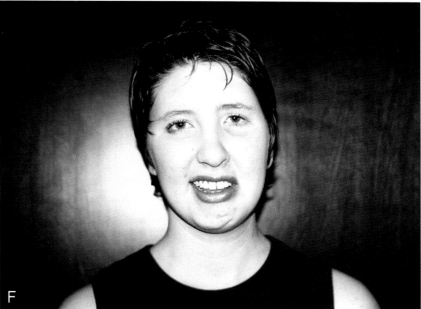

FIG 25.6 She has experienced a House grade III facial recovery (*E, F*). (The copyright to Figs. 31.6*C* and *D* belongs to Laligam N. Sekhar, M.D., F.A.C.S.)

patients after jugular foramen tumor surgery, with sensory recovery in the pharynx in two patients.

SPINAL ACCESSORY NERVE

The cranial portion of the accessory nerve innervates the vocal cords. The spinal accessory nerve supplies the sternomastoid and the trapezius muscles, although these are also innervated by 3 and 4 cervical spinal nerves. Loss of spinal accessory nerve function often results in weakness of shoulder elevation, although some patients can compensate for this partially. The spinal accessory nerve is injured in the neck after lymph node biopsies, and other cervical tumor excision, whereas the intracranial portion may be damaged after excision of jugular foramen and foramen magnum tumors. The spinal accessory nerve is a very robust nerve, with excellent functional recovery. The senior author has performed extracranial graft reconstruction in three cases, with recovery in all the three (fair recovery in one, good recovery in two). The rare procedure of intracranial-to-extracranial repair was performed in two patients with good recovery *(Fig. 25.7)*.

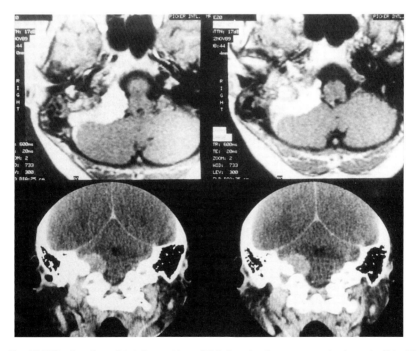

FIG 25.7 During the subtotal resection of this jugular foramen meningioma in this 43-year-old patient *(A)*

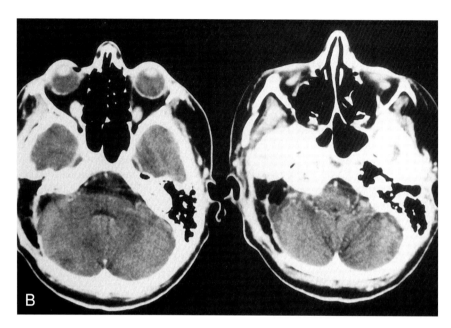

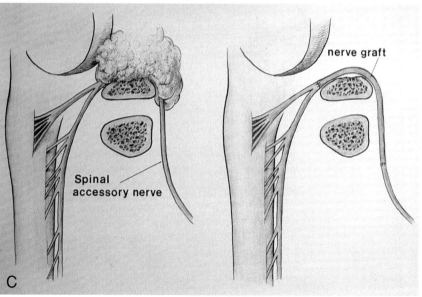

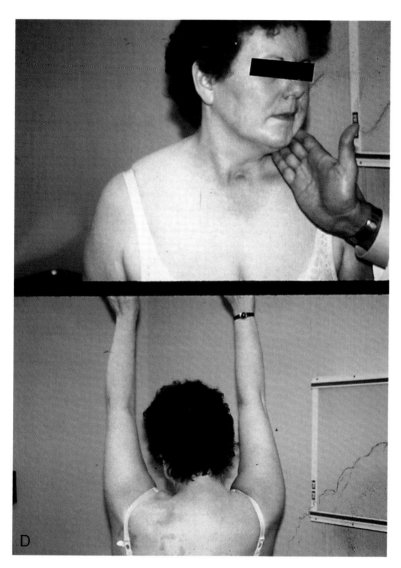

FIG 25.7 During the subtotal resection of this jugular foramen meningioma in this 43-year-old patient (*A, B*), the spinal accessory nerve was sacrificed (Part *A* see page 367). It was reconstructed by means of an intracranial-to-extracranial nerve graft anastomosis (*C*). She made an excellent recovery of trapezius and sternomastoid function (*D*). (The copyright to Fig 31.7*C* belongs to Laligam N. Sekhar, M.D., F.A.C.S.)

HYPOGLOSSAL NERVE

The hypoglossal nerve may be easily injured in the intracranial portion by tumors or operations of the foramen magnum / jugular foramen region, and in the neck during operations / tumors in the carotid triangle. Presumably because of early muscle atrophy, recovery of function of this nerve is surprisingly more difficult, even after neuropraxic injuries. The senior author performed hypoglossal reconstruction in two patients by nerve suture / graft with partial recovery being observed in one patient.

THE FUTURE OF NERVE REPAIR

The tremendous explosion in our knowledge of the mechanisms of neural regeneration bodes well for the future of cranial nerve repair *(Fig. 25.8)*. Strategies for the repair of presently unrepairable and re-

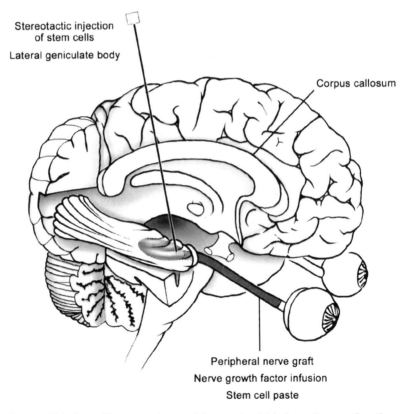

Stereotactic injection of stem cells

Lateral geniculate body

Corpus callosum

Peripheral nerve graft

Nerve growth factor infusion

Stem cell paste

FIG 25.8 This figure illustrates the possible ways in which the optic nerve function may be restored in the near future with advances in neurosciences. (The copyright for this figure belongs to Laligam N. Sekhar, M.D., F.A.C.S.)

pairable nerves include: (1) the use of nerve growth factors, e.g., brain derived neurotrophic factor (BDNF), neurotrophin-4/5; (2) peripheral nerve or cultured Schwann cell—neural tubule transplants to repair injured nerves; (3) upregulation of genes associated with neural regeneration, e.g., GAP-43, Bcl-2, c-Jun; and (4) embryonic or cultured stem cell transplants to promote nerve growth and to replace degenerated neurons. It is expected that the process of nerve regeneration may be speeded up considerably and that the problem of aberrant regeneration will be solved (1, 27).

This will open new avenues for neurosurgeons. In the twentieth century, neurosurgeons have perfected ablative (using operation, radiation, etc.) neurosurgery. Many problems being treated this way will no longer require the use of surgery in the next century, because of the powerful tools of gene technology. Instead, neurosurgeons will focus their efforts on reconstructive neurosurgery, which will require knowledge of anatomy, innovation, and the application of science and art.

REFERENCES

1. Stichel CC, Muller HW: Experimental Strategies to promote axonal regeneration after traumatic central nervous system injury. **Prog Neurobiol** 56:119–148, 1998.
2. Cho KS, Xiao YM, So KF, Diao YC, Chung SK: Synergistic effect of optic and peripheral nerve grafts on sprouting of axon-like processes of axotomized retinal ganglion cells in adult hamsters. **Neurosci Lett** 265:175–178, 1999.
3. MacLaren RE: Regeneration and transplantation of the optic nerve: Developing a clinical strategy. **Br J Ophthalmol** 82:577–583, 1998.
4. Constantine-Paton M: Trajectories of axons in ectopic VIIIth nerves. **Dev Biol (Orlando)** 97:239–244, 1983.
5. Sekhar LN: Preservation and reconstruction of cranial nerves during the removal of cranial base neoplasms, in Sekhar LN, Schramm Jr, VL (eds): *Tumors of the Cranial Base,* Mount Kisco Company, Futura Publishing Company, 1987, pp227–232.
6. Iwabuchi T, Suzuki M, Nakaoka T, et al.: Oculomotor nerve anastomosis. **Neurosurgery** 61:191–192, 1984.
7. Sekhar LN, Moller AR: Operative management of tumors involving the cavernous sinus. **J Neurosurg** 64:879–889, 1986.
8. Sandvoss G, Cervos-Navarro J, Yasargil MG: Intracranial repair of the oculomotor nerve in cats. **Neurochirurgia (Stuttg)** 29:1–8, 1986.
9. Sekhar LN, Burgess J, Akin O: Anatomical study of the cavernous sinus emphasizing operative approaches and related vascular an neural reconstruction. **Neurosurgery** 21:806–816, 1987.
10. Sekhar LN, Sen CN, Jho HD, et al.: Surgical treatment of intracavernous neoplasms: a four-year experience. **Neurosurgery** 24:18–30, 1989.
11. Sekhar LN, Linskey ME, Sen CN, et al.: Surgical management of lesions within the cavernous sinus. **Clin Neurosurg** 37:440–489, 1989.
12. Krajewski R: Oculomotor nerve repair using interposed nerve graft. **Neurosurgery** 30:591–594, 1992.
13. Sekhar, LN: Oculomotor nerve repair using interposed nerve graft. **Neurosurgery** 30:594, 1992 (Comment)

14. Sekhar LN, Lanzino G, Sen CN, Pomonis S: Reconstruction of the third through sixth cranial nerves during cavernous sinus surgery. **J Neurosurg** 76:935–943, 1992.

15. Mariniello G, Horvat A, Dolenc VA: En bloc resection of an intracavernous oculomotor nerve schwannoma and grafting of the oculomotor nerve with sural nerve. **J Neurosurg** 91:1054–1049, 1999.

16. Boghen D, Chartrand JP, Laflamme P, et al.: Primary aberrant third nerve regeneration. **Ann Neurology** 6:415–418, 1979.

17. Grimson BS, Ross MJ, Tyson G: Return of function after intracranial suture of the trochlear nerve. Case report. **J Neurosurg** 43:95–97, 1975.

18. Samii M: Reconstruction of the trigeminal nerve, in Samii M, Jennetta PJ (eds): *The Cranial Nerves.* New York, Springer-Verlag, 1981, pp 352–358.

19. Sawamra Y, Ikeda J, Miyamachi K, Abe H: Full functional recovery after surgical repair of transected abducens nerve. **Neurosurgery** 40:605–608, 1997.

20. Sekhar LN: Full functional recovery after surgical repair of transected abducens nerve. **Neurosurgery** 40:607, 1997 (comment).

21. Dott NM: Facial nerve reconstruction by graft bypassing the petrous bone. **Arch Otolaryngol** 78:426–428, 1963.

22. Samii M: Preservation and reconstruction of the facial nerve in the cerebellopontine angle, in Samii M, Jannetta PJ (eds): *The Cranial Nerves.* New York, Springer-Verlag, 1981, pp 438–450.

23. Stephanian E, Sekhar LN, Janecka IP, Hirsch B: Facial nerve repair by interposition nerve graft: results in 22 patients. **Neurosurgery** 31:73–77, 1992.

24. Samii M, Matthies C: Indication, technique and results of facial nerve reconstruction. **Acta Neurochir (Wien)** 130:125–139, 1994.

25. House JW, Brackmann DE: Facial nerve grading system. **Otolaryngol Head Neck Surg** 93:146–147, 1985.

26. Cusimano MD, Sekhar L: Partial hypoglossal to facial nerve anastomosis for reinnervation of the paralysed face in patients with lower cranial nerve palsies: Technical note. **Neurosurgery** 35: 532–534, 1994.

27. Gash DM, Zhang Z, Gerhardt G: Neuroprotective and neurorestorative properties of GDNF. **Ann Neurol** 44(Suppl 1):S121–S125, 1998.

26

Malignant Tumors Involving the Lateral Skull Base

CHANDRANATH SEN, M.D., AXXX SEN C, TRIANA A, HILTZIK D, COSTANTINO P, LAWSON W, URKEN M AND CATALANO P

A variety of malignant tumors can invade the skull base. These may arise locally from intradural or bony tissues or secondarily invade from the subcranial structures of the head and neck. Until recently, invasion of the skull base by head and neck cancers was deemed inoperable and carried a grave prognosis. Improved understanding of the anatomy, high resolution imaging modalities, innovative surgical approaches and most of all, collaboration of specialists from several disciplines have led to an improved survival of patients with diseases that are almost always ultimately fatal. Despite these advances, management of skull base malignancies remains a difficult problem. These problems are due to the biology of the tumors, the desire of the surgeon to obtain a disease-free margin following sound oncologic principles, and the presence of many important structures closely aggregated in this relatively small area that often limit the resection. In order to better understand the impact of the skull base techniques, the specific area of the skull base involved has to be taken into account in addition to the histology. For example, a squamous cell cancer invading the anterior cranial fossa has a different outlook than the same histology of the tumor involving the lateral skull base or the temporal bone. We will discuss the results of treatment of combined operative procedures for malignancies involving the lateral skull base. Chordomas and low grade chondrosarcomas are also considered malignant tumors of the skull base but have been left out of this report since they pose a completely different management problem than the cancers from the subcranial tissues.

MATERIALS AND METHODS

Reviewing the hospital and office records of 49 patients who underwent surgery at this institution for the treatment of head and neck cancers that had invaded the skull base generated this report. The data were collected and analyzed independent of the operating surgeons.

The specific aim was to assess the impact of the neurosurgical participation in this combined treatment effort, in terms of morbidity and outcome. The overall survival of the patients was tabulated and statistically analyzed using the program SPSS for Windows (release 10.00,
1999–2000). The Kaplan-Meier survival curves were plotted to determine the relative survival by tumor type and also the overall survival.
A team of a neurosurgeon, an otolaryngologist and sometimes an oro-
maxillofacial surgeon performed surgery for the resection of the tumor.

RESULTS

The age, sex distribution is noted in *Table 26.1a.*. About 50% of these tumors had recurred after prior treatment *(Table 26.1b)*. There was a large
variety of tumors, with the major groups being squamous cell cancer, ade-
nocarcinoma, adenoid cystic carcinoma, and sarcomas *(Table 26.2)*.

DISEASE CATEGORIES AND LOCATION:

There were several different types of tumors, but the most common
ones were the squamous cell carcinoma, adenoid cystic carcinoma, ade-
nocarcinoma and sarcomas. The rest were occasional cases of different
types and are listed under miscellaneous. About half the patients presented after prior resection at this or another institution. There were

TABLE 26.1A
Distribution (MSH)

• Age: mean 50.5 years (25–77 years)
• Sex: Female = 16; Male = 33

TABLE 26.1B
Distribution (MSH)

• Primary disease: 24 patients
• Recurrent disease: 25 patients

TABLE 26.2
Distribution (MSH)

	Primary	Recurrent
SCCA	3	11
Adenoid cysti	5	4
Adenocarcinoma	5	2
Sarcoma	4	2
Miscellaneous	7	6

TABLE 26.3A
Anatomical Areas Affected (MSH)

- Middle cranial fossa
- Temporal
- ICA
- Cav sinus
- Meckel's cave
- Dura
- Brain
- Jugular foramen
- Occipital condyle
- Lateral posterior fossa
- Infratemporal fossa
- TMJ
- Parapharyngeal space
- Sphenoid and ethmoid sinuses

TABLE 26.3B
Anatomical Areas Involved (MSH)

- Side: right = 30; left = 19
- 2 areas: 10 patients (20.4%)
- 3 areas: 14 patients (28.5%)
- 4 areas: 16 patients (32.6%)
- 5 areas: 7 patients (14.2%)
- 6 or more areas: 2 patients (4%)

numerous areas of the lateral skull base that were involved *(Table 26.3a)*. The tumors tend to spread into contiguous tissue planes as well as along cranial nerves. Thus the site of origin determined the areas of involvement. Since there were so many areas that could be potentially involved, the patients were stratified according to the number of areas involved in a single patient *(Table 26.3b)*. This provided a better idea of the extensiveness of the disease. Most patients had three or four areas of involvement, and could be stated to have stage 4 disease.

SURGICAL MANAGEMENT:

We looked specifically at the neurosurgical intervention that was carried out in the combined operations performed with the otolaryngology team. The range of procedures is listed in *Table 26.4a*. Most patients underwent more than one neurosurgical procedure *(Table 26.4b)*, although about 77% of patients required one or two operations. These were either planned, staged procedures or procedures related to complications or tumor recurrence.

TABLE 26.4A
Neurosurgical Interventions (MSH)

- Temporal bone partial or total: 30
- Other bone: 33
- Dura: 30
- ICA (expose, ligate, resect): 23
- Meckel's cave/V branches: 22
- Cav sinus: 15
- Ethmoid, sphenoid sinus: 7
- Transverse/sigmoid sinus: 7
- Jugular foramen: 5
- Brain: 3
- Occ condyle/lat mass C1: 2

TABLE 26.4B
Number of Operations—NS (MSH)

- Total: 49 patients
- Operations: 93
- 1 operation: 26 patients (53%)
- 2 operations: 12 patients (24.4%)
- 3 operations: 6 patients (12.2%)
- 4 operations: 3 patients (6.1%)
- 5 operations: 1 patient (2%)
- 7 operations: 1 patient (2%)

COMPLICATIONS FROM THE NEUROSURGICAL INTERVENTION:

All the patients had received radiation either prior to the Mount Sinai operation or after their operation. Some of the patients also received adjuvant chemotherapy. There were numerous complications that the patients suffered *(Tables 26.5a and 26.5b)*. However, only the neurosurgically related ones are listed. The systemic complications were assumed to be the same for this group of patients undergoing major operative procedures. Although the most common problem was cra-

TABLE 26.5A
Complications (MSH)

- Cranial nerve palsies: 30
- Cosmetic defects: 14
- CSF leaks: 9
- Dysphagia: 9
- Pain: 6
- Altered mental status (transient): 5
- Wound infection: 4

TABLE 26.5B
Complications (MSH)

- Abscess: 3
- Meningitis: 3
- Osteomyelitis: 2
- Stroke: 3
- Hematoma: 2
- Seizures: 1

nial nerve impairment, the majority of these patients underwent planned resection of the cranial nerves along with the surgical specimen. Other complications include cerebrospinal fluid leaks requiring surgical intervention, infections, meningitis, and abscess. Despite the number of patients who had substantial manipulation of the internal carotid artery at the skull base, only three patients suffered a stroke.

FUNCTIONAL STATUS AND SURVIVAL

The days of hospitalization in which there was neurosurgical intervention were tallied *(Tables 26.6a and 26.6b)*. The mean length of stay was 32.5 days but the median was 23 days because there were five patients with excessively long hospitalization. On correlating the mean length of stay with the number of anatomical areas that were involved, patients with more extensive disease stayed longer. The pre- and postoperative Karnofsky scores are listed in *Table 26.7*. Most of the patients (73.4%) dropped down in their score. There were four patients who im-

TABLE 26.6A
Length of Hospital Stay

- Total: 49 patients
- Median stay: 23 days
- Range: 4–186 days
- Mean: 32.5 days

TABLE 26.6B
Neurosurgery Intervention (MSH): Length of Stay Relative to Involved Area

Areas involved	No. of patients	Hospital days: mean
2	10	20.5
3	14	20.28
4	16	48.8 (8–186 days)
5	7	31.1 (19–62 days)
6+	2	54

TABLE 26.7
Karnofsky: Pre- and Postoperative Scores(MSH)

- Preop: mean 83.4 (100–70)
- Postop: mean 69.5 (100–40)
- Improved: 4 patients by 10 points (8%)
- Stable: 9 patients (18.3%)
- Worse: 36 patients (73.4%)
  - —10 points: 13 patients (36.1%)
  - —20 points: 12 patients (33.3%)
  - —30 points: 7 patients (19.4%)
  - —40 points: 4 patients (11.1%)

TABLE 26.8
Time to Recurrence (Mount Sinai OR)

- Total: 49 patients
- Recurrence: 24 patients
- Time to recurrence: mean 19.4 months (3–62 months)

proved in their rating. Twenty-four of the 49 patients suffered recurrences. The mean time to recurrence was 19.4 months *(Table 26.8)*. The survival of these patients was calculated using the Kaplan Meier analysis. These show that patients with recurrent disease did worse than those with primary cancers being treated for the first time *(Fig. 26.1)*.

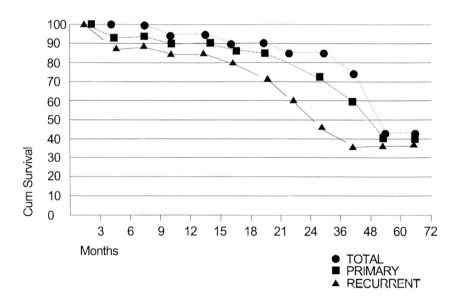

FIG. 26.1 Survival rates of patients with primary vs. recurrent disease

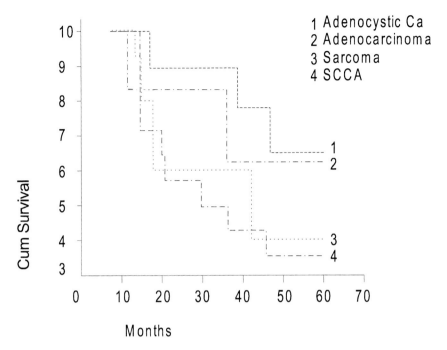

FIG. 26.2 Breakdown of disease categories

On breaking down the disease categories, patients with squamous cell carcinoma had the worst survival *(Fig. 26.2)*.

DISCUSSION

Skull base invasion by head and neck malignancies is a poor prognosticator. Since the description of Smith et al. (1) and Ketcham et al. (2) describing a standardized approach through a combined cranial and facial approach for such problems, substantial advances have occurred in improving the survival of patients. Although, anterior craniofacial approach is a well-established treatment modality for sinonasal cancers involving the anterior skull base, treatment of cancers that involve the lateral skull base continues to be a difficult problem and is still evolving.

TYPES OF TUMORS

The histological tumor type determines the results of treatment and overall survival to a large extent. It is therefore important to briefly discuss the biology of some of these tumors.

Squamous cell carcinoma (3)

These arise from the epithelial lining of the sinonasal tract. They usually attain a large size by the time of presentation. The maxillary sinus is the most common site of origin. Those that involve the temporal bone usually arise in the external ear canal, the middle ear, or the mastoid. Regional and distant metastases are quite unusual and occur in advanced disease. The temporal bone cancers extend into contiguous tissues to involve the carotid artery, jugular vein, cavernous sinus, and the infratemporal fossa. Survival rates for patients with squamous cancers vary according to the site and stage of the disease. Usually, anterior skull base tumors are more amenable to resection. The standard of treatment is combined surgery and radiation. Local failure is the most common occurrence.

Adenoid cystic carcinoma (3)

These are the most common malignancies that arise from major and minor salivary glands. They usually present in the fourth to sixth decade of life and produce symptoms by their location. They are slow growing and have a strong predilection for perineurial extension, which is the main cause of incomplete excision. Perineurial extension can occur for some distance from the main tumor site and can be seen without any significant bone destruction. Metastases are usually blood borne. These tumors are considered radiosensitive and it is not unusual to have long survivals even with metastatic disease. Surgery and radiation are recommended in their treatment.

Soft tissue and bone sarcomas (4):

Sarcomas can arise in the bone and soft tisssues of the head and neck like other regions of the body. They are classified as low grade, well-differentiated tumors or high grade, poorly differentiated tumors. Their local invasiveness, tendency to nodal, and distant metastasis is directly related to the grade of the sarcoma. In general, they are locally invasive with low tendency to distant spread. The size of the tumor at initial presentation is said to have prognostic significance. This is mainly related to the low likelihood of obtaining a clear margin around the tumor. Postoperative irradiation is usually considered in the treatment, but the value of chemotherapy is not established.

ANATOMY OF THE LATERAL SKULL BASE

The lateral and posterior skull base are composed of the greater sphenoid wing, body of sphenoid, temporal bone, and the clivus. Multiple cranial nerves and vascular structures enter and exit through numerous foramina and channels that provide an ideal avenue for the intracranial extension of head and neck cancers. The cavernous sinus, which consists of a large complex of venous channels, the internal carotid artery, and multiple cranial nerves, is often involved by intracranial extension through the middle cranial fossa. Tumors in the infratemporal fossa can extend into the jugular foramen and clivus. The proximity of the internal carotid artery, the jugular bulb, and the caudal cranial nerve IX to XI make them likely targets for invasion by the tumor. Dural and brain involvement can occur in the middle and posterior fossa. Due to the close aggregation of so many important structures in this compact area, the principles of oncologic surgery of en bloc resection can seldom be achieved. The neurosurgeon's task is to preserve as many cranial nerves as possible since this impacts on the patient's functional survival. A conflict of goals often occurs which pits the desire of preserving function against that of obtaining complete tumor excision with margins. A thorough knowledge of this complicated anatomy is therefore essential.

DISEASE CONTROL AND RECURRENCE

Anterior skull base

The role and effectiveness of the combined anterior craniofacial resection for paranasal sinus malignancies has been well established since the first systematic descriptions by Ketcham et al. (2) in 1963. The benefit of cross specialty collaboration has contributed to its effectiveness. Further progress in terms of improved imaging has allowed the surgeon to accurately assess the extent of the disease in the surgical planning. Boyle et al. (5) reviewed 115 consecutive patients who underwent craniofacial resection. They obtained local disease control in 65% of the patients while their disease-specific survival at 5 and 10 years was 58% and 48% respectively. Tumor grade and stage were important prognostic factors. In their series, the patients with esthesioneuroblastoma did better than those with squamous cell carcinoma, who in turn did better than the other types. Since it is usually difficult to obtain satisfactory confirmation of the tumor resection margins, no specific relation to surgical failure rate could be obtained from their review of the literature. Orbital and dural involvement, which indicated more extensive disease were predictive of survival. Cantu et al. (6) reporting on 123 patients who had a combined anterior craniofacial resection found a 5-year disease-free survival of 50% of T3 disease compared to 13% of T4 disease. According to their staging system, the patients with adenocarcinomas did worse than the rest. Among 65 patients who recurred, there were only 3 with distant metastases and 2 with spread to lymph nodes, underscoring the locally aggressive nature of these cancers. Janecka et al. (7) found that there was a good correlation between disease-free survival and the clear margins in a series of 50 patients with anterior skull base involvement from paranasal sinus malignancies. The overall survival at a mean of 40 months was 74%. Disease-free status at 33 months was 83% in patients with primary disease compared to 57% in patients with recurrent disease.

Lateral skull base and temporal bone

Involvement of the lateral skull base imposes many different technical difficulties and limitations compared to anterior skull base disease. En bloc resection is seldom possible and usually it is not even possible to ascertain if a disease free margin has been obtained. Bigelow et al. (8) reviewed 25 patients who underwent a lateral skull base resection for malignant stage 4 disease. In five patients the internal carotid artery was sacrificed without revascularization, while in 17 the artery was manipulated but not sacrificed. Even though en bloc resection was not possible in all cases, they were able to obtain tumor-free margins in all but three cases. Despite obtaining disease-free margins, seven patients died from the disease at a mean of 11 months after surgery. The overall disease-free survival was 25% (14% for patients with recurrent disease; 31% for patients with primary disease).

Tumors easily involve the carotid artery and the cavernous sinus through the foramina at the skull base. These structures pose the main limitation to en bloc or total resection of the cancers. This issue was specifically addressed by Saito et al. (9). Among the 25 patients treated, 10 patients had no cavernous sinus involvement, 9 of whom had no recurrence of disease in the follow-up period. In 15 patients the cavernous sinus was manipulated; among these 12 patients had extradural resection of the cranial nerves with preservation of the carotid artery, and in 3 the entire cavernous sinus with the carotid artery was resected. The more advanced the disease requiring more extensive manipulation of the cavernous sinus and carotid artery, the less was the chance of clearing the disease. The 5-year survival in the patients requiring cavernous sinus manipulation/resection was 31% while in the patients in whom the cavernous sinus was not manipulated, it was 88%. In the event that the carotid artery is involved at the skull base, the surgical options include resection of the artery without revascularization, resection of the artery with immediate revascularization and the other option is to preserve the artery but remove the tumor piecemeal around it. In the report by Brisman et al. (10), this issue was analyzed in 17 patients. Although the patient groups are not exactly comparable, those requiring carotid sacrifice had more advance disease compared to those in whom the artery was preserved; 9 patients were free of disease at average 2.1 year follow up. Patients with squamous cell cancers and those with recurrent disease did the worst. In a survey of 118 patients with malignant skull base tumors, Janecka et al. (11) found that there was a 62.5% survival without evidence of disease and 37.5% failure. In this series patients with squamous cell cancer did better than adenoid cystic cancer with respect to disease control.

Patients with temporal bone involvement face a similar course because of the many important structures in the immediate vicinity that may need to be sacrificed in order to obtain a clear margin. Manolidis et al. (12) analyzed a series of 81 patients with temporal bone involvement. The average follow-up period was 54 months at which time 31% were dead from the disease and 53% were alive and free of disease. Squamous cell and salivary gland cancers did worse. A similar outcome was reported by Sekhar et al. (13) in 20 patients who underwent total temporal bone excision. The fast growing malignancies and those that extended beyond the temporal bone had the worst outcome.

In the present series the tumor types are representative of the other series that have been reported. The overall 5-year survival was calculated at 40% with patients treated for recurrent disease doing worse than those with primary disease. Squamous cell carcinoma was the worst histologic type of disease for the purpose of prognosis for survival.

SURGICAL MORBIDITY AND COMPLICATIONS

The complications encountered in anterior skull base lesions requiring a craniofacial resection have been well described. It is important to evaluate these in terms of what complications are added as a result of the cranial portion of the operation. A recent review of the literature reported the range to be from 6% to 63% (5). These complications include cerebrospinal fluid leaks, infections, meningitis, pneumocephalus, temporary mental impairment, and visual problems. Over the years these complications have declined in their occurrence. Prior irradiation and surgery were deemed to increase the risk of complications, the majority of which were infections (14).

Complications that arise from tumor involvement of the lateral skull base and the temporal bone are related to the internal carotid artery, the cavernous sinus and the multitude of cranial nerves that serve important functions. The interval between these structures is so little that millimeters of difference can produce severe functional consequences for the patient. In addition to this, carotid artery sacrifice adds the risk of ischemic complications whether or not revascularization is performed. Often these are tumors have recurred after prior surgery and radiation which adds to the risks. Thus, by the location and the nature of the structures involved, the risks are considerably higher compared to anterior skull base surgery. In the report of Bigelow et al. (8), there were 5 (of 25 patients) patients who underwent carotid artery sacrifice. Vascular complications related to arterial rupture and ischemia were substantial. In the experience of Saito et al. (9), complication related to the carotid artery manipulation, sacrifice and revascularization were high. This included formation of a pseudoaneurysm in one patient and ischemic stroke in four patients. The other complications of infection and flap reconstruction were also seen as with the anterior skull base. The more extensive the manipulation of the cavernous sinus and the internal carotid artery, the higher were the potential risks of complications. In the report of Brisman et al. (10), the ischemic complications were the highest in the patients who underwent carotid sacrifice without revascularization. Those that had immediate revascularization with the carotid artery resection had fewer ischemic events and these were related to occlusion of the bypass, which could be attributed partly to prior irradiation or a hypercoagulable state. There was an incidence of 21% major complication rate reported by Manolidis et al. (12), these included three deaths and two strokes. In the present series, which include those patients reported by Brisman et al. (10), the highest number of complications were related to cranial nerve loss. Almost all of these were caused by planned sacrifice of these nerves at the time of tumor removal. Other risks included infections, cerebrospinal fluid leaks, and intracerebral hematomas. There were three patients with completed strokes related to carotid artery sacrifice. In a survey of 108 consecutive operations performed by Donald and his colleagues (15), there was a 50.5% incidence of complications. Although these cases were not stratified into anterior or lateral skull base, four of the six deaths in the series were related to cerebrovascular incidents. The common complications were cerebrospinal fluid leaks, meningitis and wound breakdown.

SURVIVAL AND QUALITY OF LIFE

Since majority of patients with head and neck cancers that involve the skull base die from local disease, the stage and grade of the cancer at the time of surgical intervention is very important. The more extensive the disease, the less likely it is to completely eliminate the tumor. From this and the other series reported here, squamous cell cancers appear to be worse than other tumor types. The adenoid cystic carcinoma recurred most often and had the shortest time to recurrence. The quality of life is influenced by the morbidity from the operation and the length of hospitalization as well as the functional capacity afterwards. The extent of the disease was directly proportional to the length of hospital stay. Apart from a few patients that stayed for an inordinate length of time, most of the patients followed this general rule. The preoperative and postoperative Karnofsky performance scores indicated that 73% of patients regressed in their performance. As seen from the list of complications, this drop in the Karnofsky score was predominantly due to cranial nerve impairment. In cancers that involve the lateral skull base, cranial nerves are usually sacrificed in a planned fashion in order to obtain a disease-free margin. It is difficult to confirm or sometimes even obtain a tumor-free margin. This is reflected in our series by the 50% incidence of recurrences with a mean period of appearance at 19.4 months. Many patients in our series needed multiple operations and this also impacted on the quality of life as experienced by the patient. The number of operation, an individual underwent was usually proportionate to the number of patients in each disease class. A lesser invasive way of preserving the cranial nerves and their functional capacity is to treat the area of the tumor that may be left in place around these critical structures, can be treated by radiosurgery.

The overall survival was found to be more than 40% over a 5-year follow up. Patients with recurrent disease did worse. The breakdown of this series showed that the squamous cell carcinoma was a disease with poor prognosis. Radiosurgery (16) may be an option to be considered in the event that some tumor is left on the cranial nerves or other important structures in order to preserve their integrity and function.

CONCLUSION

Head and neck cancers that invade the lateral skull base have a poor prognosis. Small invasion can be treated by surgical excision. The involvement of the cavernous sinus, the internal carotid artery and the temporal bone are unfavorable prognostic factors. This has been borne out by this paper and others. The issue of performing a craniotomy and an aggressive skull base tumor resection, certainly allow prolongation of life. Complications are higher for this group of patients. The issue of performing a major cavernous sinus excision certainly has formidable risks. However, this decision has to be made on a patient by patient basis. This should be based upon the following factors: patients age, type and extent of disease especially at the cranial aspect (whether a reasonable margin can be obtained), metastatic disease, and the general health of the patient. If carotid artery sacrifice is deemed necessary, a revascularization procedure should be planned at the same time or at a prior separate stage. Revascularization should be performed at an area away from the site of prior irradiation. Gamma knife radiosurgery may play an increasing role that could be used in conjunction with the surgical treatments.

REFERENCES

1. Smith RR, Klopp CT, Williams JM: Surgical treatment of cancer of the frontal sinus and adjacent areas. **Cancer** 7:991–994, 1954
2. Ketcham AS, Wilkins RH, Van Buren JM, et al.: A combined intracranial facial approach to the paranasal sinuses. **Am J Surg** 106:698–703, 1963
3. Snyderman, CH, Sekhar LN, Sen C, Janecka IP: Malignant skull base tumors. **Neurosurg Clin North Am** 1:243–259, 1990
4. Kraus DH, Harrison LB, O'Malley BB: Soft tissues and bone sarcomas of the head and neck, in Harrison LB, Sessions RB, Hong WK (eds): *Head and Neck Cancer.* New York, Lippincott Raven, 1999
5. Boyle J, Shah K, Shah J: Craniofacial resection for malignant neoplasms of the skull base. **J Surg Oncol** 69:275–284, 1998.
6. Cantu G, Lazzaro Solero C, mariani L, Mattavelli F, Pizzi N, Licitra L: A new classification for malignanat tumors involving the anterior skull base. **Arch. Otolaryngology Head Neck Surg** 125:1252–1257, 1999.
7. Janecka I, Sen C, Sekhar L, Curtin H: Treatment of paranasal sinus cancer with cranial base surgery: results. **Laryngoscope** 104:553–555, 1994.
8. Bigelow J, Smith P, Leonetti J, Backer R, Grubb R, Kotapka M: Treatement of malignant neoplasms of the lateral cranial base with the combined frontotemporalanterolateral approach: five-year-follow up. **Otolaryngology Head Neck Surg**. 120:17–24. 1999
9. Saito K, Fukuta K, Takahashi M, Tachibana E, Yoshida J: Management of the cavernous sinus in en bloc resections of malignant skull base tumors. **Head Neck** 21:734–742,1999.
10. Brisman M, Sen C, Catalano P: Results of surgery for head and neck tumors that involve the carotid artery at the skull base. **J Neurosurg** 86:787–792, 1997.
11. Janecka I, Sen C, Sekhar L, Ramasastry S, Curtin H, Barnes L, D'Amico F: Cranial base surgery: Results in 183 patients. **Otolaryngology Head Neck Surg** 110:539–546, 1994.
12. Manolidis S, Pappas D Jr, Von Doersten P, Gary Jackson C, Glasscock M III: The American **J Otology** 19:S1-S15, 1998.
13. Sekhar L, Pomeranz S, Janecka I, Hirsch B, Ramasastry S: Temporal bone neoplasms: A report on 20 surgically treated cases. **J Neurosurg** 76:578–587, 1992
14. Nibu K, Sasaki T, Kawahara N, Sugasawa M, Nakatsuka T, Yamada A: Complications of craniofacial surgery for tumors involving the anterior cranial base. **Neurosurgery** 42:455–462, 1998.
15. Donald PJ: Complications in skull base surgery for malignancy. **Laryngoscope** 109:1959–1966, 1999.
16. Miller R, Foote R, Coffey R, Gorman D, Earle J, Schomberg P, Kline R: The role of stereotactic radiosurgery in the treatment of malignant skull base tumors. **Int J Radiation Oncology Biol Phys** 39:977–981, 1997.

CHAPTER

27

Joint Ventures at the Skull Base

Defining the Roles of the Neurosurgeon and Non-Neurosurgeon

THOMAS C. ORIGITANO, M.D., PhD, FACS

It is a daunting task to deliver the final talk on the last day of such an inspirational Congress. My topic, Joint Ventures at the Skull Base: Defining the Roles of the Neurosurgeon and Non-Neurosurgeon, is both ethereal and politically sensitive. However, at this point, after experiencing this Congress, we should all be somewhat politically desensitized.

Being a product of Chicago and a student of human nature, I will employ my own experiences of being part of a successful Skull Base Program to try to shed some light on this provocative subject.

In forming these comments, I would ask the following caveats be remembered:

1. Like politics—which are a local phenomena—what and how we define individual roles is extremely local with past history, talent mix, opportunities, power structure, and individual relationships playing major roles. At my institution, they were part of a cultural evolution.
2. Asking individuals who themselves resist having anyone define their roles (neurosurgeons) to define other individuals' roles is much like having the fox running the hen house.
3. Defining roles is like the 10 commandments: To some they are laws of liberation and to others, laws that limit.
4. Consider, rather than assigning designated roles (a static system), creating a dynamic environment that optimizes or plays to each individual's strength.

To this end, I propose a local Chicago paradigm to illustrate my plan, which also is a Chicago historical institution—the championship Chicago Bulls basketball teams. Phil Jackson, in his book, *Sacred Hoops,*[1] re-

---

[1]Phil Jackson and Hugh Delehanty. *Sacred Hoops: Spiritual Lessons of a Hardwood Warrior.* New York: Hyperion, 1995.

lates the story and philosophy he used to forge four championship teams in the face of changing personnel, talent, and times.

Today, I offer my vision of this team management philosophy for the cranial base team: Sacred Foramen: Pragmatic Lessons for Building a Championship Skull Base Team.

The key mechanistic ingredient to the Bulls championship teams was Tex Winters' Triangle Offense. This unique system was a dynamic plan that permitted a multiple threat, ever-changing attack plan that spontaneously changed to adjust to the defensive scheme. This plan was based on a philosophy of each player adjusting his role to meet the unique challenge of a given situation rather than assigning a specific role to any individual player. This was a radical departure from the traditional "me" centered, showboat NBA play of the time.

To change the culture and therefore the philosophy of play, Phil Jackson had to have a vision of what the team could become if they, the players, could change their individualistic culture. The struggle of the leader is to get the individual members of the team who are driven by the quest for individual glory to give themselves over wholeheartedly to the group effort—a formidable task when dealing with individuals who, from birth, have been encouraged to excel as individuals.

Each team is made up of different players, each with his own personality experience, strength, weakness, and skill set. Often throughout their careers, they are groomed to play specific roles. In the case of the Bulls, many talented players were assembled: Pippen, Grant, Harper, Paxon, the three headed monster and of course, Michael Jordan, superstar (Nova). Convincing Jordan that scoring 30 points rather than 40 points per game, was the way to the championship and was one of Jackson's major challenges.

In the days when Michael was MVP, All Star, Defensive Player of the League and scoring 40 points a game, the Bulls never went deep into the playoffs! It was only when the superstar was convinced to invest his talent into making those around him better players did the championships start coming. Good teams become great teams when the members trust each other enough to surrender the "me" for the "we." This is selfless team play. Under this format, each player contributes—even the bench.

While most NBA teams played an average of 6 to 7 players a game, the Bulls averaged 10. We can all remember the many playoff games when Jordan ran down the court—drew the double team and then passed off to Paxon or Harper who were open to shoot the game winning shot. This was team play at its best.

Skull Base Surgery has many analogies to building a championship sports team. It involves the blending of multiple individual talents, all moving at full speed, interacting, integrating, and thinking as a single unit. Neurological surgeons see themselves as the Michael Jordans of the team. It is they, first and foremost, who must capture the vision of selfless team play—to choose the power of "we" over the power of "me."

The major players of the Skull Base Team include Radiology (imaging and interventional), Otolaryngology, Neurological Surgery, Plastic Surgery, Neuropathology, Anesthesiology, Radiation Oncology, and Hospital Administration. This group represents multiple talented individuals who have been taught from birth that only they can save the day. Support services include Audiology; Speech, Physical, and Occupational Therapy; Social Work; Orthotics; Neurophysiology; Rehab Services; and Nursing.

Nursing is ubiquitous: OR, Recovery, ICU, IMC, Floor, Office. Remember these valuable players and honor them; 98% of the time, patients are cared for by a nurse, *not* a doctor. Sixteen hours of brilliant technical surgery can be frustrated by a mucous plug. Their roles are indispensable for championship play. Remember also, that the referring physicians are a valuable part of the team. Educate and recognize them.

The neurosurgeon as the team leader must own the vision of selfless team play and be able to project it, understanding that technical ability is only a portion of a case. Without the non-neurosurgical colleagues, it may be impossible to have a successful championship caliber team— much like Jordan scoring 50 points a game. To forge a winning team from so many varied individually talented players, the focus must be on something greater than the individuals themselves. In our case, it is patients and their functional outcomes. The focus on the patient returning to family and work must surpass the individual surgeon's technical stardom.

The triangle offense that we use at Loyola is defined by the pathology, e.g., (1) Neurological Surgeon, Otolaryngologist, Plastic Surgeon; (2) Neurological Surgeon, Neurological Surgeon, Otolaryngologist; (3) Neurological Surgeon, Plastic Surgeon, Neurological Surgeon. The goal of each member of the team is to optimize his or her colleagues' performance. In doing so, the approach is performed with the eye on the resection and the closure facilitated by the approach and the resection. The game plan is set up front and adjusted during the case to deal with the subtleties of the pathology.

This model emphasizes inclusion and participation over "turf control" and solo performance. It is true that there are times when you do not have to work as a team. However, the more you operate as a team, the more your institutional team roles will evolve and mature. Working together on easier cases promotes the kinematics necessary for the difficult ones. The team leader must also project the vital role each primary, secondary, and ancillary individual plays on the overall outcome of the patient. Letting OR nurses and hospital administrators know about the outcome of patients bonds them back to the team. We, as neurosurgeons, must be open minded to learning the technical nuances of our non-neurosurgical colleagues. Study their instruments and approach. Read the literature. Incorporate into your own repertoire their techniques: e.g., fat graft, oversewing the ear, bifrontal orbital ridge osteotomies. This will honor them and further link your technical expertise.

The most important role you define in defining other's roles is your own. We as neurological surgeons should be selfless leaders and team advocates. Extending the continuum of oversight in the Operating Room, Recovery Room, ICU, IMC, Floor, and Rehab. Our talent and training span this spectrum like none of the other surgical specialties in cranial base. Our goal should not be to control our non-neurosurgical colleagues at the cranial base. The more you try to control, the more you lose. Rather, we must facilitate other services. The more you facilitate, the more you grow. Find ways to turn threats—whether turf or personalities—into opportunities.

The key to this is understanding, integration, and cooperation. My non-neurosurgical colleagues are not my competitors, they are my partners. They provide access to a large variety of patients and pathology (acoustic, glomus tumors, sinus cancers, and vestibular disorders). They teach my residents and I teach theirs. They care for my patients. They are part of my department. Rather than defining roles, we have adopted a system that has defined our goals. In doing so, in each case, each individual surgeon's role is optimized.

Rudyard Kipling said it best:

"The strength of the Pack is the Wolf, and the strength of the Wolf is the Pack."

Author Index

391

Subject Index

morbidity in, and decision making
on, 105–108
obliteration data, and decision
making on, 104–105
remnants after, retreatment for,
104, *106–107*
versus resection, 105
size of lesion and, 104–105, 108
staged volume, for larger lesions,
108
Sylvian fissure, *106–107*
temporal lobe, 98–99, *99*
thalamic, 101, *102,* 105
Arthrodesis. *See* Fusion, spinal
Arthroplasty, spinal disc, 84–93
Articulating disc prostheses, 88–89
Artificial blood substrates, military use
of, 176
Artificial spinal discs, 84–93
Aspartoacylase deficiency, in Canavan
disease, gene therapy for,
140–141, *141*
Astrocytes, for neural transplantation,
160–161
Astrocytomas, 3
anaplastic, 46
angiograms in patients with, 38
chemotherapy for, 50, 52, 54
resection of, histological
contamination in studies of, 13
stereotactic biopsy of, 14–15
angiograms in patients with, 38
fibrillary
age and, 21, 30–31
benign, myth of, 21
biology of, at time of recognition,
21–22
definition of tumor, 21–23
"go slow" approach in, 21
histopathology of, 22
light microscopy studies of, 22
magnetic resonance imaging of,
21–23, *23,* 25–27, *26, 28–29*
molecular-based conceptual
therapies for, 34
morphology of, 22–23
need for additional management
of, with resection, 32–33
versus oligodendroglioma, 22
radiation therapy for, 24, 24*t,*
32–33

rational surgery for, rationale for,
20–36
resection of, 21–25, 24*t,* 30–32, 32*t*
stereotactic biopsy of, 25–30, *26*
stereotactic radiosurgery for, *28,*
28–30, *29,* 33
surgery for, correct role of, 23–33
technological advances in
treatment of, 26–30
fibrillary versus pilocytic, 22
genetic alterations and, 5–6
origins of (tumorigenesis), 61–64,
63–64
pilocytic, 22, 43
supratentorial, resection of, 30–31
Autologous bone marrow rescue, after
chemotherapy for gliomas,
51–52
AVM. *See* Arteriovenous malformation
Axonal degeneration, after spinal cord
injury, *228*

B
Back pain
assessment of, instruments for, 208
with disc degeneration, 82–83
lumbar interbody fusion for, 206,
212–215
nonoperative therapeutic options in, 83
postoperative, 207
Bagan, Merwyn, *279,* 283
Ball-type disc prosthesis, 88–89
Barthel Index, 208
Basal pterional approach, for endoscopy,
294–298
Basement membrane proteins, in glioma
angiogenesis, 70–72
Batjer, Hunt, 277
Battlefield care, technology from,
174–180
Bax, 66–67
Bcl-2, 66–67
BCNU
autologous bone marrow rescue after
administration of, 51
for gliomas, 47–55, 48*t,* 75
intratumoral injection of, 53–54
intravenous versus intra-arterial
injection of, 51
polymer drug delivery of (wafers),
54–55

surgery for
  endoscopic skull-base, 301
  outcome and results of, 313–314,
    313*t*–314*t*
Microendoscopic
  laminotomy/foramenotomy
  (MED), for sports-related
  spinal injury, 254–257
Microscopic laminotomy/foramenotomy
  (ML), for sports-related spinal
  injury, 254–257
Microscopic neurosurgery
  (microsurgery), 287
  endoscope-assisted, 289–291
  endoscopy combined with, 289–290
  for meningioma resection, 321,
    327–329, 331–333, *336,* 337
  preservation of cranial nerve function
    in, 351
  and risk reduction, 288–289
Middle cranial fossa, approach to, in
  endoscopic skull-base surgery,
  299
Mierowsky, Arnold, 174
Military neurosurgery
  historical perspective on, 174–175
  technology from, 174–180
  unique mission of, 175
Misdifferentiation hypothesis, of glial
  tumorigenesis, 61–63, *64*
MK-801, in neural transplantation,
  160
ML. *See* Microscopic
  laminotomy/foramenotomy
Molecular-based therapies, for gliomas,
  34, 60, 72–78
Monoclonal antibodies, in glioma
  treatment, 77–78
Mosberg, William, 277, *279*
MRI. *See* Magnetic resonance imaging
Multiple sclerosis, myelopathy with, 263
Murine double minute 2 (MDM2) gene,
  and gliomas, 5, *62*
Musashi-1, expression of, by neural stem
  cells, 161
Muscimol, brain infusion of, for control of
  tremors, 133–134, *135*
Myelination, and cranial nerve
  regeneration, 351–352
Myelin basic protein, neural stem cells
  for replacement of, 121

Myelopathy
  diagnosis of, 262–263
  magnetic resonance imaging in,
    268–271
  non-operative/conservative
    management of, 263–264
  surgery for
    algorithm for, *265*
    lordosis and, *265,* 272
    selection of approach for, 267–272,
      268–271
Myofibroblasts, and arteriovenous
  malformation radiosurgery, 101

N
Naked-eye direct vision surgery, 287
NASCIS. *See* National Acute Spinal Cord
  Injury Studies
National Acute Spinal Cord Injury
  Studies, 230–232, 235
Natural chemotherapy agents, for
  gliomas, 48*t*
Neck pain
  with cervical spine disease, 261–264
  nonoperative therapeutic options in,
    83
  with radiculopathy, 265–266
Nelson's syndrome, ACTH-secreting
  tumors in, outcomes and
  results of surgery for, 314–315
Nepal, assistance programs in, 283
Nerve growth factor, brain infusion of
  for Alzheimer's disease, 136
  for Parkinson's disease, 132
Nerves, cranial
  avoidance of cottonoid coverings for,
    351
  function, preservation of, in surgery,
    351
  impairment of, in surgery for
    malignancies involving skull
    base, 376–377, 383, 385
  regeneration of
    nerves not presently possible in,
      352
    problems in, 351–352
  surgical repair of, 351–372
    experience and results in,
      358*t*
    future of, *370,* 370–371
    general techniques of, 352